Fundamentals of Body CT

Fundamentals of Body CT

W. RICHARD WEBB, MD
Professor of Radiology
University of California, San Francisco
San Francisco, California

WILLIAM E. BRANT, MD
Assistant Professor of Radiology
Chief of Body Computed Tomography
University of California, Davis
Sacramento, California

CLYDE A. HELMS, MD
Professor of Radiology
University of California, San Francisco
San Francisco, California

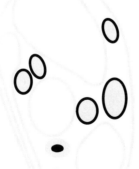
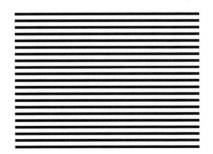

W.B. SAUNDERS COMPANY
Harcourt Brace Jovanovich, Inc.
Philadelphia London Toronto Montreal Sydney Tokyo

W. B. SAUNDERS COMPANY
Harcourt Brace Jovanovich, Inc.

The Curtis Center
Independence Square West
Philadelphia, PA 19106

Library of Congress Cataloging-in-Publication Data

Webb, W. Richard (Wayne Richard)

Fundamentals of body CT / by W. Richard Webb, William E. Brant,
Clyde A. Helms.
p.   cm.

ISBN 0–7216–3541–5

1. Tomography.   I. Brant, William E.   II. Helms, Clyde A.
   III. Title.   [DNLM: 1. Tomography, X-Ray Computed.
   WN 160 W368f] RC78.7.T6W433   1991

616.07′57—dc20

DNLM/DLC   90–8547

Editor: Lisette Bralow
Designer: Ellen Bodner
Production Manager: Ken Neimeister
Manuscript Editor: Karen Okie
Illustration Coordinator: Walt Verbitski
Indexer: Victoria Boyle

FUNDAMENTALS OF BODY CT   ISBN 0–7216–3541–5

Printed in the United States of America.

Last digit is the print number: 9   8   7   6   5   4   3

This book is dedicated to our families,
for their continuing support and tolerance.

We wish specifically to thank
Wayne, Norma, Teresa, Emma, Sonny, and Andy;
Linda, Daniel, Ryan, Jonathan, and Rachel; and
Mr. and Mrs. F. L. Helms, Glee, Caroline, Jeremy,
Allyson, Jason, and Benjamin.

Preface

Our goal is to have this book cut from the same cloth as *Fundamentals of Skeletal Radiology,* the "Cliff's notes" of skeletal radiology, recently published by Clyde Helms to great acclaim (to hear him tell it, W.R.W.).

Instead of writing a text intended to record everything that is known about body CT or even everything that we know about body CT, we have attempted to write one that *teaches* how to perform and read body CT scans. In doing this, we have tried to limit ourselves to discussing what is key to understanding body CT from a practical clinical standpoint—the key anatomy, the key concepts, the key diseases, and the key controversies. We have done this at the risk of leaving a few things out, but it isn't necessary to read about everything when you are first learning a subject. In other words, *Fundamentals of Body CT* is not intended to provide more than the best CT texts on the market do, but rather less, with a different emphasis, and in a more manageable package.

Each of us has written a different part of this book, obviously depending on our areas of expertise. Since each of us teaches in a slightly different way, each of the three sections of the book—the thorax, the abdomen, and the musculoskeletal system—is somewhat different in approach. We hope that by preserving our individual styles we have made the book more interesting to read, and for us, it certainly made this book easier to write.

W. Richard Webb
William E. Brant
Clyde A. Helms

Contents

THE THORAX

1

1

Techniques of Thoracic CT

Typically, chest computed tomography (CT) is performed using a routine technique which is valuable for the diagnosis of a variety of abnormalities; this is important, because we don't always know what we are looking for before we start the exam. However, since CT sometimes serves as a problem-solving modality in patients with chest diseases, aimed at providing a specific answer to a specific question, techniques are often modified. A certain amount of imagination may be required in selecting the specific techniques to use in specific situations, but fortunately, these are relatively few, not difficult to remember, and reasonably logical.

ROUTINE CHEST CT

In most patients, chest CT is performed using a standard protocol, and although this protocol varies slightly among different institutions, most people use approximately the same technique. This technique is designed to provide useful (although not necessarily optimal) information about the lung, mediastinum, hilum, pleura, and chest wall, and therefore is valuable in the diagnosis of a variety of conditions or diseases, and in the diagnosis of diseases such as lung cancer that can involve all of these structures.

Standard chest CT is performed using contiguous 1-cm collimation from the level of the lung apices (or suprasternal notch) to the level of the posterior costophrenic angles, which encompasses the diaphragm and upper abdomen as well. Patients are scanned supine, during suspended respiration, at full lung volume. Scans may be performed with or without the administration of contrast

1

agents, to some extent depending on your level of knowledge or confidence. For example, if you are not confident as to mediastinal vascular and node anatomy, by all means give contrast so that vessels can be distinguished from other structures. If you are experienced, contrast is not always necessary. (If you are experienced, why are you reading this book?)

How should contrast be given? The answer to this question depends partially on why you are doing CT and what you are looking for. For most routine cases, a slow drip infusion of 100 ml of contrast during scanning provides sufficient opacification for diagnosis. More rapid infusion of contrast by bolus injection is usually reserved for specific instances, and will be discussed later.

Once the scans have been performed, the scan data is reconstructed using an algorithm which determines some characteristics of the images that are produced. For routine chest imaging the "standard" or "body" algorithm is used. In chest CT, the scans must be viewed using two different window settings, which allows the evaluation of different parts of the chest. These two windows are appropriately named "lung" and "mediastinal" windows, which also describes their primary use. Lung windows typically have a window mean of approximately -600 to -700 H, and a window width of 1000 to 2000 H. (H means Hounsfield units. On the Hounsfield scale, air has a density of -1000 H, fat -40 to -100 H, water 0 H, tissue 20 to 100 H , and bone 400 to 600 H). Lung windows best demonstrate lung anatomy and lung abnormalities, contrasting soft tissue structures with surrounding air. Mediastinal windows (window mean 20 to 40 H, width 500 H) demonstrate soft-tissue anatomy in the mediastinum and other areas of the thorax, contrasting fluid density, tissue density, fat density, and, if contrast has been given, vessels. This window is also of value in providing information about consolidated lung, the hila, pleural disease, and structures of the chest wall. More specific uses of these two windows will be discussed in subsequent chapters.

VASCULAR LESIONS AND DYNAMIC CT

In some patients, CT is performed for the diagnosis of a suspected vascular lesion. (It is suspected on the basis of either clinical symptoms or radiographic findings.) Also, sometimes, a standard CT is inconclusive as to what an abnormality is, and additional scans are performed to evaluate the possibility of a vascular lesion. If this is the case, then dynamic CT is often performed with a bolus injection of contrast.

The term dynamic CT means that a sequence of scans (usually four to six) is performed, with individual scans obtained at intervals of a few seconds. Scans can be performed at the same level or at contiguous adjacent levels. Because contrast is simultaneously injected, the rapid sequence of scans will show progressive, dense opacification of vessels or vascular lesions at the levels scanned, will clearly demonstrate the vascular nature of masses, and can provide some information regarding the rapidity of flow through the abnormal area. Scans of this sort, for example, are used for the diagnosis of aortic dissection.

Dynamic CT, with scans being performed at contiguous levels (dynamic incremental CT), has also been recommended for the evaluation of the pulmonary hila. Since, in the diagnosis of hilar masses on CT, it is important to be able to distinguish hilar vessels from nodes or masses, dense opacification of the vessels can be of value in diagnosis. This can be achieved by using dynamic, bolus-enhanced CT. This technique will be discussed in detail in Chapter 5.

VOLUME AVERAGING PROBLEMS

In some areas of the thorax, and in diagnosing certain abnormalities (such as a diffuse lung disease), the volume averaging that occurs in a 1-cm slice is too much to allow a proper or correct interpretation. Volume averaging means that various densities that are present in the same slice volume (voxel) are averaged together by the computer, thus obscuring details or edges which may be important in diagnosis. In such situations, which will be mentioned in various parts of this book, using thin collimation (1, 1.5, 2 mm, or whatever your scanner can do), often called "high-resolution" scanning, can be extremely helpful.

HIGH-RESOLUTION CT

With recent improvements in scanner technology, CT is capable of imaging the lung and other intrathoracic structures with excellent anatomic detail, and has led to the development of a technique known as "high-resolution CT" (HRCT). This technique is primarily used to image the lung and is capable of demonstrating both the normal and abnormal interstitium, subtle air-space consolidation, and morphologic characteristics of localized parenchymal processes. HRCT is clearly superior to conventional CT in defining lung morphology and is an important technique in modern chest imaging. However, I would advise you to skip reading the description of the technique I have written below until you have read the chapter on lung CT and want more information, or unless you are very compulsive. (I have one or two residents in mind who I know will read it.)

High-Resolution CT Technique

High-resolution CT technique consists of using thin collimation, reconstruction using a sharp (high-spatial frequency) algorithm, targeting image reconstruction to a single lung, and often, increasing kVp and mA scan parameters.

With 1-cm collimation, volume averaging within the plane of scan significantly reduces the ability of CT to resolve small structures. Therefore, scanning with thin collimation (1 to 1.5 mm) is essential if spatial resolution is to be optimized. Scans with such thin collimation, however, are sometimes difficult to interpret without a corresponding thick section (1-cm) scan for comparison. Also, the lung cannot be completely imaged using HRCT, and some abnormalities may be missed unless conventional CT is also performed.

With conventional body CT, scan data are usually reconstructed with a relatively low spatial frequency algorithm (i.e., GE "standard" or "soft-tissue" algorithms), which smooths the image, reduces visible image noise, and improves contrast resolution. Reconstruction of the image using a high-spatial frequency algorithm (i.e., GE "bone" algorithm) reduces image smoothing and increases spatial resolution, making structures appear sharper. However, this also increases visible image noise. Since some of this noise is quantum-related, however, increasing kVp and mA settings during the scan sequence will reduce this noise and improve scan quality. Most patients we study using HRCT are scanned with kVp/mA settings of 140/170 and a scan time of 2 or 3 seconds.

Retrospectively targeting image reconstruction to a single lung, instead of the entire thorax, significantly reduces image pixel size and, thus, increases spatial resolution. However, in clinical practice, image targeting is not always done. Generally, using thin collimation and reconstruction with the bone algorithm produces most of the improvement in spatial resolution which is possible, and being able to see both lungs on the same image with a nontargeted reconstruction is often preferred.

Most patients scanned with HRCT, unless the lung disease is localized, have scans performed at 4-cm intervals from the lung apices to bases (usually five or six levels). This will provide a representative sample of disease at different levels in the lung. Scans are obtained during full inspiration with the patient in the supine position. If the lung disease being studied has a particular distribution, more scans will be obtained in the area of interest or in the area of most abnormality. Also, scans are often obtained with the patient both supine and prone at each level. Some dependent lung collapse is often seen in both normals and abnormals, and having scans in both positions allows us to differentiate this finding from true pathology. Typically, we diagnose an abnormality only when it is seen within nondependent lung.

This technique is also valuable in the detection of some mediastinal, bronchial, and pleural abnormalities.

SUGGESTED READING

Glazer GM, Francis IR, Gebarski K, et al.: Dynamic incremental computed tomography in evaluation of the pulmonary hila. J Comput Assist Tomogr, 7:59–64, 1983.

Mayo JR, Webb WR, Gould R, et al.: High-resolution CT of the lungs: An optimal approach. Radiology, 163:507–510, 1987.

2

Mediastinum— Introduction and Normal Anatomy

CT is commonly used in patients suspected of having a mediastinal mass or vascular abnormality (for example, an aortic aneurysm), because its ability to image mediastinal anatomy is far superior to that of conventional radiographic techniques such as plain films or tomograms. In general, CT of the mediastinum is obtained in two situations.

First, CT is almost always performed in patients who have an abnormality visible on plain radiographs which is suggestive or diagnostic of mediastinal pathology. It is quite unusual in current medical practice for a patient with a mediastinal abnormality visible on plain films to have surgery or even mediastinoscopy without having a CT first. In patients with a visible mass, CT can be helpful in confirming the presence of a significant lesion (because mediastinal contour abnormalities seen, or imagined, on plain films do not always reflect a real abnormality), defining its location, determining the relationship of the lesion to vascular or nonvascular structures from which it may be arising or is involving, showing other, unrecognized mediastinal lesions, and characterizing the mass as solid, cystic, vascular, enhancing, calcified, inhomogeneous, fatty, etc. Although CT may not be able to diagnose a lesion with certainty, it may be possible to limit the differential diagnosis to a few entities, and this may determine the most appropriate next step, be it percutaneous biopsy, mediastinoscopy, surgery, arteriography, or nothing.

Second, CT is often used to evaluate the mediastinum in patients who have normal chest radiographs but for whom there is clinical suspicion of mediastinal disease. Again, chest films are relatively insensitive to mediastinal abnormalities. One example would be a patient with lung cancer in whom mediastinal nodes might be detected using CT despite a normal chest radiograph. Another example would be a patient with myasthenia gravis who, therefore, has a significant chance (approximately 15%) of having a thymoma which may be detected on CT.

If you think about it, since we should obtain CT in patients who have an abnormal chest radiograph suggesting mediastinal disease, and since we may obtain CT in patients with a normal chest radiograph if we are suspicious, we can justify obtaining CT in almost anyone! If you are suspicious, get CT. Sometimes you will find something, sometimes you won't. I think it is always better to have more information than you need, rather than less than you need. Don't be afraid to get a CT because you think it might turn out to be normal.

NORMAL ANATOMY

The mediastinum can be thought of as the tissue compartment situated between the lungs, marginated on each side by the mediastinal pleura, anteriorly by the sternum and chest wall, and posteriorly by the spine and chest wall. It contains the heart, great vessels, trachea, esophagus, thymus, considerable fat, and a number of lymph nodes grouped together in specific regions. Many of these structures can be reliably differentiated because of differences in location, appearance, and density.

In general, the mediastinum can be conceptualized as consisting of three almost equal divisions, the first beginning at the thoracic inlet and the third ending at the diaphragm. Each of these three is made up of about seven or eight contiguous 1-cm slices in adults. For lack of official names, these can be remembered as the *supra-aortic mediastinum*, from the thoracic inlet to the top of the aortic arch, the *subaortic mediastinum* from the aortic arch to the level of the heart, and the *paracardiac mediastinum* from the heart to the diaphragm. In each of these compartments, certain structures are consistently seen, which need to be evaluated in every patient.

Although very detailed mediastinal anatomy can be seen using modern CT scanners, I will limit my description of normal anatomy to structures which I can remember having been of some diagnostic value over the last 10 or 12 years. If you desire a more detailed knowledge of mediastinal anatomy, I could refer you to a number of excellent atlases of cross-sectional anatomy, but I don't think that a more detailed knowledge is usually needed in interpreting CT. Some additional structures will be mentioned, where appropriate, in discussing various abnormalities. My main goal in this section is to give you an approach to viewing the mediastinum using CT.

Supra-aortic Mediastinum

In evaluating a CT scan of this part of the mediastinum, it is a good idea to localize the trachea before you do anything else; it can always be recognized with certainty on CT scans (Fig. 2—1A). If you cannot find the trachea in looking at a scan of this part of the mediastinum, I would recommend giving up right now. The trachea is easy to recognize because it contains air, is seen in cross section, and has a reasonably consistent round or oval shape. It is relatively central in the mediastinum, from front to back and from right to left, and it serves as an excellent reference point. Many other mediastinal structures maintain a consistent relationship to it.

At or near the thoracic inlet, the mediastinum is relatively narrow from front to back. The esophagus lies posterior to the trachea at this level (Fig. 2—1A), but depending on the position of the trachea relative to the spine, the esophagus can be displaced to one side or the other. It is usually collapsed and appears as a flattened soft-tissue density, but small amounts of air or air and fluid may sometimes be seen in its lumen.

In the supra-aortic mediastinum, the great arterial branches of the aortic arch and the great veins are the most important structures to recognize. At or near the thoracic inlet, the brachiocephalic veins are the most anterior and lateral vascular branches visible, lying immediately behind the clavicular heads (Fig. 2–1A). Although they vary in size, their positions are relatively constant. The great arterial branches (innominate, left carotid, and left subclavian arteries) are posterior to the veins and lie adjacent to the anterior and lateral walls of the trachea. They can be reliably identified by their relative positions.

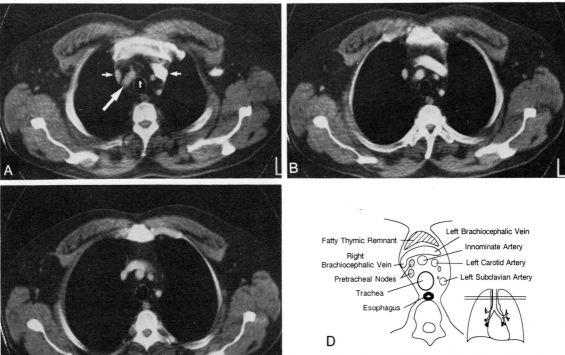

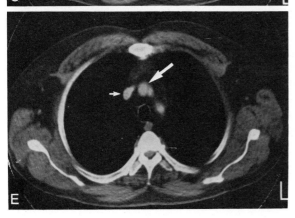

FIGURE 2–1. Normal Mediastinal Anatomy. These illustrations are largely from a single normal patient who had a contrast-enhanced CT of the thorax. Some structures indicated in the accompanying diagrams are not visible in the patient scanned. **Supra-aortic mediastinum.** *(A)* In the upper part of the supra-aortic mediastinum, the trachea (t) is clearly seen, with the air-filled esophagus posterior to it. The right and left brachiocephalic veins (small arrows) are anterior and lateral. The left brachiocephalic vein is densely opacified by contrast material, as is the left axillary vein. The great arterial branches (innominate, left carotid, and left subclavian arteries) are posterior to the veins, lying adjacent to the anterior and lateral walls of the trachea. The innominate artery (large arrow) appears elliptical because of its orientation in the plane of the scan. *(B)* In this section taken 1 cm below *A*, the opacified left brachiocephalic vein is visible crossing the mediastinum from left to right. The left subclavian artery is most posterior and is situated lateral to the left tracheal wall, at approximately 3 or 4 o'clock relative to the tracheal lumen. The left carotid artery is anterior to the left subclavian artery, at about 1 or

2 o'clock, and is somewhat variable in position. The innominate artery is usually anterior to and somewhat to the right of the tracheal midline. *(C)* One cm lower, the left brachiocephalic vein joins the right brachiocephalic vein, forming the superior vena cava. The major aortic branches are again clearly seen. *(D)* Diagram of supra-aortic anatomy at the level of *C*. The location of pretracheal lymph nodes is shown, although these are not visible in the patient scanned. Also shown here, although not well seen in *C*, is the location of the thymic remnant. The approximate level of scan is shown. *(E)* At a level just above the aorta, the superior vena cava (small arrow) is visible abutting the right mediastinal pleura. The origins of the aortic arterial branches are visible. The innominate artery (large arrow) and left carotid artery are very close. Streaky density in the anterior mediastinum represents residual thymus.

Below the thoracic inlet, anterior to the arterial branches of the aorta, the left brachiocephalic vein crosses the mediastinum from left to right (Fig. 2–1B) to join the right brachiocephalic vein, thus forming the superior vena cava (Fig. 2–1C,D). The left subclavian artery is most posterior and is situated adjacent to the left side of the trachea, at approximately 3 or 4 o'clock relative to the tracheal lumen. The left carotid artery is anterior to the left subclavian artery, at about 1 or 2 o'clock, and is somewhat variable in position. The innominate artery is usually anterior and somewhat to the right of the tracheal midline (11 o'clock), but it is the most variable of all the great vessels and can have a number of different appearances in different patients, or in the same patient at different levels.

Near its origin from the aortic arch, the innominate artery is usually oval in shape, being somewhat larger than the other aortic branches (Fig. 2–1E). As it ascends toward the thoracic outlet, it may become more elliptical in shape because of its orientation or because of the way it begins to divide into the right subclavian and carotid arteries. Also, this vessel can be quite tortuous and can appear double if both limbs of a U-shaped part of the vessel are imaged on the same slice. Usually, these vessels can be traced from their origin at the aortic arch to the point where they leave the chest, if there is any doubt as to what they represent.

Other than the great vessels, trachea, and esophagus, little is usually seen in the supra-aortic mediastinum. Some lymph nodes are sometimes visible, but more about these later. Small vascular branches, particularly the internal mammary veins, can sometimes be seen in this part of the mediastinum, but are rarely important in diagnosing disease. In some patients, the thyroid gland may extend into this portion of the mediastinum, and the right and left thyroid lobes may be visible on each side of the trachea. This appearance is not abnormal and does not imply thyroid enlargement or "substernal thyroid." On CT, the thyroid can be distinguished from other tissues or masses because its density is greater than that of soft tissue (because of its iodine content).

Subaortic Mediastinum

Like the supra-aortic region, the subaortic mediastinum consists of approximately seven scans in adults, extending from the aortic arch to the upper heart (Fig. 2–2). While the supra-aortic region largely contains arterial and venous branches of the aorta and vena cava, this compartment contains many of the undivided mediastinal great vessels which we must concern ourselves with, such as the aorta, superior vena cava, and pulmonary arteries. This compartment also contains most of the important lymph node groups which become abnormal in patients with lung cancer, infectious diseases, or lymphoma. In other words, on most CT studies of the mediastinum, this is where the action is. There are a few key levels in this part of the mediastinum which need to be discussed in detail.

Aortic Arch Level

In the upper portion of this compartment, the aortic arch is visible and has a characteristic but somewhat variable appearance (Fig. 2–2A,B). The anterior aspect of the arch is seen anterior to the trachea, with the arch itself passing to the left of the trachea, and the posterior arch usually lying anterior and lateral to the spine. Usually the aortic arch is about the same diameter in its anterior and midportion as it is posteriorly, although the posterior arch is typically smaller. The position of the anterior and posterior aspects of the arch can vary in the presence of atherosclerosis and aortic tortuosity, with the anterior arch moving more anteriorly and to the right, and the posterior aorta moving laterally and posteriorly, in a position to the left of the spine. At this level, the superior vena cava is visible anteriorly and to the right of the trachea, usually being oval in shape (Fig. 2–2A,B). The esophagus appears the same as at higher levels and, again, is variable in position. Often it lies somewhat to the left of the midline of the trachea (and of course is behind the trachea).

The aortic arch on the left, the superior vena cava and mediastinal pleura on the right, and the trachea posteriorly serve to define a roughly triangular space (with the apex of the triangle directed anteriorly) which can be called the *pretracheal* or *anterior paratracheal space* (Fig. 2–2A,B). This fat-filled space is important because it contains middle mediastinal lymph nodes in the pretracheal chain which are commonly involved in various lymph node diseases. Whenever you view the mediastinum for the diagnosis of lymphadenopathy, you should look here first. Other mediastinal node groups are closely related to this group both spatially and in regard to lymphatic drainage. It is not uncommon to see a few normal-sized lymph nodes (diameter < 1 cm) in this compartment, but this will be discussed in detail when we cover mediastinal lymphadenopathy.

Anterior to the great vessels (aorta and superior vena cava) at this level is another roughly (very roughly) triangular space called the *prevascular space* (Fig. 2–2A,B). This compartment, which is anterior mediastinal, primarily contains lymph nodes, the thymus gland, and fat. The apex of this triangular space represents the anterior junction line which can sometimes be seen on chest radiographs.

In young patients, usually in their teens or early twenties, CT shows the thymus to be of soft tissue density, and of a bilobed or arrowhead shape, with each of the two lobes (the right and left) contacting the mediastinal pleura. Each lobe will usually measure 1 to 2 cm in thickness (measured perpendicular to the pleura), but this is variable (Fig. 2–2C). In adulthood, the thymus involutes, with soft tissue elements being replaced by fat. Thus, in patients in their thirties, forties, and older, the prevascular space will appear to be primarily fat filled, with thin wisps of tissue passing through the fat. Most of this, including the fat, actually represents the thymus. At higher levels, the thymus is sometimes visible anterior to the brachiocephalic arteries and veins, again within the prevascular space.

Azygos Arch and Aorticopulmonary Window Level

At a level slightly below the aortic arch, the ascending aorta and descending aorta are visible as separate structures. Characteristically, the descending aorta is slightly smaller (20 to 30 mm) than the ascending aorta (25 to 35 mm), because the subclavian, carotid, and innominate arteries have arisen. Several additional anatomic features are visible at this level which can be very important in the interpretation of thoracic CT.

At or near this level, the trachea bifurcates into the right and left main bronchi. Near the carina, the trachea commonly assumes a somewhat triangular shape (Fig. 2–2F), which is quite normal. The carina itself is usually visible on CT. On the right side, the arch of the azygos vein (azygos, incidentally, means "unpaired") arises from the posterior wall of the superior vena cava, passes over

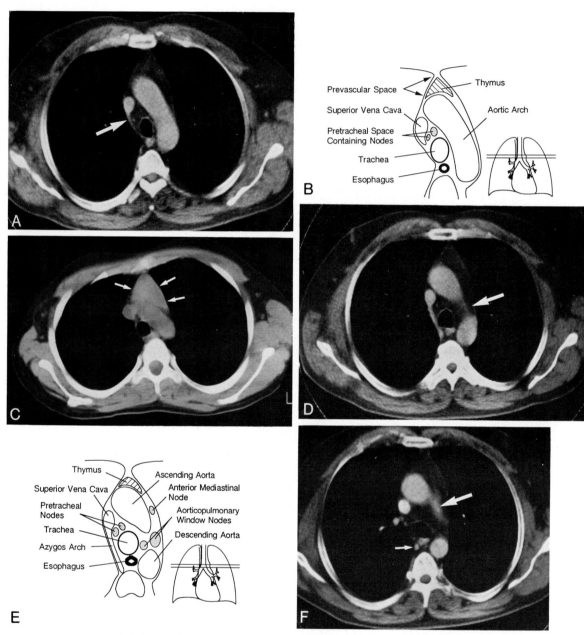

FIGURE 2–2. Subaortic Mediastinum. *(A)* **Aortic arch level.** The aortic arch extends from a position anterior to the trachea, to its left, with the posterior part of the arch usually lying anterior and lateral to the spine. The most cephalad aspect of the azygos arch (arrow) is also seen. *(B)* The locations of the pretracheal node-bearing space and the prevascular space, containing the thymic remnant, are indicated. The locations of the thymus and pretracheal nodes are shown, although they are not seen in *A*. *(C)* A large normal thymus (arrows) in a young patient occupies most of the prevascular space. *(D)* **Azygos arch and aorticopulmonary window level.** At the level of the aorticopulmonary window, the azygos arch is visible contacting the right mediastinal pleura and forming the lateral margin of the pretracheal space. Fat visible under the aortic arch (arrow) is in the aorticopulmonary window. *(E)* The locations of lymph nodes in the pretracheal space, aorticopulmonary window, and anterior mediastinum at this level are shown, although they are not visible in *D*. *(F)* At the tracheal carina, the trachea assumes a somewhat triangular shape. The posterior azygos vein is now visible (small arrow). The upper aspect of the left pulmonary artery (large arrow), which defines the margins of the caudal aspect of the aorticopulmonary window, should not be confused with a mass lesion.

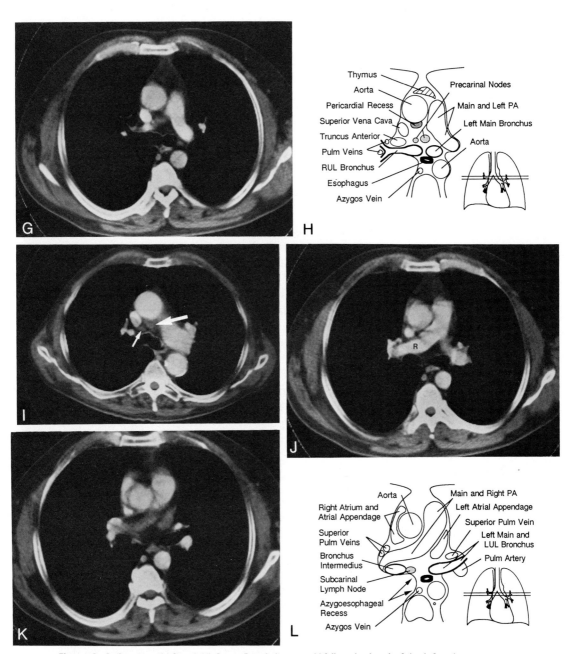

Figure 2–2 *Continued* (*G* and *H*) Scan *G* and diagram *H* fall at the level of the left pulmonary artery and right upper lobe bronchus. The superior pericardial recess posterior to the aorta is indicated in *H*, although it is not visible in *G*. (*I*) In another normal patient, the superior pericardial recess has a typical crescent shape (large arrow). A small pretracheal lymph node is also seen (small arrow). (*J*) **Main pulmonary arteries, subcarinal space, and azygoesophageal recess level.** Slightly below the tracheal carina, the right pulmonary artery (R) is visible crossing the mediastinum, filling the pretracheal and precarinal space. A small amount of fat is visible in the subcarinal space, slightly anterior to the esophagus and the azygos vein. (*K* and *L*) Scan *K* and diagram *L* are at the level of the azygoesophageal recess. The recess appears concave laterally, with the mediastinal pleura closely related to the azygos vein and esophagus.

the right main bronchus (thus we see it at a higher level than the bronchus itself), and continues posteriorly along the mediastinum, to lie to the right and anterior to the spine (Fig. 2–2D,E). (Below the level of the azygos arch, the azygos vein is seen in this position, as long as it is visible.) The azygos arch is often visible on one or two adjacent slices and sometimes appears nodular. However, its characteristic location is usually sufficient to correctly identify this structure. When the azygos arch is visible, it marginates the right border of the pretracheal space.

On the left side of the mediastinum, we are now under the aortic arch, but not yet down far enough to see the main pulmonary artery. This is the region of the *aorticopulmonary window*, which contains fat, lymph nodes (middle mediastinal), the recurrent laryngeal nerve, and the ligamentum arteriosum (the latter two are usually invisible) (Fig. 2–2D–F). These lymph nodes freely communicate with those in the pretracheal space, and, in fact, it may be difficult to distinguish nodes in the medial aorticopulmonary window from those in the left part of the pretracheal space. In some patients, the aorticopulmonary window is not well seen, with the main pulmonary artery lying immediately below the aortic arch. In such patients, it is usually difficult to distinguish lymph nodes from volume averaging of the adjacent aorta and pulmonary artery (Fig. 2–2F). If this is the case, all I can say is "Good luck." However, sometimes scans with thin (1.5 mm) collimation are helpful in distinguishing nodes and volume averaging.

At or slightly below the aorticopulmonary window, the level at which the ascending aorta is first clearly seen in cross section (i.e., it is round or nearly round), a portion of the pericardium, usually containing a small amount of pericardial fluid, extends up from below, into the pretracheal space, immediately behind the ascending aorta. This part of the pericardium is called the *superior pericardial recess* (Fig. 2–2G – I). Although it can sometimes be confused with a lymph node, its typical location immediately behind and contacting the aortic wall, its oval or crescent shape, and its relatively low (water) density allow it to be distinguished from a significant abnormality. Another part of the pericardial recess can sometimes be seen anterior to the ascending aorta and pulmonary artery.

Main Pulmonary Arteries, Subcarinal Space, and Azygoesophageal Recess

Below the level of the carina and azygos arch (Fig 2–2J–L), the medial aspect of the right lung tucks into the posterior aspect of the middle mediastinum, in close association with the azygos vein and esophagus. This part of the mediastinum, reasonably called the *azygoesophageal recess*, is important because of the adjacent subcarinal lymph nodes, which can become enlarged in a variety of diseases, particularly lung cancer, and its close relationship to the esophagus and main bronchi. The contour of the azygoesophageal recess is concave laterally in the large majority of normals, and a convexity in this region should alert you to the presence of underlying pathology. However, a convexity in this region may be produced by a normal esophagus or azygos vein. Of course, the great value of CT is that we do not need to rely on contours, as we do on plain radiographs, to make a diagnosis of mediastinal disease. If a contour abnormality is detected (usually on lung window scans, which best show mediastinal contours), a close look at the mediastinal windows should be sufficient to delineate the cause of the abnormal contour. If the contour abnormality does not reflect the esophagus or azygos vein, then it is abnormal and subcarinal node enlargement is the usual culprit.

In many subjects, the azygoesophageal recess is somewhat posterior to the node-bearing subcarinal space, which lies between the main bronchi. Normal nodes are commonly visible in this space, being larger than normal nodes in other parts of the mediastinum, and up to 1.5 cm in diameter. The esophagus usually is seen immediately behind the subcarinal space, and distinguishing nodes and esophagus may be difficult, unless the esophagus contains air or contrast material. At levels below the subcarinal space, the appearance of the azygoesophageal recess is relatively constant, although it narrows somewhat in the retrocardiac region.

Also at or near this level, the main pulmonary artery (PA) divides into its right and left branches. The left pulmonary artery (Fig. 2–2G–I) is somewhat higher than the right, usually being seen 1 cm above it, and appears as the continuation of the main pulmonary artery, directed posterolaterally and to the left. The right pulmonary artery arises at an angle of nearly 90 degrees to the main and left PA, and crosses the mediastinum from left to right, anterior to the carina or main bronchi. In this location, the right PA effectively fills in the pretracheal space. At the point where the main bronchi and pulmonary arteries exit the mediastinum, we enter the pulmonary hila. Their anatomy will be discussed in detail in Chapter 5.

Paracardiac Mediastinum

As we progress caudally through the mediastinum, the origins of the great vessels from the cardiac chambers can be seen to a variable degree. Although CT is not commonly used to diagnose cardiac abnormalities (magnetic resonance or angiography are much better), some simple understanding of cardiac anatomy on CT can be helpful in diagnosis.

The main pulmonary artery is most anterior, arising from the right ventricle, which can be seen at lower levels to be anterior and to the right of the left ventricle (Fig. 2–3A,B). The superior vena cava enters the right atrium, which is elliptical or crescent shaped. The right atrial appendage extends anteriorly from the upper atrium, bordering the right mediastinal pleura.

Between the right atrium and the main pulmonary artery or pulmonary outflow tract, the aortic root enters the left ventricle. At this level it is common in adults to see some coronary artery calcification (Fig. 2–3C), and, occasionally, the uncalcified coronary arteries are visible, surrounded by mediastinal fat. The left atrium is posteriorly located, appearing larger than the right. The left atrial appendage extends anteriorly and to the left and is visible below the left pulmonary artery, bordering the pleura. On each side, superior and inferior pulmonary veins can be seen entering the left atrium (Fig. 2–3A,B,D,E). These will be discussed further when we review hilar anatomy.

Near the level of the diaphragm, the inferior vena cava is visible as an oval structure extending caudally from the posterior right atrium (Fig. 2–3F,G). It is easy to identify.

The only other structures of consequence at this level that we need to mention are the esophagus, which lies in a retrocardiac location, the azygos vein, which is often still visible in the same relative position as it is at higher levels, and the hemiazygos vein, which is usually smaller than the azygos and on the opposite side, behind the descending aorta. Paravertebral nodes lie in association with the azygos and hemiazygos veins, but are not normally visible.

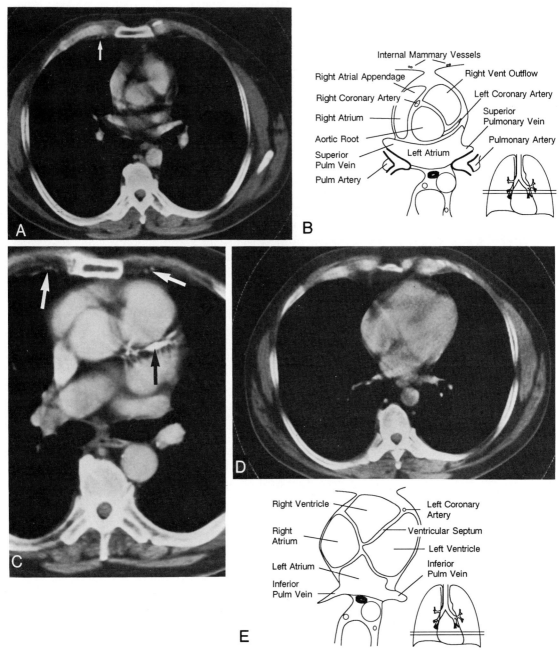

FIGURE 2–3. Paracardiac Mediastinum. *(A)* Being most cephalad, the origins of the aorta and pulmonary artery are visible, with the aortic root being central. The pulmonary outflow tract or main pulmonary artery is anterior and to the left of the aortic root at this level. The right atrium, with its appendage extending anteriorly, borders the right mediastinal pleura. The superior pulmonary veins enter the upper aspect of the left atrium at this level. Anteriorly, the right internal mammary vessels are visible (arrow). *(B)* Diagram shows the level of A. The left and right coronary arteries are shown. *(C)* In another subject, calcification of the left coronary artery (black arrow) is easily seen. The left coronary artery arises from the posterolateral aortic root. The internal mammary vessels (white arrows) are also visible. *(D and E)* At a lower level, the right and left atria and ventricles are visible. The right ventricle is now located anterior and to the right of the left ventricle. At this level, the inferior pulmonary veins enter the left atrium.

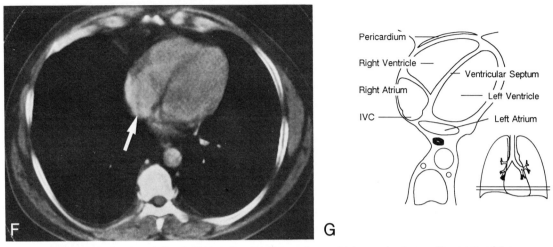

Figure 2–3 Continued (F and G) Near the diaphragm, the ventricles are best seen. The origin of the inferior vena cava (arrow) is indicated.

Normal Cardiac Anatomy

Without the injection of contrast, little cardiac anatomy is discernible on CT, but some differentiation of cardiac chambers is possible because of the presence of epicardial fat collections. When contrast is given, additional features of cardiac anatomy are visible, depending on the amount and rapidity of contrast injection; the myocardium opacifies less than the intracardiac blood and is sometimes visible as a relatively low density band following rapid infusion of a large contrast bolus. The interventricular septum is usually visible if contrast has been infused; it is typically oriented at an angle of about 2 o'clock to the vertical (Fig. 2–3). However, other segments of the myocardium may be difficult to appreciate as distinct from the opacified cardiac chambers on clinical scans. (On routine scans, the contrast bolus is usually too slow or is not properly timed to optimize cardiac opacification—usually we are more interested in the upper mediastinum.) The lateral or "free" left ventricular wall is about three times thicker than the right ventricular wall (it is about 1 cm), and is better seen.

Cardiac anatomy is easiest to understand if we start with a scan near the cardiac apex (and diaphragm). At this level, the left ventricle is elliptical in shape, with its long axis directed laterally and anteriorly (Fig. 2–3F,G). Being the highest pressure chamber, it dominates cardiac anatomy, and the other cardiac chambers mold themselves to its shape. The right ventricle, which is anterior and to the right, is triangular in shape. On scans at this level or slightly above, the line of the interventricular septum, if continued posteriorly and to the right, separates the lower right atrium anteriorly (and in contiguity with the right ventricle), from the lower left atrium posteriorly. The mitral and tricuspid valves are located at or near this level, but are not normally visible.

At higher levels (Fig. 2–3A,B), the left ventricular outflow tract and aortic valve are centrally located within the heart. The right ventricular outflow tract is directed toward the left and is visible anterior or to the left of the left ventricular outflow tract. In other words, because of twisting of the heart during development, the left ventricular outflow tract is directed rightward, and the right ventricular outflow tract is directed leftward. This accounts for the location of the aorta on the right and the pulmonary artery on the left. The aortic and pulmonary valves are located near this level, and are invisible in normals.

The Normal Pericardium

The normal pericardium (the visceral and parietal pericardium and pericardial contents) is visible as a 1-to 2-mm stripe of soft tissue density paralleling the heart and is outlined by mediastinal fat (outside the pericardial sac) and epicardiac fat. It is best seen near the diaphragm, along the anterior and lateral aspects of the heart, where the fat layers are thickest (Fig. 2–3F,G). As stated above, extensions of the pericardium into the mediastinum can also be seen in normals.

The Retrosternal Space

In a retrosternal location, the internal mammary arteries and veins are normally visible 1 or 2 cm lateral to the sternum, on good CT scans (Fig. 2–3A–C). These vessels are not of much diagnostic significance, although the veins commonly enlarge in patients with superior vena caval obstruction, but they are important because they serve to localize the internal mammary chain of lymph nodes. Although normal nodes can be seen in several areas of the mediastinum (most notably the pretracheal space, aorticopulmonary window, and subcarinal space), I don't think that normal internal mammary nodes are large enough to be recognized as such. A lymph node in this region which is large enough to be visible should be regarded as abnormal. Internal mammary node enlargement is most common in patients with breast cancer or lymphoma.

SUGGESTED READING

Francis I, Glazer GM, Bookstein FL, et al.: The thymus: Reexamination of age-related changes in size and shape. Am J Roentgenol, 145:249–254, 1985.

Glazer HS, Aronberg DJ, Sagel SS: Pitfalls in CT recognition of mediastinal lymphadenopathy. Am J Roentgenol, 144: 267–274, 1985.

Zylak CJ, Pallie W, Pirani M, et al.: Anatomy and computed tomography: A correlative nodule on the cervicothoracic junction. Radiographics, 3:478–530, 1983.

3

Mediastinum—Vascular Abnormalities

On any thoracic CT study in a patient with a mediastinal mass, the first objective is to prove that the mass is or isn't vascular in origin.

AORTIC ABNORMALITIES

A variety of aortic arch and great arterial abnormalities are visible on CT, and CT is commonly used to diagnose aortic disease when it is suspected clinically or when chest radiographs are abnormal.

Congenital Anomalies

Congenital abnormalities of the aorta and its mediastinal branches are easily diagnosed using CT, and no other study is usually needed unless the anomaly is complex or associated with congenital heart disease.

Anomalous Right Subclavian Artery

This relatively common anomaly (1 in 200 people) does not usually produce a recognizable mediastinal abnormality on chest radiographs, and thus is usually detected incidentally on CT scans obtained for another reason. Its main significance is that it should not be misinterpreted as something else. In patients with this anomaly, the aortic arch is usually somewhat higher than normal. The anomalous artery arises from the medial wall of the aorta, as its last branch (Fig. 3–1). It passes toward the right, behind the esophagus, and then ascends on the right toward the thoracic outlet. In the supra-aortic mediastinum it lies much more posterior than is normal for the subclavian artery, often anterolateral to the spine. At its point of origin, the artery may be dilated, or if you wish to think of it in a more complicated way, the artery may arise from an aortic diverticulum (diverticulum of Kommerell). This may cause compression of the esophagus and symptoms of dysphagia. In some patients, the diverticulum dilates further, resulting in a focal aneurysm.

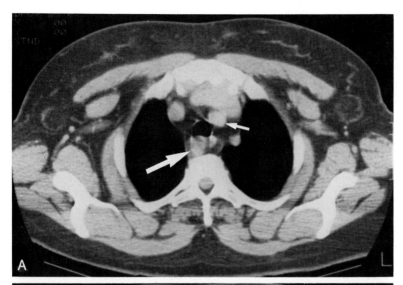

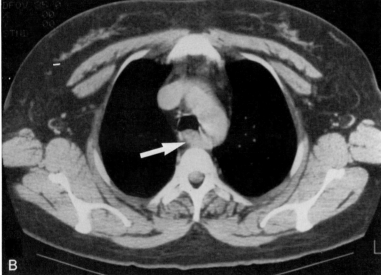

FIGURE 3–1. Anomalous right subclavian artery. *(A)* An anomalous right subclavian artery (large arrow) is visible in a retrotracheal location. Its relatively large size is characteristic. In this patient, the right and left carotid arteries share a common origin (small arrow). *(B)* At a lower level, the anomalous artery (arrow) arises from the posteromedial aortic arch.

Right Aortic Arch

There are two main types of right aortic arch—*mirror image right arch* and *right arch associated with anomalous left subclavian artery*. Mirror image right arch is relatively uncommon and is almost always associated with congenital heart disease (usually complex anomalies such as tetralogy of Fallot). The CT appearance of a mirror image arch is well described by its name—it is the mirror image of a normal left arch, with a left innominate artery being present. Right arch with an anomalous left subclavian artery is present in about 1 in 1000 subjects. It is the reverse of a left arch with an anomalous right subclavian artery, although the presence of an aortic diverticulum is more common with a right arch (Fig. 3–2). With this anomaly, there is a low frequency (about 5 to 10%) of associated congenital heart lesions, and they are usually simple, such as atrial septal defect. With both types of right arch the descending aorta is usually left sided, crossing from right to left in the lower mediastinum.

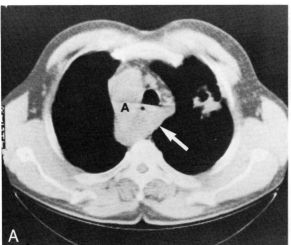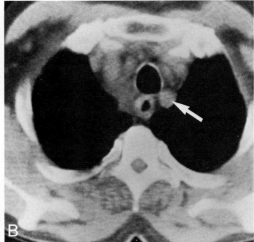

FIGURE 3–2. Right aortic arch with anomalous left subclavian artery. *(A)* In a patient with no evidence of congenital heart disease and with a right aortic arch (A), an anomalous left subclavian artery arises from a retroesophageal aortic diverticulum (arrow). The position of the esophagus is marked by air in its lumen. *(B)* At a higher level, the anomalous left subclavian artery (arrow) is visible.

Double Arch

Double aortic arches are relatively uncommon, but because the plain radiograph shows a mediastinal abnormality they are often evaluated using CT. This anomaly is usually unassociated with congenital heart disease, but because a complete vascular ring is present, symptoms of dysphagia are not uncommon. In this anomaly, the ascending aorta splits into right and left halves. The right arch, which is usually higher and larger than the left, passes to the right of the trachea and esophagus, crosses behind these structures, and rejoins the left arch, which occupies a relatively normal position (Fig. 3–3). Each arch is smaller than normal, and smaller than the descending aorta. Also, each arch gives rise to a subclavian and a carotid artery, and no innominate artery is present. This results in a symmetric appearance to the great vessels in the supra-aortic mediastinum which is virtually diagnostic.

Coarctation and Pseudocoarctation

Coarctation, and its variant pseudocoarctation, can be diagnosed using CT, but even if this is possible, catheterization is usually necessary in order to measure intra-arterial pressures and, thus, the significance of the vascular obstruction. Some feel that the use of the term pseudocoarctation is inappropriate, considering this lesion to be a coarctation and not "pseudo," but the CT and clinical findings in these two entities are somewhat different. I will consider them separately, if for no other reason than because the term pseudocoarctation is in common usage.

The site of narrowing in coarctation is generally at the aortic isthmus, distal to the origin of the left subclavian artery, and near the ligamentum arteriosum (juxtaductal coarctation). On CT, the narrowed segment is often visible, being decidedly smaller than the aorta above and below this level (Fig. 3–4). This size difference reflects not only the narrowed segment at the coarctation, but also some dilation of the prestenotic and poststenotic aorta.

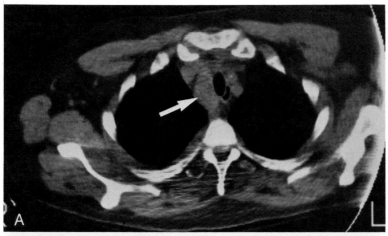

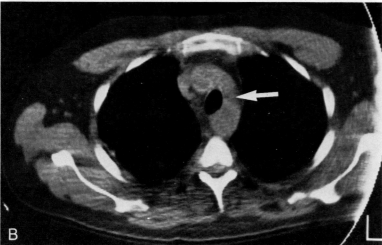

FIGURE 3–3. Double aortic arch. *(A)* The right arch (arrow) is visible at the level of the junction of the brachiocephalic veins. The left carotid and subclavian arteries, which arise from the left arch, are visible to the left of the trachea. *(B)* At a lower level, the left arch (arrow) is visible. Both right and left aortic arches appear smaller than normal.

Reformatted CT in the plane of the aortic arch can show the coarctation to better advantage, but the resolution of reformatted scans is limited by scan thickness. Also, the degree of narrowing at the site of coarctation may be overestimated if the reformatted plane is slightly off the sagittal plane of the aorta. A long narrowing of the aortic arch (hypoplasia) is less common.

In pseudocoarctation, the aortic arch is kinked anteriorly, and its lumen is somewhat narrowed, but a significant pressure gradient across the kink, and collateral vessels, are not present. The CT appearance of this anomaly is characteristic, but sometimes confusing. The aortic arch is higher than normal and initially descends in an abnormally anterior position, well in front of the spine. At a level near the carina, however, it again angles posteriorly, forming a second arch, and assumes its normal position anterolateral to the spine. This anomaly is usually unassociated with symptoms and is usually detected incidentally on chest radiographs. Its plain film appearance is also characteristic, but it may be mistaken for a soft tissue mass.

Both coarctation and pseudocoarctation are associated with congenital bicuspid aortic valve (from 30 to 85% of patients with coarctation), which may produce aortic stenosis. In some patients, CT shows aortic valve calcification, allowing this diagnosis to be suggested.

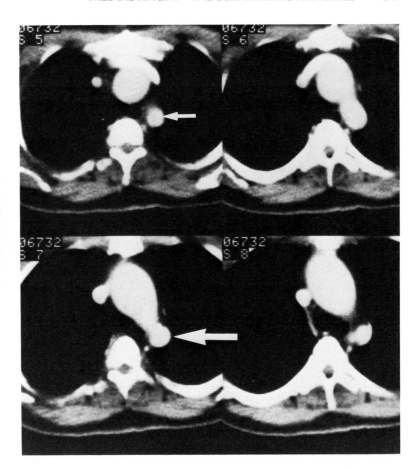

FIGURE 3–4. Aortic coarctation. CT with bolus contrast enhancement at four levels in a patient with coarctation. The proximal descending aorta, at the level of the coarctation (large arrow), is significantly smaller than the ascending aorta. The coarctation is distal to the origin of the left subclavian artery (small arrow), which is large because of collateral blood flow.

Aortic Aneurysm

CT is of great value in diagnosing aortic aneurysm and distinguishing it from soft tissue mediastinal mass. If the aorta measures more than 4 cm in diameter, it is probably dilated. Although a diagnosis of "aortic dilatation" as opposed to "aortic aneurysm" is somewhat arbitrary, I use "aortic dilatation" or "ectasia" to refer to a generalized dilatation of relatively mild degree (5 cm), with the implication that it is not necessarily a serious problem. "Aneurysm," on the other hand, is used to refer to a more focal lesion, or more severe dilatation of the entire aorta.

In some patients with an (atherosclerotic) aortic aneurysm, the diagnosis can be made, and the aneurysm distinguished from a solid mass, because of peripheral intimal calcification visible on unenhanced scans. In most patients, however, this diagnosis requires contrast infusion, and the best opacification is achieved if a rapid bolus of contrast is given with dynamic scanning at one or more levels in the area of abnormality. With a bolus technique, the lumen of the aorta and the aneurysm, and the thickness of its wall, can be clearly defined (Figs. 3–5,3–6).

With atherosclerotic aneurysms, the aortic wall is thickened and calcification is commonly visible. There may be visible areas of plaque or thrombus in the lumen of the aorta which (very) occasionally show some calcification as well. The plaque may appear low in density relative to soft tissue or aortic wall

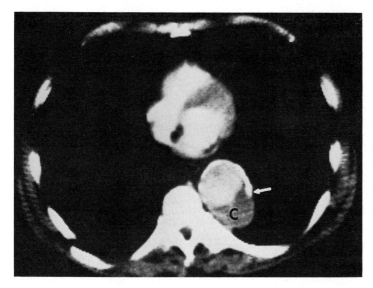

FIGURE 3–5. Aortic aneurysm. Clot (C) fills a focal aneurysm of the descending aorta on this contrast-enhanced scan. Calcification marks the location of the aortic wall. (Reproduced with modification. From CE Putnam and CE Ravin. *Textbook of Diagnostic Imaging.* Philadelphia, W.B. Saunders, 1988.)

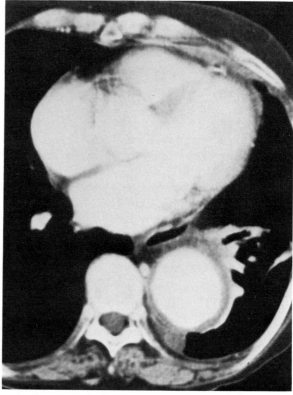

FIGURE 3–6. Aortic aneurysm. A layer of thrombus lines a fusiform aneurysm of the descending aorta.

because of its fat content or because of some opacification of the aortic wall itself. Mycotic aneurysms are usually focal and may be associated with periaortic inflammation or abscess, and air bubbles within soft tissues may be seen.

Trauma

CT has no real role in the diagnosis of acute aortic injuries, such as aortic rupture or laceration. Aortography should be done in these cases to show the area of the aortic tear. Although CT is good for demonstrating chronic false aneurysms, or mediastinal hematoma which occurs in association with laceration, the tear itself is usually below the resolution of this technique. Post-traumatic false aneurysms are usually located in the region of the aorticopulmonary window, below the takeoff of the left subclavian artery (Fig. 3–7). Because these represent contained aortic rupture, and they are not marginated by aortic wall, peripheral calcification is unusual. Aneurysmal dilatation of the ductus or ductus diverticulum (ductus aneurysm) can occur in the same region.

Dissection

CT has revolutionized the diagnosis of dissection, and to a large extent has replaced arteriography. The goal in diagnosing dissection, using any technique, is the demonstration of an intimal flap, displaced inward from the edge of the aorta, lying between the true and false channels. CT is ideally suited to this because of its cross-sectional format.

Two schemes for the classification of dissections have been proposed by Daily and DeBakey. Daily's classification is most frequently used in my experience because of its simplicity and relevance to treatment.

Using this classification, aortic dissections are divided into types A and B. Type A dissections involve the ascending aorta (Fig. 3–8); approximately two-thirds of acute dissections are type A. Because of the possibility of retrograde dissection and rupture into the pericardium (resulting in tamponade) or occlusion

FIGURE 3–7. Post-traumatic false aneurysm. Contrast-enhanced CT in a patient with a past history of a motor vehicle accident. Aneurysmal dilatation of the aorta distal to the left subclavian artery is consistent with a post-traumatic false aneurysm. This was confirmed at surgery.

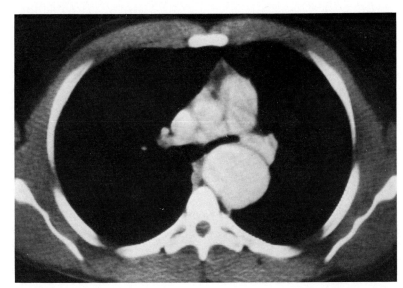

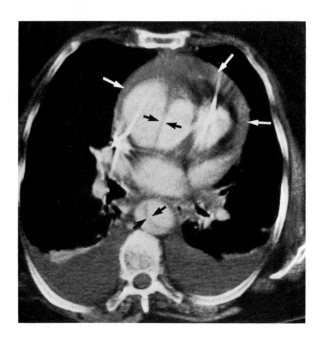

FIGURE 3–8. Type A aortic dissection. A patient with acute chest pain shows a type A dissection involving the ascending and descending aorta. The intimal flaps (black arrows) are lower in density than the contrast-opacified blood. The ascending aorta is also dilated. Pleural and pericardial hemorrhage (white arrows) are present as a complication of the dissection. Streak artifacts reflect the presence of a catheter in the superior vena cava and pulmonary artery.

of the cephalic arteries, these dissections are usually treated surgically with grafting of the region of the tear. Type B dissections do not involve the aortic arch, but typically arise distal to the left subclavian artery (Fig. 3–9). These are generally treated medically instead of surgically.

DeBakey's classification has three types. Type I (involvement of the entire aorta, both ascending and descending) is most common. Type II dissections, which are often associated with Marfan's syndrome, involve the ascending aorta only, and along with type I correspond to Daily's type A. Type III dissections involve the descending aorta only.

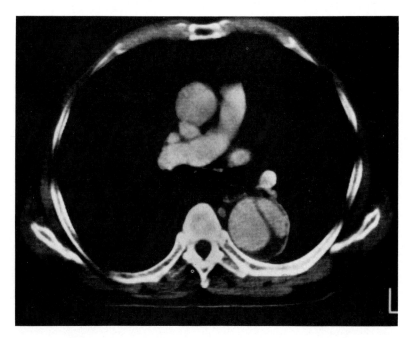

FIGURE 3–9. Type B aortic dissection. A well-defined intimal flap is visible in the dilated proximal descending aorta on this contrast-enhanced scan.

Because CT is quite accurate in diagnosing dissection and in determining its location and type (it is at least as good as arteriography), CT is an excellent screening procedure in patients with a suggestive clinical presentation. CT is the only imaging procedure performed in most patients with suspected dissection, although an aortogram may be obtained prior to surgery, depending on the surgeon's preference, in patients shown to have a type A dissection. Also, CT is commonly used to follow patients with dissection after treatment to watch for redissection or extension of the dissection.

Occasionally, intimal dissection can be diagnosed on unenhanced scans, if the intima is calcified and visibly displaced inward from the aortic wall. However, there is no real rationale for obtaining unenhanced CT in patients with a suspicion of dissection. In patients with suspected dissection, CT should be performed with bolus contrast enhancement and dynamic scanning.

Sequential scans are usually obtained at three levels during rapid infusion of contrast. These levels are 1) the aortic arch, 2) the proximal aortic root and descending aorta near the level of the right pulmonary artery, and 3) the more distal descending thoracic aorta. If there is a dissection present, it will involve one of these levels. Generally the injection of 25 ml of contrast at each level will be sufficient, if rapid infusion is used along with sequential dynamic scanning. After scanning these levels, and if a dissection is present, the remainder of the aorta, including its major abdominal branches, can be studied using a drip infusion of contrast and scans every 1 or 2 cm.

In a patient with dissection, the intimal flap may be clearly delineated by contrast filling both the true and false channels. Slow flow in one of the channels, usually the false channel, may require that images late in the sequence be used to make this diagnosis. In some patients, the false channel may not opacify because it is filled with clot. In such cases, dissection may be difficult to distinguish from a clot-filled atherosclerotic aneurysm. However, dissections are usually longer than typical clot-filled aneurysms. Other findings which can be associated with dissection are an abrupt change in aortic caliber, with a long dilated segment, and thickening of the aortic wall, but these are nonspecific and insufficient to make a definite diagnosis.

Streak artifacts, arising because of motion or vascular pulsations, may mimic an intimal flap. They are usually seen in the descending aorta, adjacent to the left heart border. Typically they are less sharply defined than a true intimal flap, extend beyond the edges of the aorta, and are inconsistently seen from one level to the next. If any question exists as to the reality of an intimal flap, repeating the scan with a reinfusion of contrast is all that is usually necessary.

SUPERIOR VENA CAVA

Congenital Abnormalities

Azygos Lobe

An azygos lobe is a common anomaly and is present in about 1 in 200 patients. Azygos lobe results in a typical appearance on plain radiographs and CT which is easily recognized, and it produces a characteristic alteration in normal mediastinal anatomy.

In patients with this anomaly, the azygos arch is located more cephalad than normal, at or near the junction of the brachiocephalic veins. Above this

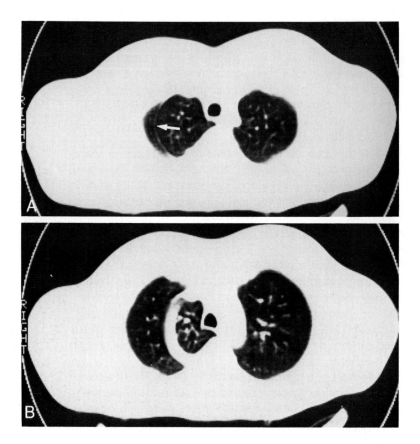

FIGURE 3–10. Azygos lobe. *(A)* Within the upper lung, the azygos fissure (arrow) distinguishes the azygos lobe medially from the remainder of the upper lobe. *(B)* At a lower level, the azygos arch passes from anterior to posterior. The posterior azygos vein is more laterally placed than normal.

level, the azygos fissure is visible within the lung, marginating the azygos lobe (Fig. 3–10).

Persistent Left Superior Vena Cava

The only other frequent venous anomaly is persistent left superior vena cava (SVC), representing failure of the embryonic left anterior cardinal vein to regress. This anomaly is difficult to recognize on plain films, but in some patients, there is a slight prominence of the left superior mediastinum. It is present in 0.3% of normal subjects, approximately the same frequency as an azygos lobe, and is usually without symptoms or associated abnormalities. It is, however, seen in 4.4% of patients with congenital heart disease.

On CT in patients with this anomaly, the left superior vena cava is positioned lateral to the left common carotid artery in the supra-aortic mediastinum (Fig. 3–11). It descends along the left mediastinum, passing downward, anterior to the left hilum, to enter the coronary sinus posterior to the left atrium. In most subjects, a right vena cava is also present, and the two vessels will be about the same size and in the same relative position, on opposite sides of the mediastinum. In 65% the left brachiocephalic vein is absent. If it is also present, joining the right and left SVCs, the right SVC will be larger than the left.

A left SVC will densely opacify after contrast injection into the left arm. If contrast is injected on the right, and the vein does not opacify, its tubular shape and characteristic position are usually enough for a definite diagnosis.

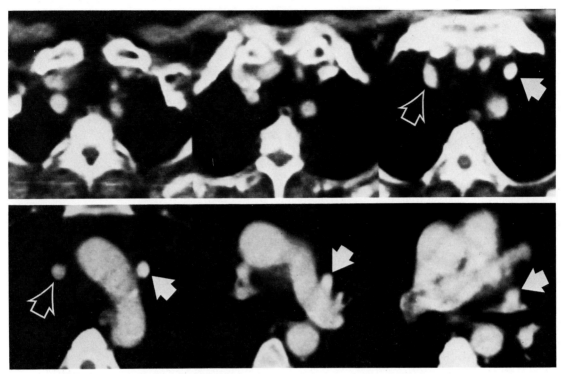

FIGURE 3–11. Persistent left superior vena cava. In a patient with this anomaly, the course of the left superior vena cava (white arrow) is visible at different levels, following contrast infusion into the left arm. The right vena cava (open arrow) is similar in size and there is no evidence of a connecting left brachiocephalic vein anteriorly. The left vena cava passes anterior to the left hilum and eventually enters the coronary sinus posterior to the heart. Reproduced with permission. From Webb WR et al.: Computer tomographic demonstration of mediastinal venous anomalies. Am J Roentgenol, 139:157–161, 1982.)

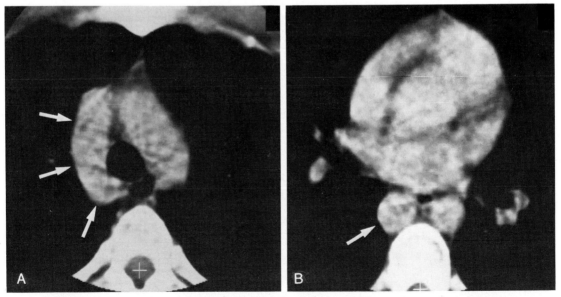

FIGURE 3–12. Azygos continuation of the inferior vena cava. *(A* and *B)* The azygos arch (arrows, *A),* and the posterior azygos vein (arrow, *B)* are markedly dilated. (Reproduced with permission. From Webb WR et al.: Computer tomographic demonstration of mediastinal venous anomalies. Am J Roentgenol, 139:157–161, 1982.)

Azygos or Hemiazygos Continuation of the Inferior Vena Cava

The embryogenesis of the inferior vena cava (IVC) is one of the most complicated sequences I know of, and several vessels must develop and regress for it to form normally. Suffice it to say that during fetal development, the vessels which form the azygos and hemiazygos veins normally communicate with the suprarenal IVC, but this communication usually breaks down. If it does not, then azygos or hemiazygos continuation of the IVC is said to be present. These lesions may be associated with other congenital anomalies, including polysplenia (in patients with hemiazygos communication) or asplenia (with azygos communication), or they may be isolated abnormalities. Typical findings include marked dilatation of the azygos arch and posterior azygos vein (Fig. 3–12). If hemiazygos continuation is present, the dilated azygos vein will be seen to cross the mediastinum, from right to left, behind the descending aorta, to communicate with a dilated hemiazygos vein. A normal-appearing IVC is very often visible at the level of the heart and diaphragm, draining the hepatic veins. Either anomaly may be associated with duplication of the abdominal IVC. Rarely, a dilated hemiazygos vein drains into the left brachiocephalic vein instead of joining the azygos.

Superior Vena Cava Syndrome

Obstruction of the superior vena cava, or either of the brachiocephalic veins, is not an uncommon clinical occurrence, and symptoms of venous obstruction may lead to CT. Also, in some patients having CT for the diagnosis of mediastinal mass, CT will show findings of vena cava obstruction. CT has replaced other methods of making this diagnosis, because it shows not only the vascular abnormality, but also the responsible mass, if one happens to be present.

Superior vena cava obstruction can be seen in a variety of diseases, most commonly bronchogenic carcinoma, although in some parts of the country, granulomatous mediastinitis as a result of histoplasmosis is a very common cause. Because of the frequent use of subclavian catheters in modern medicine, venous thrombosis resulting in obstruction can also be seen.

On CT in patients who have brachiocephalic vein (Fig. 3–13) or SVC obstruction (Fig. 3–14), a number of characteristic findings are present. Beginning peripherally as the contrast bolus is injected, it is common to see opacification of a number of small venous collaterals in the shoulder, upper chest wall, and upper mediastinum. However, this finding is not always abnormal; some filling of small veins in the chest wall and axilla can be seen in the absence of a venous abnormality (perhaps because of poor positioning of the patient's arm for injection). Unless other evidence of venous obstruction is present, this finding should not be of great concern.

In patients with SVC obstruction, contrast flow from the arm into the great veins will be delayed, and the scan sequence must be delayed accordingly, or opacification will be poor. Some characteristic collaterals are often seen in patients with SVC obstruction. These include a number of veins which drain into the azygos system, and thus bypass the area of obstruction. These veins commonly include the internal mammary veins, left superior intercostal vein (which results in the "aortic nipple" sometimes visible on chest radiographs), intercostal veins, and the hemiazygos vein. In addition to dilatation of these veins because of increased flow, they opacify after contrast infusion.

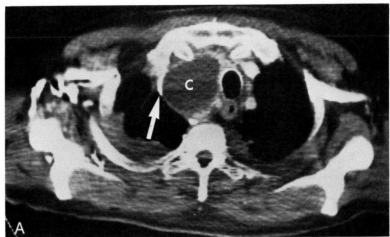

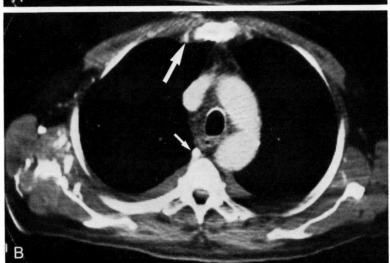

FIGURE 3–13. Brachiocephalic vein obstruction. *(A)* This patient has a bronchogenic cyst (C) obstructing the opacified right brachiocephalic vein (arrow). *(B)* At a lower level, there is opacification of a number of veins in the right chest wall, the internal mammary vein (large arrow) and the right superior intercostal vein (small arrow), a branch of the azygos system.

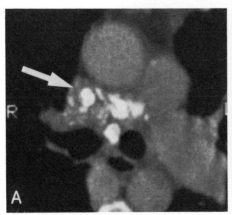

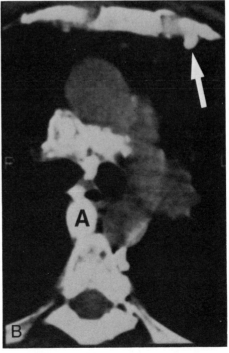

FIGURE 3–14. Superior vena cava syndrome. *(A)* A CT without contrast in a patient with granulomatous mediastinitis from histoplasmosis shows calcified mediastinal lymph nodes. The superior vena cava appears to contain calcified clot (arrow). (Reproduced with modification. From CE Putman and CE Ravin. *Textbook of Diagnostic Imaging.* Philadelphia, W.B. Saunders, 1988.) *(B)* Following contrast infusion, there is opacification of a dilated azygos vein (A) and an internal mammary vein (arrow).

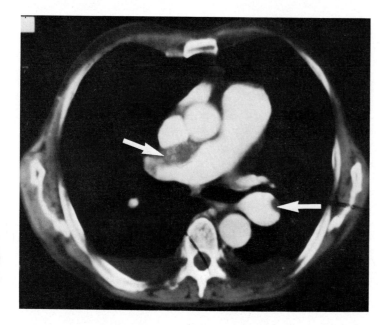

FIGURE 3–15. Pulmonary Embolism. A contrast-enhanced CT shows clots (arrows) within the anterior right and descending left pulmonary arteries.

In patients with thrombosis of the SVC or brachiocephalic veins, thrombus is sometimes visible in the vessel lumen, outlined by contrast. One word of caution, however—if contrast is injected into only one arm, streaming of unopacified blood from one brachiocephalic vein into the SVC can mimic the appearance of vena cava clot. This problem can be avoided by injecting contrast into both arms at the same time.

PULMONARY ARTERY ABNORMALITIES

Pulmonary artery anomalies are very rare, but some may be diagnosed using CT. Dilatation of the pulmonary artery as a result of pulmonic stenosis or pulmonary hypertension is much more common than congenital lesions. With pulmonic stenosis, the main and left pulmonary arteries will be dilated, while the right pulmonary artery is relatively normal in size. With pulmonary hypertension, both pulmonary arteries will be large.

CT can be used to diagnose pulmonary embolism or thrombosis involving central pulmonary arteries (Fig. 3–15). This is most often done in patients with chronic emboli and pulmonary hypertension. Quite simply, a filling defect is visible in the pulmonary artery, often appearing to be adherent to one wall of the pulmonary artery. These can be accurately diagnosed in the main right and left pulmonary arteries and within the largest hilar arteries, but attempting to diagnose emboli in smaller branches is risky.

SUGGESTED READING

Bechtold RE, Wolfman NT, Karstaedt N, et al.: Superior vena caval obstruction: Detection using CT. Radiology, 157:485–487, 1985.

Webb WR, Gamsu G, Speckman JM, et al.: CT demonstration of mediastinal aortic arch anomalies. J Comput Assist Tomogr, 6:445–451, 1982.

Webb WR, Gamsu G, Speckman JM, et al.: CT demonstration of mediastinal venous anomalies. Am J Roentgenol, 159:157–161, 1982.

White RD, Dooms GC, Higgins CB: Advances in imaging thoracic aortic disease. Invest Radiol, 21:761–778, 1986.

4

Mediastinum—Lymph Node Abnormalities and Masses

The detection and diagnosis of mediastinal lymph node enlargement is important in the evaluation of a number of thoracic diseases, particularly bronchogenic carcinoma. Mediastinal lymph nodes are generally classified by location, and most descriptive systems are based on a modification of Rouvière classification of lymph node groups.

LYMPH NODE ANATOMY

Anterior Mediastinal Nodes

Internal Mammary Nodes. These nodes are located in a retrosternal location near the internal mammary artery and veins (Fig. 4–1). They drain the anterior chest wall, anterior diaphragm, and medial breasts.

Paracardiac Nodes. These surround the heart on the surface of the diaphragm and communicate with the lower internal mammary chain (Fig. 4–2). As with internal mammary nodes, they are most commonly enlarged in patients with lymphoma and metastatic carcinoma, particularly breast cancer.

Prevascular Nodes. These lie anterior to the great vessels (Fig. 4–3). They may be involved in a variety of diseases, notably lymphoma, but their involvement in lung cancer is unusual.

Middle Mediastinal Nodes

Lung diseases (i.e., lung cancer, sarcoidosis, tuberculosis, fungal infections) which secondarily involve lymph nodes typically involve middle mediastinal lymph nodes.

Pre- or Paratracheal Nodes. These occupy the pretracheal (or anterior paratracheal) space (Fig. 4–4A,B). The most inferior node in this region is the

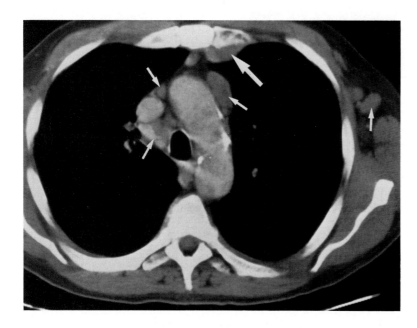

FIGURE 4–1. Internal mammary node enlargement from Hodgkin's lymphoma. A left internal mammary node (large arrow) is enlarged, as are pretracheal, prevascular, and axillary nodes (small arrows).

FIGURE 4–2. Paracardiac node enlargement. In a patient with lymphoma, enlargement of paracardiac nodes (large arrows) is visible. The pericardium (small arrows) and inferior vena cava (V) are also seen. (Reproduced with modification. From Webb WR. Diseases of the mediastinum. *In* CE Putman and CE Ravin (eds). *Textbook of Diagnostic Imaging.* Philadelphia, W.B. Saunders, 1988.)

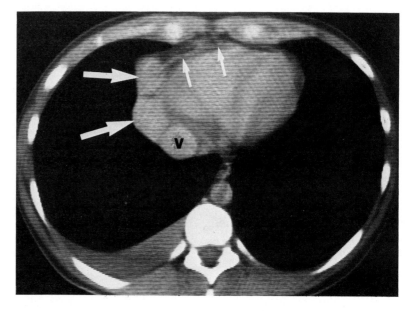

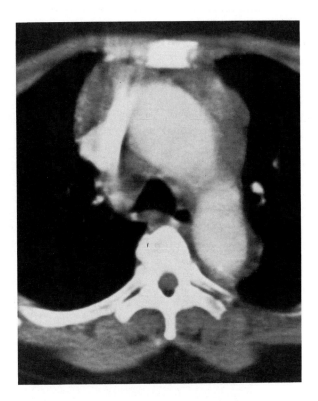

FIGURE 4–3. Prevascular node enlargement. Anterior mediastinal or prevascular node enlargement is present in this patient with sarcoidosis. This is considered an atypical location in sarcoidosis, but nodes in this location are commonly seen on CT scans.

so-called azygos node. These nodes form the final pathway for lymphatic drainage from most of both lungs (excepting the left upper lobe). Because of this, they are commonly abnormal regardless of the location of the lung disease.

Aorticopulmonary Nodes. These are considered by Rouvière to be in the anterior mediastinal group, but because they serve the same function as right paratracheal nodes, I prefer to consider them as middle mediastinal (Fig. 4–4C). The left upper lobe drains via this node group.

Subcarinal Nodes. These are located in the subcarinal space (Fig. 4–4D), and drain the inferior hila and lower lobes on both the right and left. They communicate in turn with the right paratracheal chain.

Tracheobronchial Nodes. They surround the main bronchi on each side. They will be considered along with the hilar nodes (bronchopulmonary nodes) in the chapter on hilar CT. They can be difficult to distinguish from true hilar nodes on CT.

Posterior Mediastinal Nodes

Paraesophageal or Inferior Pulmonary Ligament Nodes. These nodes are associated with the esophagus and descending aorta, and lie medial to the inferior pulmonary ligament. They drain the medial lower lobes, esophagus, pericardium, and posterior diaphragm. On the right, they are impossible to distinguish from subcarinal nodes, unless they are near the diaphragm.

Paravertebral Nodes. These nodes lie lateral to the vertebral bodies, posterior to the aorta on the left. They drain the posterior chest wall and pleura. They are most commonly involved contiguous with retroperitoneal abdominal nodes in patients with lymphoma or metastatic carcinoma.

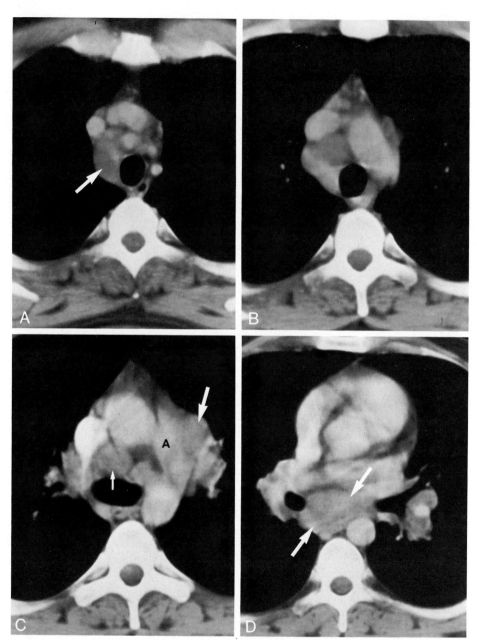

FIGURE 4–4. Lymph node enlargement in a patient with sarcoidosis. *(A and B)* **Pre- or Paratracheal nodes.** *(A)* Enlarged nodes (arrow) are anterolateral relative to the trachea, and posterior to the brachiocephalic veins. *(B)* At a lower level, they displace the vena cava anteriorly. *(C)* **Aorticopulmonary, precarinal, and tracheobronchial nodes.** Extensive mediastinal adenopathy is present. The superior aspect of the left pulmonary artery *(A)* mimics adenopathy (large arrow) in the aorticopulmonary window. A large precarinal node (small arrow) is also visible. Tracheobronchial nodes lie adjacent to the main bronchi. *(D)* **Subcarinal nodes.** A large convex mass (arrows) is present in the azygoesophageal recess and subcarinal space. The right pulmonary artery anterior to the mass is slightly compressed.

NORMAL LYMPH NODES

Lymph nodes are generally visible as discrete, round or elliptical, soft-tissue density structures, surrounded by mediastinal fat, and distinguishable from vessels by location. They often occur in clusters of a few nodes of similar size (Fig. 4–5A, B). In some locations, nodes which contact vessels may be difficult to identify without contrast infusion.

Internal mammary nodes, paracardiac nodes, and paravertebral nodes are not usually seen on CT in normals, but in other areas of the mediastinum, normal nodes are often visible. The expected size of normal nodes varies with their location, and a few general rules apply. Subcarinal nodes can be quite large in normal patients. Pretracheal nodes are also commonly visible, but these nodes are typically smaller than normal subcarinal nodes. Nodes in the supra-aortic mediastinum are usually smaller than lower pretracheal nodes, and left paratracheal nodes are usually smaller than right paratracheal nodes.

LYMPH NODE SIZE AND THE DIAGNOSIS OF LYMPH NODE ENLARGEMENT

There has been a great deal of controversy regarding the seemingly simple question of how mediastinal lymph nodes should be measured, and therefore, what the upper limits of normal node size should be. For a number of years, most investigators have used the largest or longest node diameter as the measurement of choice, with 1 cm being considered the upper limits of normal in most parts of the mediastinum. However, it has been suggested that the least (or smallest) node diameter is a better measurement, more closely reflecting

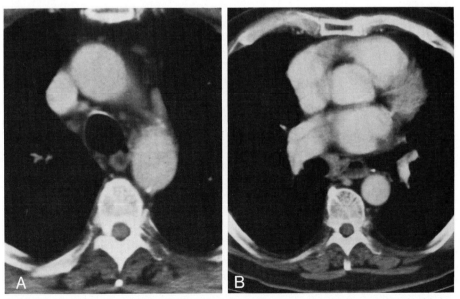

FIGURE 4–5. Normal mediastinal nodes. *(A)* Small lymph nodes are visible in the pretracheal and prevascular spaces and in the aorticopulmonary window. A lymph node in the lateral aorticopulmonary window measures 20 x 7 mm. With a node of this shape, least node diameter is the best measurement to use. *(B)* A normal subcarinal lymph node is visible. Subcarinal nodes larger than 1 cm are commonly seen.

actual node diameter when nodes are obliquely oriented relative to the scan plane, and showing less variation among normal patients. Using least node diameter, different values for upper limits of normal node size have been suggested for different mediastinal node groups (Table 4–1).

Despite this controversy, I think it is reasonable to continue using 1 cm as the upper limit of normal node size in those areas of the mediastinum where we normally see nodes, although in the subcarinal space, 1.5 cm is a better upper limit to use. It has not been clearly shown that using the least diameter *significantly* improves diagnostic accuracy.

If you use greatest node diameter for your measurements, it is important to consider the shape of the node. If the node appears elliptical rather than round and is much longer than it is wide (in other words, if it is shaped like a hot dog), measuring the long axis or largest diameter will give you a false impression of the node's actual size and significance. A node which appears much longer than it is wide may, in fact, be oriented longitudinally in the plane of scan rather than perpendicular to it, or may represent two separate nodes lying very close together, which cannot be resolved. In this situation, you should be wary of calling the node abnormal (Fig. 4–5A).

Enlarged mediastinal lymph nodes are usually easy to identify on CT. In most cases, they are outlined by fat and are visible as discrete structures. However, several nodes can be matted together in the presence of inflammation or neoplastic infiltration of the node capsule, giving the appearance of a single large mass. Furthermore, some neoplastic or inflammatory diseases, which break out of nodes and involve mediastinal tissues, may not show discrete node enlargement. Rather, they show infiltration and replacement of mediastinal fat by soft tissue density on CT; this diagnosis may be difficult to make unless the density of mediastinal soft tissues (which should be the same as fat) is compared to the density of subcutaneous fat on the same scan.

The significance given to the presence of an enlarged lymph node seen on CT must be tempered by a knowledge of the patient's clinical situation. For example, if the patient is known to have lung cancer, then an enlarged lymph node has a likelihood of about 70% of being involved by tumor. However, the same node in a patient without lung cancer is much less likely to be of clinical significance. In the absence of a known disease, an enlarged node must be regarded as likely to be hyperplastic or postinflammatory.

DIFFERENTIAL DIAGNOSIS OF MEDIASTINAL LYMPH NODE ENLARGEMENT

Lung Cancer

The most common cause of mediastinal node enlargement is metastatic lung cancer, and the use of CT in making this diagnosis will be discussed in detail.

Approximately 30% of patients diagnosed with lung cancer have mediastinal node metastases. Lung cancer most often involves the middle mediastinal node groups. Left upper lobe cancers typically metastasize to aorticopulmonary window nodes, while tumors involving the lower lobes on either side tend to metastasize to the subcarinal and right paratracheal chains. Right upper lobe tumors typically involve paratracheal nodes.

TABLE 4–1. Approximate Upper Limits of Normal for Least Node Diameter

Node Location	Diameter (mm)*
Supra aortic pretracheal	7
Subaortic pretracheal	9
Aorticopulmonary window	9
Subcarinal	12
Prevascular space	8
Paraesophageal	8

*Mean normal node diameter plus two standard deviations

Mediastinal Staging of Lung Cancer

Because large mediastinal masses in patients with lung cancer are considered unresectable, a patient who has a mediastinal mass visible on plain radiographs (indicating its large size) usually does not require CT, but mediastinoscopy or biopsy should usually be performed to confirm the presence of mediastinal disease. On the other hand, plain radiographs are relatively insensitive for the detection of mediastinal adenopathy, and normal chest films certainly do not exclude the presence of lymph node enlargement.

A large number of studies evaluating the accuracy of CT in differentiating mediastinal node metastases from bronchogenic carcinoma have been performed. These studies cannot easily be compared because of the different criteria used in different studies for determining a mediastinal lymph node to be abnormal, different scanners and techniques, different methods for confirming or ruling out the presence of lymph node metastases (i.e., mediastinoscopy, palpation, total nodal dissection), and differences in the population of patients studied. Not surprisingly, the results of these studies vary, but often in a predictable fashion. First, the larger the node diameter which is used to distinguish malignant nodes from benign, the more specific but less sensitive CT becomes in detecting metastases. (We will be more accurate in predicting that a large node will be involved by tumor but will detect fewer involved nodes). On the other hand, using a small node diameter to distinguish malignant from benign tumors increases sensitivity, but at the expense of specificity.

Despite these difficulties in evaluating the accuracy of CT in diagnosing mediastinal lymph node metastases from lung cancer, most investigators consider CT to be quite helpful. Although CT cannot be considered accurate enough to determine with certainty that mediastinal lymph nodes are, or are not, involved by tumor, it can provide information of value in guiding therapy and invasive diagnostic procedures.

Generally speaking, lymph nodes less than 1 cm in diameter can be considered benign, with an accuracy of approximately 70%. In such patients, thoracotomy without prior mediastinoscopy is often performed, with a mediastinal node exploration conducted at surgery. Although some patients will be found to have microscopic or small intranodal metastases, their presence does not necessarily indicate that surgery should not have been performed. A growing body of literature suggests that some patients with intranodal mediastinal metastases can be cured following surgical excision of nodes and radiation.

On the other hand, mediastinal lymph nodes measuring more than 1.5 cm in diameter are involved by tumor in about 70 to 80% of patients; hyperplasia of mediastinal lymph nodes accounts for the 20 to 30% of large nodes that are not involved by tumor. For this reason, patients with large mediastinal nodes should not be denied an attempt at surgical cure without confirmation of node metastases, and enlarged nodes should be sampled at mediastinoscopy or by CT-guided needle biopsy. Lymph nodes measuring between 1 and 1.5 cm may or may not be involved by tumor (the likelihood is about 50%), and should be considered suspicious; they should probably be biopsied before surgery.

Mediastinoscopy Versus CT for Diagnosing Node Metastases

Although mediastinoscopy is generally regarded as the gold standard of preoperative mediastinal evaluation in patients with lung cancer, the mediastinoscope cannot evaluate all mediastinal compartments or lymph node groups, and a significant percentage (up to 25%) of patients with bronchogenic carcinoma, who have a negative mediastinoscopy, are proved to have mediastinal nodal metastases at surgery. Through a standard cervical approach, the mediastinoscopist can evaluate pretracheal lymph nodes, nodes in the anterior subcarinal space, and lymph nodes extending anterior to the right main bronchus. Lymph nodes in the anterior mediastinum (prevascular space), aorticopulmonary window, and posterior portions of the mediastinum (posterior subcarinal space, azygoesophageal recess, etc.) are inaccessible using this technique, although some can be evaluated using a left parasternal mediastinoscopy. CT, on the other hand, allows evaluation of all these areas, shows where any enlarged nodes are, and can serve to guide needle aspiration biopsy or parasternal mediastinotomy if enlarged lymph nodes are visible in areas which cannot be evaluated using a standard approach.

The accuracies of CT and mediastinoscopy have been compared in large groups of patients with lung cancer. Simply stated, both mediastinoscopy and CT have the same reasonably high sensitivity for detecting mediastinal node metastases (about 70 to 80%). However, as would be expected, mediastinoscopy was 100% specific (no normals were called abnormal), while CT has a lower specificity. Thus, overall, mediastinoscopy was the more accurate study. In light of this, how should CT be used in evaluating and staging mediastinal nodes in lung cancer? Should mediastinoscopy be done instead of CT?

First, it is important to consider your surgeon's approach. Some thoracic surgeons consider many patients with mediastinal node metastases (in particular those with squamous cell carcinoma who have low mediastinal nodes) to be treatable using radical surgery, including resection of mediastinal nodes along with the primary tumor. In this setting, neither mediastinoscopy nor CT may be considered of much value, but in fact, CT is often used by such surgeons in their preoperative assessment of patients or as a guide to their surgical resections.

Others suggest that positive lymph nodes found at mediastinoscopy rule out effective surgical treatment. In such patients, survival following surgical resection is poor compared to that for patients who have had a negative mediastinoscopy but have positive nodes found at surgery. However, despite this and the fact that mediastinoscopy is more accurate than CT, CT is usually obtained (in addition to mediastinoscopy) in these patients. If CT shows abnormally enlarged lymph nodes, it is used to guide mediastinoscopy and biopsy. However, biopsy should not be limited to nodes which appear abnormal on CT; other nodes may be the ones involved by tumor.

In patients with small, peripheral lung nodules, mediastinal metastases are uncommon, and thoracotomy may be warranted without prior CT or mediastinoscopy, but this remains controversial. Among those surgeons who favor the use of mediastinoscopy because of its prognostic significance, CT and mediastinoscopy are recommended in all patients with lung cancer, even those with small nodules.

Mediastinal Invasion by Lung Cancer

In addition to mediastinal node metastasis, bronchogenic carcinoma can involve the mediastinum by direct extension—so-called mediastinal invasion. In current surgical practice, invasion of the mediastinal pleura does not preclude surgery. However, significant invasion of mediastinal fat or other mediastinal structures, such as the trachea or esophagus, does preclude resection (Fig. 4–6).

How accurate is CT in predicting mediastinal invasion? Obviously, you can be sure that a lung nodule which does not contact the mediastinum is not invasive, and this is an important use of CT. On the other hand, a definite diagnosis of invasion can be more difficult to make, unless the invasion is gross.

Only when there is significant replacement of mediastinal fat by soft – tissue density tumor, or compression or displacement of mediastinal vessels by tumor, can mediastinal invasion by a bronchogenic carcinoma be diagnosed with a high degree of accuracy on CT.

Specific CT signs which can be relied upon to make this diagnosis in more subtle cases have been difficult to find. However, some findings which can indicate mediastinal invasion include 1) obliteration of the fat plane which is normally seen adjacent to the descending aorta or other mediastinal vessels (Fig. 4–7); (2) tumor contacting more than one-fourth of the circumference of the aortic wall (Fig. 4–7), or (3) tumor contacting more than 3 cm of the mediastinum (Fig. 4–7). If none of these findings is present, the tumor is likely to be resectable. Thickening of the mediastinal pleura, as seen on CT, can indicate pleural invasion, but even if present, it does not rule out surgery.

Lymphoma and Leukemia

Most patients with lymphomas present with cervical adenopathy, and mediastinal lymph nodes are also commonly involved. A small percentage of

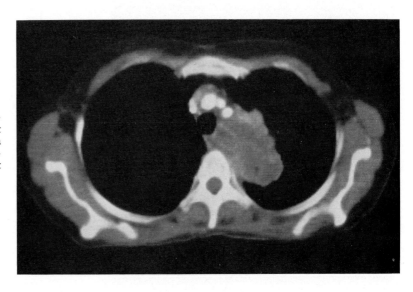

FIGURE 4–6. Mediastinal invasion from lung cancer. A patient with a left upper lobe carcinoma has contiguous mediastinal invasion. Fat is replaced by dense soft tissue.

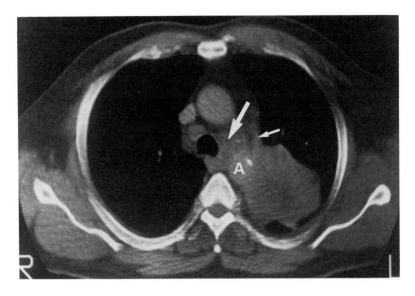

FIGURE 4–7. Mediastinal invasion from lung cancer. The fat plane adjacent to the descending aorta (A) is obliterated, suggesting invasion, and soft tissue extends anteriorly within mediastinal fat (small arrow). Soft tissue mass (large arrow) fills the medial aorticopulmonary window. Pretracheal node enlargement is also present. (Reprinted with permission. From Aspen Publishers, Inc, © January, 1987. Webb WR: Plain radiography and computed tomography in the staging of bronchogenic carcinoma: A practical approach. J Thorac Imaging, 2(1):57-65.)

patients are first recognized because of mediastinal masses noted on chest films, but these patients will often have systemic signs and symptoms, including fever, night sweats, weight loss, weakness, and fatigue.

Hodgkin's Disease

Hodgkin's disease has a predilection for thoracic involvement, both at the time of diagnosis and if the disease recurs. Hodgkin's disease occurs at all ages, but with peaks in the third and fifth decades.

It is estimated that more than 85% of patients with Hodgkin's lymphoma eventually develop intrathoracic disease, typically involving the superior medias-

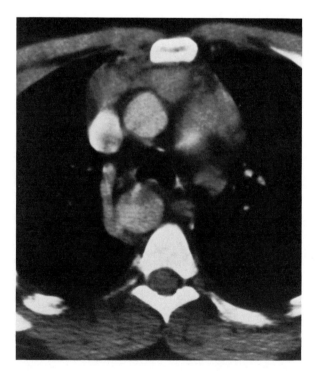

FIGURE 4–8. Hodgkin's lymphoma with anterior mediastinal adenopathy. Lymph node masses were limited to the anterior mediastinum in this patient. Also note the presence of a right aortic arch.

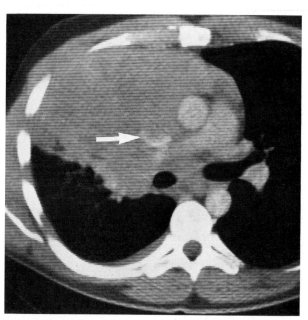

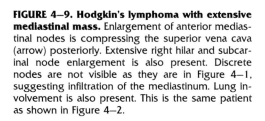

FIGURE 4–9. Hodgkin's lymphoma with extensive mediastinal mass. Enlargement of anterior mediastinal nodes is compressing the superior vena cava (arrow) posteriorly. Extensive right hilar and subcarinal node enlargement is also present. Discrete nodes are not visible as they are in Figure 4–1, suggesting infiltration of the mediastinum. Lung involvement is also present. This is the same patient as shown in Figure 4–2.

tinal (prevascular, pretracheal, and aorticopulmonary) lymph nodes (Figs. 4–1, 4–2, 4–8, 4–9). In fact, it has been suggested that the absence of involvement of these mediastinal nodes in patients with intrathoracic adenopathy should prompt the radiologist to question the diagnosis of Hodgkin's lymphoma. Subcarinal nodes and hilar nodes are involved in almost half of patients. In one study, it was uncommon for CT to show evidence of mediastinal adenopathy if the chest radiograph was normal, but if it was abnormal, CT detected additional sites of adenopathy in many (Table 4–2). CT was most helpful in diagnosing subcarinal, internal mammary, and aorticopulmonary window node enlargement. Cardiophrenic angle (paracardiac) lymph nodes are present in about 10% of patients, and are well seen on CT. Adenopathy in this location is unusual in other diseases. In a significant percentage of patients, the additional node involvement shown by CT changes therapy.

Enlargement of a single node group can be seen with Hodgkin's disease, most commonly in the prevascular mediastinum (Fig. 4–8). This often indicates the presence of nodular sclerosing histology, which accounts for 50 to 80% of adult Hodgkin's disease. In patients with lymphoma, mediastinal lymph nodes may become matted, being visible as a single large mass rather than individual discrete nodes (Fig. 4–9). Mediastinal nodes or masses in patients with Hodgkin's lymphoma can appear cystic or fluid filled on CT.

TABLE 4–2. Mediastinal Node Enlargement in Hodgkin's Disease

Site	Percentage Abnormal	Percentage Visible on	
		Radiographs	CT
Paratracheal	70–80	60–70	70–80
Pretracheal	65–80	60–70	65–80
AP window	60–80	50–60	60–80
Subcarinal	25–40	5–10	25–40
Internal mammary	35	5	35
Posterior mediastinal	5–15	2–10	12
Paracardiac	10–15	1–5	10

Non-Hodgkin's Lymphoma

Non-Hodgkin's lymphoma is a diverse group of diseases that vary in radiologic manifestation, clinical presentation, course, and prognosis. In comparison to Hodgkin's disease, these tumors are less common and occur in an older group (40 to 70 years). At the time of presentation the disease is often generalized (85% are stages III or IV) and chemotherapy is most appropriate. Because of this, precise anatomic staging is less crucial than with Hodgkin's disease.

In one series, 43% had intrathoracic disease, and 40% had involvement of only one node group—much more common than in patients with Hodgkin's. Also, posterior mediastinal nodes were more frequently involved. Lung involvement was present in only 4%; in some patients lung infiltration may be rapid.

CT can show evidence of intrathoracic disease when it is unrecognizable on plain radiographs as in patients with Hodgkin's, and can affect management in patients with localized (stages I or II) disease.

Leukemia

Leukemia, particularly the lymphocytic varieties, can cause hilar or mediastinal lymph node enlargement, pleural effusion, and occasionally infiltrative lung disease. Lymphadenopathy is generally confined to the middle mediastinum, and the larger masses seen with some lymphomas generally do not occur.

Metastases

Extrathoracic primary tumors can result in mediastinal node enlargement, either with or without hilar or lung metastases. Node metastases can be present because of inferior extension from neck masses (thyroid carcinoma, head and neck tumors), extension along lymphatic channels from below the diaphragm (testicular carcinoma, renal cell carcinoma, gastrointestinal malignancies), or dissemination by other routes (breast carcinoma, melanoma). Middle mediastinal (paratracheal) or paravertebral mediastinal nodes are most commonly involved when the tumor is subdiaphragmatic. With breast carcinoma, internal mammary node metastases occur. Rarely, lymph node metastases can appear cystic (Fig. 4–10).

Sarcoidosis

Mediastinal lymph node enlargement is very common in patients with sarcoidosis, occurring in 60 to 90 of cases. Typically, node enlargement is extensive, involving the hila as well as the mediastinum, and masses appear bilateral and symmetrical in the large majority of patients (Fig. 4–4); this usually allows the differentiation of sarcoidosis from lymphoma. Also, lymph nodes can be quite large in patients with sarcoidosis, but large isolated masses, as seen in some patients with lymphoma, do not occur. Paratracheal lymph nodes are typically involved. Even though it is commonly stated that sarcoidosis does not involve anterior mediastinal lymph nodes, this is often visible on CT; paravertebral node enlargement is occasionally seen.

Infections

A variety of infectious agents can cause mediastinal lymph node enlargement during the acute phase of disease. These include a number of fungal

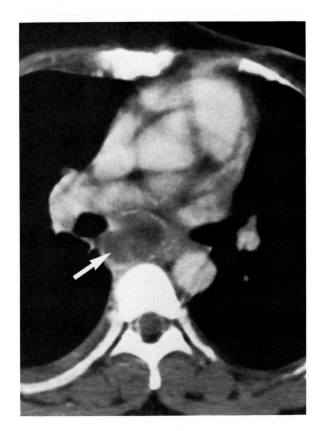

FIGURE 4–10. Cystic lymph node metastasis. In a patient with metastatic carcinoma, a subcarinal node mass (arrow) is cystic, with an enhancing rim and low density contents.

infections (commonly histoplasmosis and coccidioidomycosis), tuberculosis, bacterial infections, and viral infections. Typically, there will be symptoms and signs of acute infection, and chest radiographs will show evidence of pneumonia.

The lymph node enlargement will often be asymmetric, involving hilar and middle mediastinal nodes. In patients with acute infection, particularly with TB, cystic areas of necrosis within nodes can be seen following contrast injection. Lymph node calcification occurs in patients with chronic fungal or tuberculous infection (Fig. 3–14).

Benign Lymph Node Hyperplasia (Castleman's Disease)

This unusual disease of unknown cause is characterized by enlargement of hilar or mediastinal lymph nodes, predominantly in the middle and posterior mediastinal compartments. It appears on CT as a smooth or lobulated solitary node mass, which can be large. This lesion is typically quite vascular, and on CT it may densely opacify following contrast injection.

DIAGNOSIS OF MEDIASTINAL MASSES

Some General Principles

The differential diagnosis of a mediastinal mass on CT is usually based on several characteristics of the mass and on the presence or absence of several findings. These include mass location, whether it is single or multifocal (involves several areas of the mediastinum [Fig. 4–1]), its shape (round or lobulated), whether it appears cystic (Fig. 4–10), its density (fatty, fluid, solid, or a combination of these, the presence of calcification and its character and amount), and additional findings such as pleural effusion.

The density of a mass (or densities, if it is inhomogeneous) can be very helpful in differential diagnosis. The variety of mediastinal mass densities and their frequency are shown in Table 4–3.

LOCALIZATION OF MEDIASTINAL MASSES

Mediastinal masses result in alterations of normal mediastinal contours, and displacement or compression of mediastinal structures; recognizing these findings can be valuable in diagnosis and in suggesting the site of origin of the mass. Although most mediastinal masses can occur in different parts of the mediastinum, most have characteristic locations.

Prevascular Space

Masses in this compartment, when large, tend to displace the aorta and great arterial branches posteriorly (see Figs. 4–9, 4–13, 4–14), but distinct compression or narrowing of these relatively thick walled structures is unusual. Within the supra-aortic mediastinum, displacement, compression, or obstruction of the brachiocephalic veins is not uncommon (Fig 3–13A). In the subaortic mediastinum, posterior displacement or compression of the SVC is typical only with right-sided masses. On the left, compression of the main pulmonary artery can be seen. Mediastinal contours in this region are not particularly helpful in diagnosing masses. The anterior junction line is rather variable in thickness, and cannot be relied upon as abnormal unless grossly thickened. The lateral medias-

TABLE 4–3. Density of Mediastinal Masses

Type	Air	Fat	Fluid	Solid	>Solid	Calcification
Thymoma	N	N	O	A	N	O
Thymolipoma	N	A	N	C	N	N
Lymphoma (Thymus)	N	N	O	A	N	R
Dermoid/Teratoma	N	O	O	A	N	O
Germ-cell	N	N	R	A	N	R
Thyroid	N	N	O	A	C	C
Lipoma	N	A	N	N	N	N
Hygroma	N	C	C	C	N	N
Cysts (Congenital)	R	N	C	O	N	R
Hernia	O	O	N	O	N	N
Metastatic tumor (Nodes)	N	N	R	A	N	N
TB/Fungus (Nodes)	N	N	O	A	N	C
Sarcoid (Nodes)	N	N	N	A	N	R
Neurogenic	N	N	N	A	N	O
Neurenteric cyst	R	N	A	N	N	N
Meningocele	N	N	A	N	N	N
Hematopoiesis	N	N	N	A	N	N

"ACORN"—A = always; C = common; O = occasionally; R = rare; N = never. ("Never" doesn't mean it never happens, but that it is so unlikely you should "never" consider the diagnosis, and if you turn out to be wrong, you will "never" be blamed.)

tinal pleural contours are often convex laterally, although a marked convexity may suggest a mass. The differential diagnosis of masses arising in this area includes thymoma and other thymic tumors, cysts, lymphoma, germ-cell tumors, thyroid masses, parathyroid masses, fatty masses, and lymphangioma (hygroma).

Thymic Tumors

Tumors of various histology arise from cells of thymic origin and therefore can be called "thymomas." However, it is most appropriate to reserve the term thymoma for tumors derived from thymic epithelial or lymphocytic tissues. Other thymic tumors include thymic carcinoid, thymolipoma, thymic cyst, lymphoma, and leukemia.

Thymoma

Thymoma is a common anterior mediastinal mass occurring primarily in adults. Occasionally these lesions arise in the middle or posterior mediastinum. It is extremely difficult to determine if thymomas are benign or malignant by histologic criteria. Local invasion is a much more reliable sign of malignancy. Approximately 30% of thymomas are pathologically and surgically invasive.

From 10 to 30% of patients with myasthenia gravis will be found to have a thymoma, while a larger percentage of patients with thymoma (30 to 50%) have myasthenia. Other syndromes associated with thymoma include red cell hypoplasia and hypogammaglobulinemia.

On CT, thymomas are usually visible in the prevascular space (Fig. 4–11) but can also be seen in a paracardiac location. They are detected as a localized bulge or mass distorting the normally arrowhead-shaped thymus. Typically they are unilateral. Calcification and cystic degeneration can be present. Bilaterality, large size, lobulated contour, or poor definition of the tumor's margin on CT suggests malignancy, but a definite diagnosis may be difficult to make.

In patients suspected of having a thymoma because of myasthenia gravis, who have been studied using both plain radiographs and CT, it is clear that CT can demonstrate tumors that are invisible using conventional techniques. However, very small thymic tumors may not be distinguished from a normal or hyperplastic gland with CT.

Thymic carcinoid tumors are usually malignant and aggressive. This lesion does not differ significantly from thymoma in its CT appearance.

Thymolipoma

Thymolipoma is a rare, benign thymic tumor, consisting primarily of fat but also containing strands or islands of thymic tissue. The tumor is generally unaccompanied by symptoms and can be large when first detected, usually on routine chest radiographs. Because of its fatty content and pliability, it tends to drape around the heart and can simulate cardiac enlargement. On CT, its fatty composition, with wisps of soft tissue within it, can permit a preoperative diagnosis (Fig. 4–12).

Thymic Cyst

Thymic cysts, either congenital or acquired, can be diagnosed using CT if the contents have a density close to that of water, but in some cases they will show soft tissue density. Calcification of the cyst margin can occur. It is important to note that thymoma can have cystic components, but will also demonstrate solid areas or a thick or irregular wall.

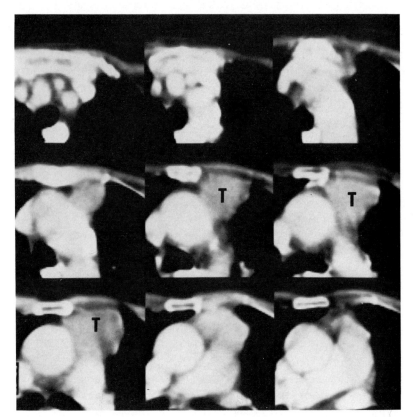

FIGURE 4–11. Thymoma. Benign thymoma (T) is seen in the prevascular mediastinum at contiguous levels.

FIGURE 4–12. Thymolipoma. The large anterior mediastinal mass is composed primarily of fat, but it also contains strands of soft tissue.

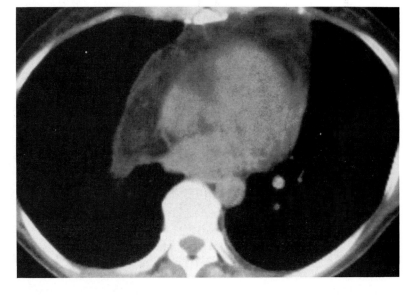

(An important general rule in diagnosing mediastinal masses is that cysts can appear solid, and solid [malignant] masses can have cystic or necrotic components. A true cyst will have a very thin wall; a mass with cystic degeneration will usually have a thick irregular wall.)

Thymic Hyperplasia and Thymic Rebound

The thymus may appear enlarged and relatively dense (containing little fat) in patients with thymic hyperplasia, but in some, it may appear quite normal. In young patients, the thymus may show a significant rebound hyperplasia, 3 months to 1 year after cessation of chemotherapy for malignancy. This can result in a distinctly enlarged thymus.

Lymphoma

Anterior mediastinal lymph node enlargement or lymphoma involving the thymus is present in more than half of patients with Hodgkin's disease. On CT, lymphoma involving the anterior mediastinum typically presents as a lobulated mass or one projecting to one or both sides (Figs. 4–8, 4–9). In some cases it may appear as a single spherical mass. In either case, it is usually indistinguishable from thymoma or other causes of prevascular mass. However, if it is multifocal (indicating its origin from nodes) or is associated with other sites of lymph node enlargement, the diagnosis is more easily made. Cystic areas of necrosis may be visible at CT (Fig. 4–13). Except in rare cases, calcification does not occur in the absence of radiation.

Germ-Cell Tumors

Several different tumors, originating from rests of primitive germ cells, can occur in the anterior mediastinum. These include dermoid cysts, teratoma,

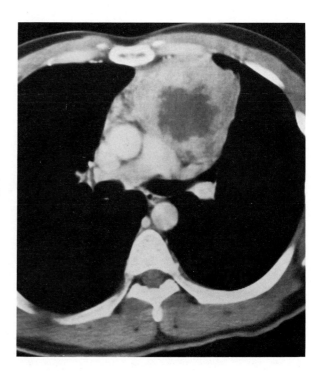

FIGURE 4–13. Cystic or necrotic Hodgkin's lymphoma. The anterior mediastinal mass contains an irregular area of cystic necrosis.

seminoma, choriocarcinoma, and endodermal sinus tumor. These are somewhat less common than thymoma. Approximately 80% of germ-cell tumors are benign.

Dermoid Cyst and Teratoma

These tumors can be cystic or solid and are most commonly benign. Dermoid cyst is a tumor derived from epidermal tissues, whereas a teratoma contains tissues of ectodermal, mesodermal, and endodermal origins.

These tumors occur in a distribution similar to that of thymomas; rarely they originate in the posterior mediastinum. Benign lesions are often round, oval, and smooth in contour; as with thymoma, an irregular, lobulated, or ill-defined margin suggests malignancy. On the average, these tumors are larger than thymomas but can be any size. Calcification can be seen but is nonspecific except in the unusual instance when a bone or tooth is present within the mass. They may appear cystic or composed of visible fat, a finding of great value in differential diagnosis (Fig. 4–14).

Other Germ-Cell Tumors

Seminoma, choriocarcinoma, and endodermal sinus (yolk sac) tumors are other cell types of anterior mediastinal germ-cell tumors. They are malignant lesions occurring primarily in young men. They have no distinguishing characteristics on CT.

Thyroid Masses

A small percentage of patients with a thyroid mass have some extension of the mass into the superior mediastinum, and, rarely, a completely intrathoracic mass can arise from ectopic mediastinal thyroid tissue. In most patients, such masses represent a goiter (Fig. 4–15), but other diseases (Graves' disease, thyroiditis) and neoplasms can result in an intrathoracic mass. Most patients with intrathoracic goiter are asymptomatic, but symptoms of tracheal or esophageal

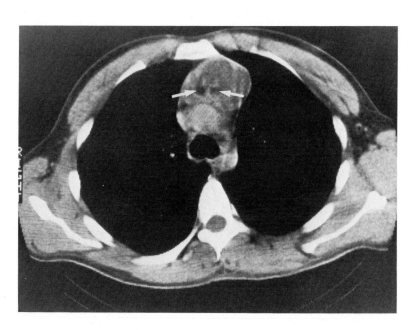

FIGURE 4–14. Teratoma. A lobulated anterior mediastinal mass contains areas of fat (arrows). This appearance strongly suggests teratoma as the diagnosis. (Reproduced from Webb WR. Radiol Clin North Am, 21:723-739, 1983.)

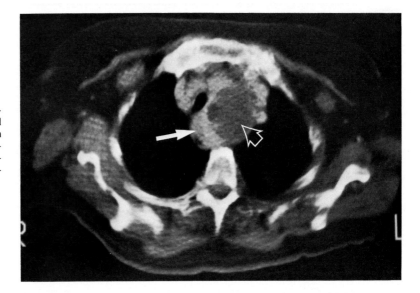

FIGURE 4–15. Mediastinal goiter. The mass, which is both solid (white arrow) and cystic (open arrow), is located lateral and posterior to the trachea. The brachiocephalic vessels are displaced anteriorly and laterally.

compression can be present. CT generally shows anatomic continuity with the cervical thyroid gland. The location of the mass at CT is somewhat variable, and they can be anterior or posterior to the trachea. Masses anterior to the trachea splay the brachiocephalic vessels, whereas masses that are primarily posterior and lateral to the trachea displace the brachiocephalic vessels anteriorly (Fig. 4–15). A location anterior to the great vessels is unusual. Calcifications and low-density cystic areas are common in patients with goiter. Also, because of their iodine content, the CT density of goiters, Graves' disease, and thyroiditis can be greater than that of soft tissue and thyroid tumors, but less dense than normal thyroid tissue.

Mesenchymal Masses

Lipomatosis and Lipoma

A diffuse accumulation of unencapsulated fat in the mediastinum, so-called mediastinal lipomatosis, can occur in patients with Cushing's syndrome, long-term steroid therapy, or occasionally as a result of exogenous obesity. It produces no symptoms. CT shows a generalized increase in anterior mediastinal fat surrounding the great vessels, with some lateral bulging of the mediastinal pleural reflections. On CT, fat has a characteristic low density, measuring from -50 to -100 H.

As with other mesenchymal tumors, lipomas can occur in any part of the mediastinum but are most common anteriorly. Because of their pliability, they rarely cause symptoms. A lipoma, although of the same density as lipomatosis, is localized. Most fatty masses are benign. Liposarcoma, teratoma, and thymolipoma, other masses which can contain fat, also contain soft-tissue elements and thus can be distinguished from lipoma or lipomatosis.

Lymphangioma (Hygroma)

Lymphangiomas are classified histologically as simple, cavernous, and cystic. Simple lymphangiomas are composed of small, thin-walled lymphatic channels with considerable connective tissue stroma. Cavernous lymphangiomas consist of dilated lymphatic channels, while cystic lymphangiomas (hygromas) contain single or multiple cystic masses filled with serous or milky fluid and have little if any communication with normal lymphatics. Most commonly, these lesions are detected in children and may extend into the neck. However, they can be seen in adults as well. On CT, the mass can appear to envelop, rather than displace, mediastinal structures. Discrete cysts may not be visible; calcification does not occur.

Pretracheal Space

Masses which occupy this compartment characteristically replace or displace the normal pretracheal fat. Since the pretracheal space is limited by the relatively immobile aortic arch anteriorly and to the left, large masses extend preferentially to the right, displacing and compressing the SVC anteriorly and laterally (see Figs. 4–1, 4–4B, 4–19). In the presence of a pretracheal mass, the SVC will appear crescent-shaped, convex laterally, with its concave aspect moulding itself to the convex contour of the adjacent mass. This lateral displacement of the SVC results in most of the mediastinal widening visible on plain films. Very large masses also displace the trachea posteriorly, but this is somewhat more difficult to recognize because the tracheal cartilages prevent much tracheal narrowing. Masses in this compartment are almost always of lymph node origin.

The Trachea

The trachea extends inferiorly from the thoracic inlet for a distance of 8 to 10 cm before bifurcating into the right and left main bronchi. As stated above, the trachea is usually round, or more often oval, and is approximately 2 cm in diameter. In some patients, the trachea can appear somewhat triangular in shape, with the apex of the triangle directed anteriorly. This appearance is particularly common at the level of the carina and proximal main bronchi. In some patients, the tracheal cartilage is visible as a relatively dense horseshoe-shaped structure within the tracheal wall, with the open part of the horseshoe being posterior. These can calcify in older patients, particularly women. The tracheal wall should measure no more than 2 or 3 mm in thickness.

Tracheal abnormalities are uncommon and may be asymptomatic unless the tracheal lumen is reduced to a few millimeters in diameter. Thus, do not expect patients with tracheal lesions to have symptoms. A high degree of suspicion must be maintained if tracheal abnormalities are to be correctly interpreted.

Saber-sheath trachea is a relatively common tracheal abnormality, occurring in patients with chronic obstructive pulmonary disease, probably because of the repeated trauma of coughing. In this condition, there is side-to-side narrowing of the intrathoracic trachea, with the anterior-to-posterior tracheal diameter being preserved or increased (Fig. 4–16); the extrathoracic trachea is normal. A focal segment at the thoracic inlet may be involved first. In severe cases, the tracheal walls may touch each other, and appear slightly thickened. Saber-sheath trachea should be distinguished from several diseases which produce concentric tracheal narrowing and also involve the extrathoracic trachea. These include amyloidosis, tracheobronchopathia osteochondroplastica (both of which show thickening and irregular calcification of the tracheal wall), polychondritis, and scleroma. These are very rare and will not be described further.

Tracheal stenosis occurring because of previous intubation is a relatively common abnormality. Narrowing of the tracheal lumen may be associated with intratracheal soft tissue masses of reactive (granulation) tissue or collapse of the

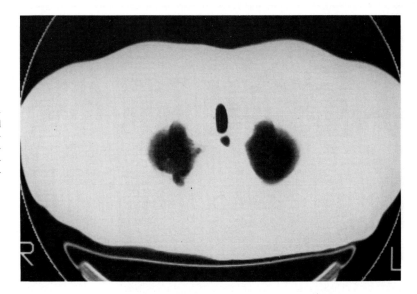

FIGURE 4–16. Saber-sheath trachea. The trachea is narrowed from side to side, while the sagittal diameter is normal or increased. In this patient, the air-filled esophagus is visible posterior to the trachea.

tracheal wall because of destruction of the tracheal rings and associated fibrosis. Identifying the shapes of the tracheal cartilages (and therefore the tracheal wall) may be helpful in distinguishing these two types of tracheal stenosis, and this may affect treatment. Although CT can show the cross-sectional appearance of the trachea to great advantage in such cases, narrowing because of thin webs cannot be accurately diagnosed.

Primary tracheal tumors are rare. The most common primary malignancies, occurring in approximately equal numbers, are squamous cell carcinoma (Figs. 4–17, 4–18) and cylindroma (adenoid cystic carcinoma). In patients with either of these, CT can be helpful in choosing treatment. If there is no mediastinal invasion (as evidenced by a mediastinal mass), then the lesion may be curable with a partial tracheal resection.

The trachea may be compressed, displaced, or invaded by a variety of malignant mediastinal tumors. Unless tumor can be seen within the tracheal

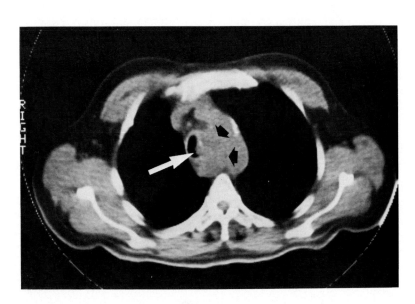

FIGURE 4–17. Tracheal carcinoma (squamous cell). There is narrowing of the tracheal lumen and an intraluminal mass (large arrow), associated with a significant mediastinal mass (small arrows), in a patient with invasive carcinoma. (Reproduced with permission. From Gamsu G, Webb WR: Computed tomography of the trachea: Normal and abnormal. Am J Roentgenol, 139:321-326, 1982.)

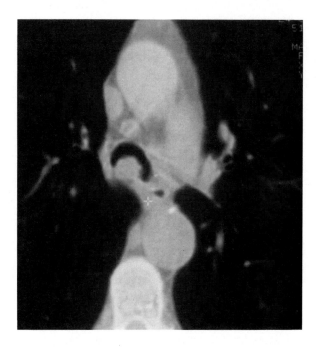

FIGURE 4–18. Tracheal carcinoma (squamous cell). An In intraluminal mass is visible in a patient with squamous cell carcinoma involving the trachea. (Reprinted with permission. From Webb WR. Aspen Publishers, Inc, © January, 1987. J Thorac Imaging, 2(1):57-65.)

lumen, tracheal invasion is difficult to diagnose. The trachea is commonly involved by tumor as a result of direct extension of a main bronchus carcinoma to the carina or distal trachea. Thickening of the carina or tracheal wall contiguous with a bronchial lesion suggests this diagnosis, but bronchoscopy is usually required for a definite diagnosis.

Subcarinal Space

Large masses in this location often produce a convexity of the azygoesophageal recess, but as stated above, the subcarinal space is anterior to the azygoesophageal recess, and a subcarinal mass need not produce an abnormality of this contour. Large subcarinal masses may splay the carina or displace the carina anteriorly, but these findings are often easier to recognize on plain radiographs. The esophagus may be displaced to the left. Subcarinal masses extending anteriorly from the subcarinal space commonly displace the right pulmonary artery anteriorly and compress its lumen (Fig. 4–4D). The most common masses involving this compartment are lymph node masses or cysts.

Esophageal Lesions

Esophageal lesions are discussed in Chapter 15.

Bronchogenic and Esophageal Cysts

Congenital bronchogenic cysts result from anomalous budding of the foregut during development. Most commonly, they are visible in the subcarinal space, but they can occur in any part of the mediastinum. They appear as single smooth, round, or elliptical masses (Fig. 4–19) and occasionally show calcification of their walls or contents. Air-fluid levels occurring because of communication with the trachea or bronchi are rare. When large, bronchogenic cysts can produce

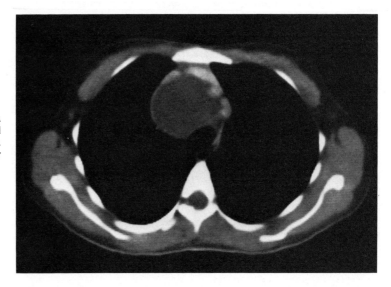

FIGURE 4–19. Bronchogenic cyst. A low density, thin-walled pretracheal mass represents a bronchogenic cyst. This mass is displacing the superior vena cava anteriorly.

symptoms by compression of mediastinal structures. A rapid increase in size can occur because of infection or hemorrhage.

Esophageal cysts are indistinguishable from bronchogenic cysts. They usually appear as well-defined solitary masses and can also contain an air-fluid level when they communicate with the esophagus.

CT can be of great value in diagnosing a mediastinal cyst. If a mass is thin walled and is of fluid density (0 H), it can be assumed to represent a benign cyst. However, high CT numbers (40 to 80 H), suggesting a solid mass, can also be found in patients with foregut duplication cysts. These cysts contain blood or a rather thick gelatinous material. In such patients surgery is usually required for diagnosis, but MR may sometimes help.

Aorticopulmonary Window

Masses in this region typically replace mediastinal fat and, when large, displace the mediastinal pleural reflection laterally (Fig. 4–4C). Displacement or compression of the aorta, pulmonary artery, and trachea are usually difficult to recognize. AP window masses are almost always the result of lymph node enlargement.

Retrosternal Mediastinum

Enlargement of internal mammary nodes results in a convexity in the expected position of this node chain (Fig. 4–1). Other than lymph node enlargement, masses in this region are unusual.

Paravertebral Space

Paravertebral masses may be seen to replace paravertebral fat. On the left, the normal concave mediastinal pleural reflection, posterior to the aorta,

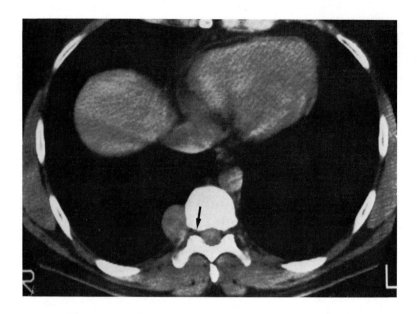

FIGURE 4–20. Neurofibroma. A smooth paravertebral, posterior mediastinal mass is visible. The neural foramen (arrow) is normal. (Reproduced with modification. From W.R. Webb. Diseases of the mediastinum. *In* CE Putman and CE Ravin (eds). *Textbook of Diagnostic Imaging,* Philadelphia, W.B. Saunders, 1988.)

becomes convex in the presence of a significant mass. On the right a paravertebral convexity is visible in a region where little tissue normally exists (Fig. 4–20).

Neurogenic Tumors

Neurogenic tumors are divided into three groups—those arising from peripheral nerves (neurofibroma, neurilemmoma), sympathetic ganglia (ganglioneuroma, neuroblastoma), and paraganglionic cells (pheochromocytoma, chemodectoma). Tumors in each of these three groups may be benign or malignant. Although neurogenic tumors can occur at any age, they are most common in young patients. Neuroblastoma and ganglioneuroma are most common in children, whereas neurofibroma and neurilemmoma more frequently affect young adults.

Radiographically, neurogenic tumors appear as well-defined, round or oval soft-tissue masses, typically in a paravertebral location (Fig. 4–20). Although the different tumors are by no means always distinguishable, ganglioneuromas tend to be elongated, lying adjacent to the spine, while neurofibromas are smaller and more spherical. Calcification can occur, particularly in neuroblastoma; the presence of calcium does not help in distinguishing benign from malignant lesions.

A neurofibroma arising in a nerve root can be dumbbell-shaped, part being inside and part outside the spinal canal. In such cases, the intervertebral foramen may be enlarged. CT can be helpful in determining the extent of the mass and associated vertebral abnormalities and can distinguish the mass from an aortic aneurysm or another vascular lesion if an intravenous contrast agent is given. CT following injection of myelographic contrast may be useful in demonstrating intraspinal extension.

Anterior or Lateral Thoracic Meningocele

This entity represents anomalous herniation of the spinal meninges through an intervertebral foramen or a defect in the vertebral body. It results in a soft tissue mass visible on chest radiographs. In most patients, this abnormality is associated with neurofibromatosis; most are detected in adults.

Meningoceles are described as lateral or anterior, depending on their relationship to the spine. They are slightly more common on the right. Findings that suggest the diagnosis include rib or vertebral anomalies at the same level or in association with scoliosis. The mass is often visible at the apex of the scoliotic curve. CT following intraspinal contrast injection shows filling of the meningocele and is diagnostic (Fig. 4–21).

Neuroenteric Cyst

This rare cyst is composed of both neural and gastrointestinal elements and frequently is attached to both the meninges and gastrointestinal tract. They appear as homogeneous posterior mediastinal masses but rarely contain air because of communication with abdominal viscera. As with meningocele, they are frequently associated with vertebral anomalies or scoliosis. They rarely fill with myelographic contrast. As opposed to meningocele, they frequently cause pain and are generally diagnosed at a young age.

Diseases of the Thoracic Spine

Tumors, either primary or malignant, infectious spondylitis, or vertebral fracture with associated hemorrhage can produce a paravertebral mass. Frequently, the abnormality is bilateral and fusiform, allowing it to be distinguished from solitary masses such as a neurogenic tumor. Associated abnormalities of the vertebral bodies or discs assist in diagnosis and should be sought.

Extramedullary Hematopoiesis

This can result in a paravertebral mass in patients with severe anemia, usually congenital hemolytic anemias or thalassemia. These masses are of unknown origin but perhaps arise from lymph nodes, veins, or an extension of rib marrow. Masses can be multiple and bilateral and are most commonly associated with the lower thoracic spine. They have no specific CT characteristics.

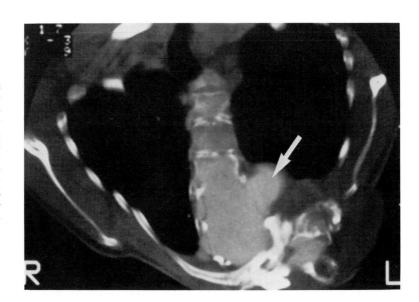

FIGURE 4–21. Lateral thoracic meningocele. In a patient with neurofibromatosis and scoliosis, a meningocele (arrow) is associated with a large foraminal defect. Myelographic contrast material opacifies the meningocele. (Reproduced with modification. From Webb WR. Diseases of the mediastinum. *In* CE Putman and CE Ravin (eds). *Textbook of Diagnostic Imaging.* Philadelphia, W.B. Saunders, 1988.)

Fluid Collections

Occasionally, posterior pleural fluid collections can simulate a paravertebral mediastinal mass. Mediastinal extension of a pancreatic pseudocyst through the aortic or esophageal hiatus can occur, but this is rare.

Vascular Abnormalities

Posteriorly located aortic aneurysms can occupy this part of the mediastinum. Also, azygos and hemiazygos vein dilatation (Fig. 3–12) will produce abnormalities in this region. Dilated azygos or hemiazygos veins, since they are visible on a number of contiguous slices, are easily distinguished from a focal mass.

GENERALIZED MEDIASTINAL ABNORMALITIES

Mediastinitis

Mediastinal infections can be acute or chronic. Acute mediastinitis results from bacterial infection, has a rapid onset and acute symptoms, and is sometimes fatal.

Chronic mediastinitis is usually granulomatous in origin and often is asymptomatic, coming to attention only because of a radiographic abnormality. Chronic sclerosing mediastinitis unassociated with infection is rare but results in similar findings.

Acute Mediastinitis

This usually results from esophageal perforation or the spread of infection from adjacent tissue spaces, including the pharynx, lungs, pleura, and lymph nodes. The primary symptoms are substernal chest pain and fever. CT shows mediastinal widening and replacement of normal fat by fluid density and can detect the presence of gas bubbles (Fig. 4–22). Prognosis is particularly poor in patients with esophageal perforation.

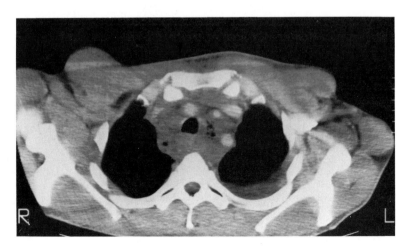

FIGURE 4–22. Acute mediastinitis. A patient with a retropharyngeal abscess developed secondary mediastinitis. This shows mediastinal widening, increased density of mediastinal fat as a result of abscess or inflammation, and small bubbles of air.

Granulomatous Mediastinitis

In patients with sarcoidosis, tuberculosis, and histoplasmosis, chronic mediastinal lymph node enlargement and an associated fibrotic response can result in so-called granulomatous mediastinitis. In these patients, the large nodes and associated fibrous tissue form a mediastinal mass that can compress the superior vena cava, pulmonary arteries or veins, bronchi, and esophagus (Fig. 3–14).

The node enlargement tends to be asymmetric except in patients with sarcoidosis. Fibrosis can replace normally visible mediastinal fat. Calcification of the nodes can be seen in some patients, indicating the benign nature of the disease process. Compression of the main bronchi or pulmonary arteries can sometimes be recognized.

Sclerosing Mediastinitis

In some patients, a similar mediastinal fibrosis is unassociated with obvious granulomatous disease. In a few, this is associated with a similar fibrosis elsewhere (retroperitoneal fibrosis). Symptoms and radiographic findings are similar to those in granulomatous mediastinitis, but calcification does not occur.

Mediastinal Hemorrhage

Mediastinal hemorrhage usually results from trauma such as venous or arterial laceration, from aortic rupture or dissection, or as a result of anticoagulation therapy. Superior mediastinal widening is usually present, associated with blurring of normal mediastinal contours. Blood can dissect extrapleurally over the lung apex, resulting in a so-called apical cap. In some patients, blood will also be present in the left pleural space. CT is rarely of value in diagnosing the site of bleeding unless a dissection is present.

HEART AND PERICARDIUM

CT is not used much in clinical practice for the evaluation of cardiac abnormalities, but some knowledge of cardiac anatomy on CT is necessary for the proper interpretation of scans, and for the identification of paracardiac abnormalities or masses and the effect they have on the heart. Only occasionally are incidental cardiac abnormalities detected on CT. CT, on the other hand, is excellent for evaluating pericardial abnormalities.

Cardiac Pathology

Although CT can show a number of abnormalities in patients with ischemic heart disease or other cardiac abnormalities, it does not usually play a significant role in the clinical evaluation of patients with cardiac pathology. Echocardiography, MRI, and angiography are more commonly used.

As stated above, coronary artery calcification can be clearly identified on CT scans at the level of the aortic root. CT is also very sensitive in detecting valve or annular calcification.

In patients with an acute myocardial infarction (MI), following the bolus injection of contrast, infarcted myocardium can show less opacification than normal myocardium, and to some degree, infarct size can be quantitated. Ventricular thrombus can also be shown in patients with an acute MI.

In patients with prior infarct, CT can be valuable in showing ventricular aneurysms and associated thrombus. In patients who have had coronary artery bypass grafts, graft patency can be determined with an accuracy of about 90%, by performing dynamic, sequential bolus-enhanced CT. However, significant stenoses of patent grafts are difficult to see.

Intracardiac tumors can be shown with contrast-enhanced CT (Fig. 4–23), but are rare and usually evaluated using other techniques. Myocardial wall thickening can be seen in some patients with myocardopathy.

Pericardial Abnormalities

Pericardial Effusion, Thickening, and Fibrosis

Pericardial effusion results in thickening of the normal pericardial stripe. When fluid begins to accumulate, it accumulates first in the dependent portions of the pericardium, typically posterior to the left ventricle (Figs. 3–8, 4–24). As the effusion increases in size, it is visible lateral and anterior to the right atrium and ventricle and, when large, as a concentric density surrounding the heart. Large effusions can also extend into the superior pericardial recess in the mediastinum. The presence of tamponade, associated with pericardial effusion, may be more directly related to the speed at which the fluid accumulates and the distensibility of the pericardium than to the size of the effusion alone.

Pericardial thickening or fibrosis, usually as a result of inflammation, can

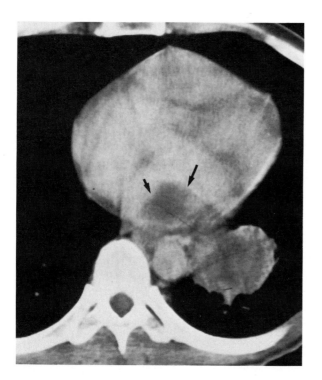

FIGURE 4–23. Left atrial metastasis. In a patient with renal cell carcinoma and a left hilar mass, a mass within the opacified left atrium (arrows) represents a large metastasis.

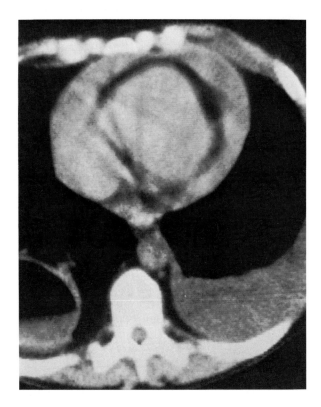

FIGURE 4–24. Pericardial thickening. In a patient with rheumatoid pericarditis, marked pericardial thickening is seen concentrically at the level of the ventricles.

produce a similar thickening of the pericardial stripe. With contrast infusion, the thickened pericardium may be seen to enhance, thus distinguishing it from effusion. Also, pericardial thickening may be denser than fluid collections that also may be present, even without contrast infusion. Thickening may be smooth or focal and nodular. Calcification can occur, particularly as a result of TB, purulent pericarditis, or hemopericardium.

In the presence of symptoms of constrictive pericarditis, the CT appearance of a normal pericardium rules out the diagnosis, while a thickened pericardium allows a presumptive diagnosis of constriction to be made. In the presence of pericardial metastases, CT can show an effusion, or nodular masses may be visible, particularly after contrast infusion.

Paracardiac Masses

Compression of the atria or right ventricle can be seen in the presence of a paracardiac mass, but left ventricular compression is uncommon because of the thickness of it wall and the relatively high pressure of its contents.

Anterior Cardiophrenic Angle Masses

Although a number of the mediastinal masses already described can occur inferiorly to the level of the anterior cardiophrenic angle, the differential diagnosis of lesions occurring in this location includes several additional entities. These include pericardial cyst, large epicardiac fat pad, Morgagni's hernia, and enlargement of paracardiac lymph nodes (discussed above).

Pericardial Cyst

Very commonly, these occur in the anterior right cardiophrenic angle, but approximately one-third are found in other locations. Most patients are asymptomatic. The cysts typically appear as smooth, round, homogeneous masses touching the right anterior chest wall and diaphragm. They range in size up to 15 cm in diameter. As with other mediastinal cysts, their density may be that of water or soft tissue.

Fat Pad

Deposition of fat in either cardiophrenic angle is not uncommon, particularly in obese patients, and fat deposits can simulate a mass on plain radiographs. CT, of course, is diagnostic.

Morgagni's Hernia

Hernias of abdominal contents through the anteromedial diaphragmatic foramen of Morgagni can result in a cardiophrenic angle mass; 90% of these occur on the right. Hernia contents are usually omentum or liver, but they can be bowel. When the hernia contains fat, CT can confirm its benign nature but does not allow its differentiation from a fat pad. When it contains liver, CT may allow diagnosis by showing hepatic vessels or bile ducts. If bowel is present in the hernia sac, gas is usually visible.

SUGGESTED READING

Bashist B, Ellis K, Gold RP: Computed tomography of intrathoracic goiters. Am J Roentgenol, 140:455–460, 1983.

Glazer HS, Aronberg DJ, Sagel SS: Pitfalls in CT recognition of mediastinal lymphadenopathy. Am J Roentgenol, 144:267–274, 1985.

Glazer GM, Gross BH, Quint LE, et al.: Normal mediastinal lymph nodes: Number and size according to American Thoracic Society mapping. Am J Roentgenol, 144:261–265, 1985.

Glazer HS, Kaiser LR, Anderson DJ, et al.: Indeterminate mediastinal invasion in bronchogenic carcinoma: CT evaluation. Radiology, 173:37–42, 1989.

Hopper KD, Diehl LF, Lesar M, et al.: Hodgkin disease: Clinical utility of CT in initial staging and treatment. Radiology, 169:17–22, 1988.

Levitt RG, Husband JE, Glazer HS: CT of primary germ-cell tumors of the mediastinum. Am J Roentgenol, 142:73–78, 1984.

Pugatch RD, Faling LJ, Robbins AH, et al.: CT diagnosis of benign mediastinal abnormalities. Am J Roentgenol, 134:685–694, 1980.

Staples CA, Müller NL, Miller RR, et al.: Mediastinal nodes in bronchogenic carcinoma: Comparison between CT and mediastinoscopy. Radiology, 167:367–372, 1988.

5

The Pulmonary Hila

There are not many things in chest radiology which are as difficult as accurately evaluating the pulmonary hila on chest radiographs. The hila have extremely complex and somewhat variable silhouettes as seen on the frontal or lateral films. It is often difficult to decide if a hilum is normal or abnormal, and if abnormal, what the abnormal finding represents. CT, in allowing the hila to be imaged tomographically in cross section, with opacification of the vessels, has revolutionized the radiographic evaluation of the pulmonary hila. It has completely (or almost completely) replaced conventional hilar tomography, and if it hasn't yet, it should.

CT is very helpful in the diagnosis of endobronchial lesions, hilar and parahilar masses, and hilar vascular lesions. The sensitivity and specificity of CT in diagnosing hilar mass or adenopathy in patients with lung cancer average between 80% and 90%, and are highest when bolus contrast enhancement is used.

TECHNIQUE

In general, we examine the hila in combination with the remainder of the chest and mediastinum. As stated above, most patients with hilar abnormalities are being scanned because of lung cancer, and the diagnostic information we obtain regarding the presence of mediastinal abnormalities is most important in determining treatment. However, it is best to think of the examination of the hila as a separate and distinct part of the chest CT study. Unless this is done, the technique may not be optimal.

Scans 1 cm thick are routinely performed. Contrast medium is given by bolus injection, and often scans are obtained dynamically at successive levels (dynamic incremental CT). Although the method of contrast infusion and scanning sequences which are used can be varied, it is important to keep in mind that the more rapidly the contrast is given, the better the vascular opacification will be, and the easier it is to distinguish normal hilar vessels from masses or enlarged lymph nodes.

When dynamic incremental CT of the hilum is performed, we give an intravenous bolus injection of approximately 50 ml of contrast, with the scanner positioned at the level of the upper lobe bronchus. Midway through the bolus, rapid (2-second) sequential scanning is performed at 1-cm intervals to the level of the inferior hila. If the patient cannot hold his breath for the entire sequence (which is typical), the bolus and scanning sequence can be divided as necessary. In patients who cannot hold their breath for more than one or two slices, we obtain hilar sequences during the slow infusion of contrast. As with the different parts of the mediastinum, described in Chapter 2, it takes about seven contiguous slices to image the hila.

Scans are viewed with a mean window level of −600 H and a window width of 1000 H or 2000 H (lung window) for accurate assessment of hilar contours and bronchial anatomy. Scans are also viewed at a mean window value of 0 to 50 H and a window width of 500 H (mediastinal window) in order to obtain additional information about hilar structures and masses, as well as a more accurate assessment of bronchial narrowing. This window is also necessary in order to observe vascular opacification.

Thin sections (1 to 5 mm) are sometimes valuable in the diagnosis of questionable hilar or bronchial abnormalities seen with 1-cm collimation. However, thin sections are not used routinely.

DIAGNOSIS OF HILAR MASS OR ADENOPATHY

A detailed understanding of cross-sectional hilar anatomy is necessary in order to identify hilar abnormalities on CT.

Lobar and segmental bronchi (Fig. 5–1) are consistently seen on CT, reliably identify successive hilar levels, and are the key to interpreting the pulmonary hila. In general, hilar anatomy and contours at the same bronchial levels are relatively constant from one patient to the next. The bronchi should be looked at first, whenever you read a CT scan of the hila.

In some locations, normal hilar contours are consistent enough that a diagnosis of hilar adenopathy or mass can be made on the basis of an abnormality

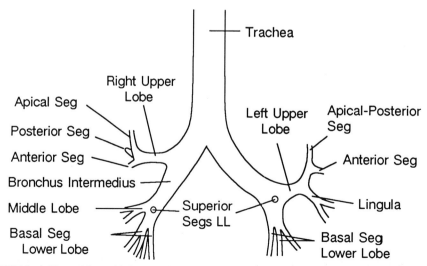

FIGURE 5–1. Normal bronchial tree. All the bronchi shown are visible on CT in most patients. Those bronchi that appear horizontal (such as the right upper lobe) or nearly vertical are usually better seen than those that have an oblique course relative to the plane of scan (such as right middle lobe or lingular bronchi).

in hilar contour alone, seen using lung windows. In other locations, however, contours can vary according to the size and position of the hilar pulmonary arteries and veins. In these locations, contrast opacification of the pulmonary vessels is essential to accurate diagnosis. Also, in any location, contrast infusion can be helpful, if you are uncertain as to the presence of a mass. It is wise to always perform hilar CT with contrast infusion.

A hilar mass or lymph node enlargement may be indicated by a local or generalized alteration in hilar contour; bronchial narrowing, obstruction, or displacement; and thickening or obliteration of the walls of bronchi which normally contact lung. At mediastinal window settings, any nonenhancing hilar area larger than 5 mm has been considered abnormal, but this is not always the case. A normal soft tissue collection larger than this, representing fat and normal nodes, is sometimes visible (see below and Fig. 5–7).

Normal and Abnormal Hilar Anatomy

With one or two exceptions, rather than describe the anatomy of each hilum separately, I will illustrate normal anatomy for both hila as seen on the same scan, at the same time. Although this will seem somewhat more compli-cated at first, it is actually easier, and is, in fact, the best way to read hilar CT. Looking at both hila at the same time allows you to compare one to the other. Although the hila are not symmetric structures, they have a number of similarities, and identifying these can be of value. These similarities will be emphasized in the following description. In order to reinforce the normal appearances and their significance, and expected alterations in anatomy occurring because of mass of node enlargement, abnormal findings will be shown at each hilar level described.

Please note that there is some variation among patients in the relative levels of the hila, and therefore in the levels at which right and left hilar structures are visible on CT. The right-to-left relationships illustrated in Figure 5–1 and described in the following text may or may not be present in individual cases, although variation will usually be minor (1 or 2 cm).

Upper Hila

CT at the level of the distal trachea or carina will show the apical segmental bronchus of the right upper lobe in cross section, surrounded by several vessels of similar size (Fig. 5–2). On the left, the apical posterior segmental bronchus and associated arteries and veins have a similar appearance. On either side, a mass or lymphadenopathy is easily recognizable. Anything larger than the expected pulmonary vessels is abnormal (Fig. 5–3). Comparing with the opposite side at this level is very helpful.

Right Upper Lobe Bronchus and Left Upper Lobe Segments

Right Hilum. Approximately 1 cm distal to the carina, the right upper lobe bronchus is usually visible along its length, with its anterior and posterior segmental branches both generally seen at the same level (Fig. 5–4). The anterior segment, usually lying in or near the scan plane, is very commonly seen over a length of 2 to 3 cm. The posterior segmental bronchus usually angles slightly cephalad, out of the plane of scan, and may not be as well seen. If not, look for

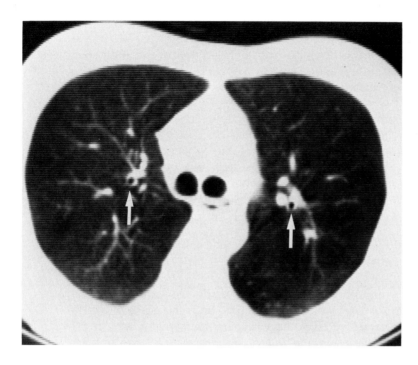

FIGURE 5–2. Upper hilar level. Normal anatomy. CT at the level of the carina shows the apical segmental bronchus (arrow) of the right upper lobe in cross section, with several adjacent vessels of similar size. On the left, the apical posterior segmental bronchus (arrow) of the left upper lobe and associated arteries and veins have a similar appearance. Note that this same patient is also used to illustrate normal anatomy at lower levels.

it on the next highest level. In some normals, the origin of the apical segment can be seen at this level as a round lucency, usually at the point of bifurcation (or, in this case, trifurcation) of the right upper lobe bronchus.

Anterior to the right upper lobe bronchus, the truncus anterior produces an oval density of variable size, but often about the same size as the right main bronchus visible at the same level. An upper lobe vein branch (posterior vein), lying in the angle between anterior and posterior segmental branches, is present and visible in almost all patients. The posterior wall of the upper lobe bronchus is usually outlined by lung, and appears smooth and 2 to 3 mm thick.

Within the anterior right hilum at this level, a mass or lymph node enlargement can be identified if a soft-tissue density larger than the expected size of the truncus anterior is visible (Fig. 5–5). This, of course could be confirmed by contrast injection. Laterally, in the angle between the anterior and posterior segmental bronchi, anything larger than the expected vein is abnormal (Fig. 5–5). This vein should not be significantly larger than it is at the level 1 cm above. Posteriorly, thickening of the wall of the upper lobe bronchus or main bronchus, or a focal soft tissue density behind it, will almost always be abnormal (Fig. 5–5A).

Left Hilum. On the left side, at or near this level, the apical-posterior and anterior segmental bronchi of the left upper lobe are usually visible (Fig. 5–4). The apical-posterior segmental bronchus is seen in cross section as a round lucency, while the anterior segmental bronchus is directed anteriorly, roughly in the plane of scan, at an angle of about 1 o'clock. These bronchi lie lateral to the main branch of the left pulmonary artery, which produces a large convexity in the posterior hilum at this level, and to the superior pulmonary vein, which results in an anterior convexity. In a number of normals, the artery supplying the anterior segment of the left upper lobe is seen medial to the anterior segmental bronchus. Lymphadenopathy can be seen in relation to all these structures, most easily recognized after contrast infusion (Fig. 5–5B).

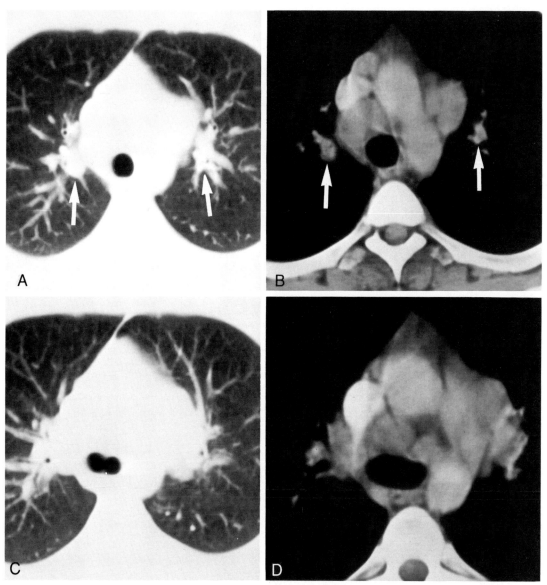

FIGURE 5–3. Abnormal upper hila (adenopathy). In a patient with sarcoidosis and bilateral hilar adenopathy, contrast-enhanced scans at two levels through the upper hila have been photographed with lung *(A and C)* and mediastinal *(B and D)* window settings. *(A and B)* This scan level is slightly above that illustrated in Figure 5–2. Note that two small bronchial branches are visible on each side, rather than a single apical or apical-posterior bronchus. Enlarged nodes (arrows) adjacent to the bronchi are too large to represent normal vessels, and they appear unopacified on the mediastinal window scan. *(C and D)* At a level 1 cm below *A* and *B,* extensive hilar lobulation is visible, reflecting the adenopathy.

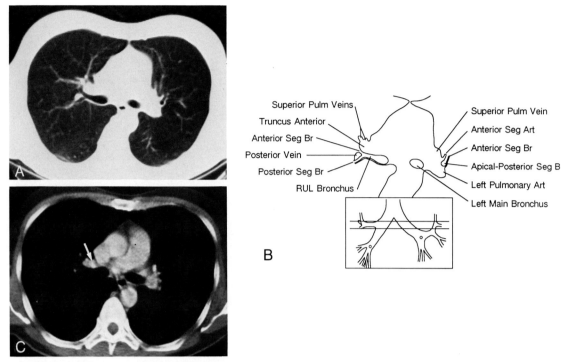

FIGURE 5–4. Right upper lobe bronchus and left upper lobe segments level. Normal anatomy.
(A, B, and *C)* Right hilum: The right upper lobe bronchus is visible along its length, along with its anterior and posterior segmental branches. The truncus anterior (arrow, *C)* is anterior to the right upper lobe bronchus. An upper lobe vein branch (posterior vein) lies in the angle between anterior and posterior segmental branches; the superior pulmonary veins result in some lobulation anterior to the truncus anterior. The posterior wall of the upper lobe bronchus appears smooth and is 2 to 3 mm in thickness. Left hilum: On the left side, the apical-posterior and anterior segmental bronchi of the left upper lobe are visible. The apical-posterior segment is seen in cross section as a round lucency, while the anterior segment is directed anteriorly. These bronchi lie lateral to the main branch of the left pulmonary artery, which produces a large convexity in the posterior hilum, and to the superior pulmonary vein, which results in an anterior convexity. The artery supplying the anterior segment of the left upper lobe is seen medial to the anterior segmental bronchus.

A small vein is visible lateral to the apical-posterior bronchus in about 40% of individuals. In this location, mass or adenopathy can be recognized when a mass larger than the normal vein is present within the lateral hilum (Fig. 5–6).

Right Bronchus Intermedius

Below the level of the right upper lobe bronchus, the bronchus intermedius is visible as an oval lucency at two or three adjacent levels (Figs. 5–7, 5–14). Its posterior wall is sharply outlined by lung. Anterior and lateral to the bronchus, the hilar silhouette may vary in appearance, primarily because of variations in the sizes and positions of pulmonary veins. Mass involving the posterior hilum can be readily diagnosed without contrast injection, because of thickening of the posterior bronchial wall (Figs. 5–8, 5–9, 5–15); thickening of the posterior wall of the bronchus intermedius is a common finding in patients with a right hilar mass, particularly one resulting from lung cancer.

The diagnosis of anterior or lateral hilar masses at this level generally requires contrast administration (Figs. 5–8, 5–10, 5–15). Even contrast-enhanced scans can be difficult to interpret at this level. A collection of fat and

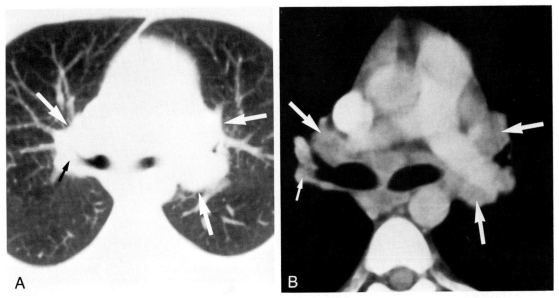

A   B

FIGURE 5–5. Hilar adenopathy. *(A* and *B)* In the patient with sarcoidosis illustrated in Figure 5–3, there is extensive adenopathy (arrows) at this level. On the right, nodes are visible as unopacified structures anteriorly and laterally in the angle of the bifurcation of the right upper lobe bronchus into its anterior and posterior segments (small arrows). The soft tissue density seen in the position of the posterior vein on the right (small arrow) is too large to represent a vessel. The posterior wall of the right upper lobe bronchus is thickened; this is best seen at the lung window setting *(A).* On the left side, there are enlarged nodes (arrows) in both the anterior and posterior hila, which are distinguishable from the opacified left pulmonary artery in *(B).*

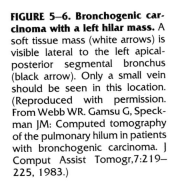

FIGURE 5–6. Bronchogenic carcinoma with a left hilar mass. A soft tissue mass (white arrows) is visible lateral to the left apical-posterior segmental bronchus (black arrow). Only a small vein should be seen in this location. (Reproduced with permission. From Webb WR, Gamsu G, Speckman JM: Computed tomography of the pulmonary hilum in patients with bronchogenic carcinoma. J Comput Assist Tomogr,7:219–225, 1983.)

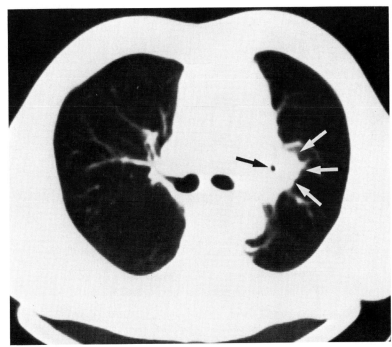

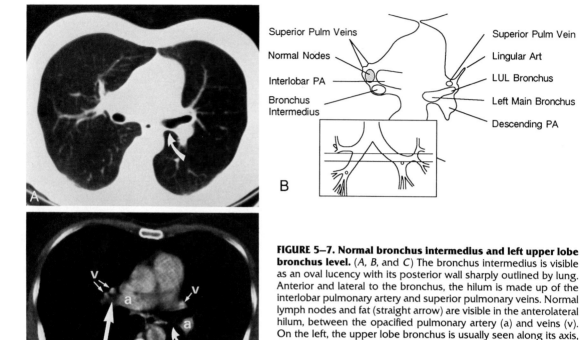

FIGURE 5–7. Normal bronchus intermedius and left upper lobe bronchus level. (*A, B,* and *C*) The bronchus intermedius is visible as an oval lucency with its posterior wall sharply outlined by lung. Anterior and lateral to the bronchus, the hilum is made up of the interlobar pulmonary artery and superior pulmonary veins. Normal lymph nodes and fat (straight arrow) are visible in the anterolateral hilum, between the opacified pulmonary artery (a) and veins (v). On the left, the upper lobe bronchus is usually seen along its axis, extending anteriorly and laterally from its origin. The left superior pulmonary vein (v) is anterior and medial to the bronchus, and the descending branch of the left pulmonary artery (a) forms an oval soft tissue density posterior and lateral to it. The left posterior bronchial wall (curved arrow) is outlined by lung at this level.

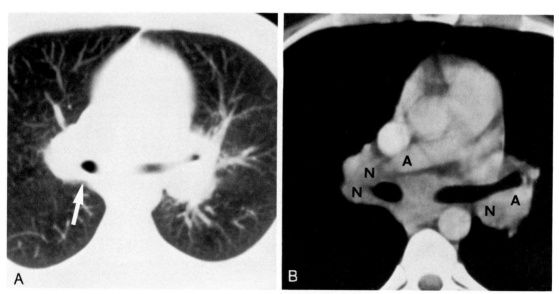

FIGURE 5–8. Abnormal bronchus intermedius and left upper lobe bronchus level. (*A* and *B*) In the patient with sarcoidosis, there is lymph node enlargement (N) in the lateral right hilum, distinguishable from the opacified pulmonary artery (A) at a mediastinal window setting. Thickening of the posterior wall of the bronchus intermedius (arrow) is also seen. On the left, there are large nodes (N) posterior to the left bronchus and medial to the pulmonary artery (A). These nodes obscure the posterior wall of the left bronchus. Subcarinal node enlargement is also present.

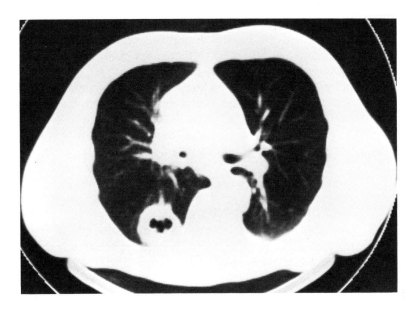

FIGURE 5–9. Thickening of the posterior wall of the bronchus intermedius. In a patient with a cavitary lung cancer in the posterior lower lobe, there is thickening of the posterior wall of the bronchus intermedius and narrowing of its lumen.

normal-sized nodes, sometimes measuring more than 1 cm in diameter, is commonly seen at the level of the bifurcation of the right pulmonary artery, anterior and lateral to the bronchus intermedius (Fig. 5–7C). This normal soft tissue should not be mistaken for a hilar mass.

Left Upper Lobe Bronchus and Right Middle Lobe Bronchus

I have taken some liberty with anatomy in describing these two levels at the same time—the left upper lobe bronchus is usually visible 1 cm above the right middle lobe bronchus. However, I feel justified in doing this because the right and left hila are nearly symmetric at these two levels and are sometimes seen on the same scan.

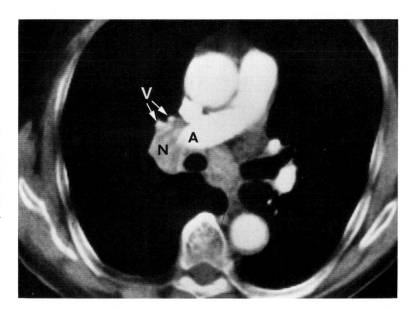

FIGURE 5–10. Abnormal bronchus intermedius level. In a patient with bronchogenic carcinoma and right hilar adenopathy (N), the soft tissue mass is clearly distinguished from the opacified artery (A). Veins (V) are displaced anteriorly. Note that this mass is much larger than the normal collection of nodes and fat that can be seen in this location (Fig. 5–7).

Left Upper Lobe Bronchus. The left upper lobe bronchus is usually seen along its axis, extending anteriorly and laterally from its origin, at an angle of approximately 10 to 30 degrees (Fig. 5–7). The left superior pulmonary veins are anterior and medial to the bronchus at this level, and the descending branch of the left pulmonary artery forms an oval soft-tissue density posterior and lateral to it. Because only the oval artery occupies the lateral hilum, lobulation of the lateral hilum (more than one convexity) indicates lymphadenopathy (Figs. 5–8, 5–11, 5–12). The superior segment bronchus of the left lower lobe can arise at this level.

Although lung contacts and sharply outlines the posterior wall of the bronchus intermedius at several levels, the left posterior bronchial wall is usually outlined only at this level, that is, at the level of the left upper lobe bronchus. In approximately 90% of individuals, lung sharply outlines the posterior wall of the left main or upper lobe bronchus, medial to the descending pulmonary artery (Figs. 5–7, 5–9). As on the right, the bronchial wall should measure 2 to 3 mm in thickness. Thickening of this stripe of density, or a focal soft tissue density behind it, indicates lymph node enlargement or bronchial wall thickening (Figs. 5–8, 5–13). In 10 percent of normal individuals, however, lung does not contact

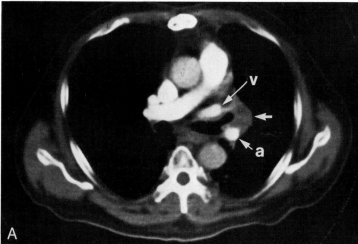

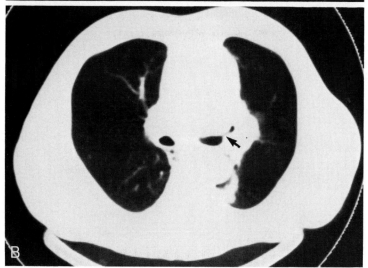

FIGURE 5–11. Left hilar adenopathy (left upper lobe bronchus level). *(A)* In a patient with left hilar adenopathy from lung cancer, lateral left hilar lymph nodes (arrow) are distinguishable from artery (a) and vein (v) following contrast injection. *(B)* At a lung window setting, the upper lobe bronchus appears narrow (arrow). The lateral hilum is lobulated. (Reproduced with permission. From Webb WR, Gamsu G, Speckman JM: Computed tomography of the pulmonary hilum in patients with bronchogenic carcinoma. J Comput Assist Tomogr, 7:219–225, 1983.)

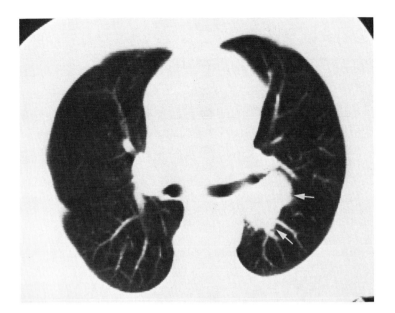

FIGURE 5–12. Left hilar adenopathy (left upper lobe bronchus level). Lobulation of the posterior left hilum reflects adenopathy; only one convexity would be normal. (Reproduced with permission. From Webb WR, Glazer GM, Gamsu G: CT of the abnormal pulmonary hilum. J Comput Assist Tomogr, 5:485–490, 1981.)

the bronchial wall because the descending pulmonary artery is medially positioned against the aorta. This should not be misinterpreted as abnormal.

Lingular Bronchus. The lingular bronchus is usually visible at a level near the undersurface of the left upper lobe bronchus; its two segments (superior and inferior) can sometimes be seen. The pulmonary artery and veins appear the same as at the level of the left upper lobe bronchus (Fig. 5–14). At this level as well, lobulation of the lateral hilar contour indicates mass or adenopathy (Fig. 5–15).

Right Middle Lobe Bronchus. The appearance of the right hilum at the level of the middle lobe bronchus is quite similar to that of the left hilum at the level of the left upper lobe bronchus.

On the right, at the level of the lower bronchus intermedius, the middle

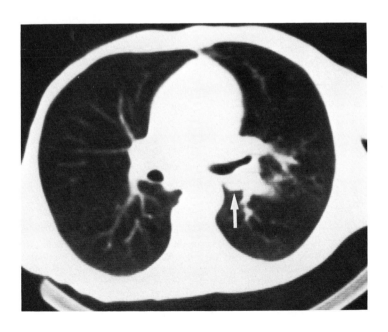

FIGURE 5–13. Left hilar adenopathy (left upper lobe bronchus level). In a patient with metastatic breast carcinoma, an enlarged lymph node is visible posterior to the left bronchus (arrow). A convexity in the azygoesophageal space also reflects adenopathy.

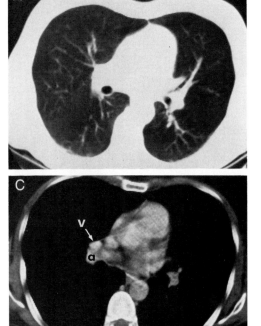

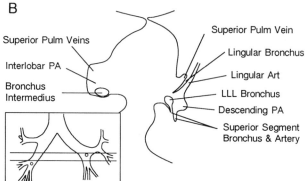

FIGURE 5–14. Normal lingular and lower lobe bronchi. (*A, B,* and *C*) The lingular bronchus is visible slightly below the level of the upper lobe bronchus, with its accompanying artery branch. The left lower lobe bronchus and the superior segmental branch of the lower lobe are also seen at this level. As at the level 1 cm above, the descending pulmonary artery appears oval in shape. On the right, the bronchus intermedius appears similar to the level above. The pulmonary veins (v) are anterior to the pulmonary artery (a).

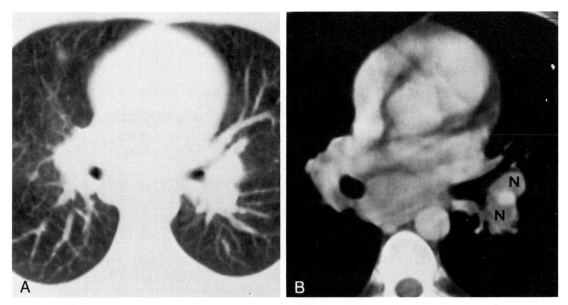

FIGURE 5–15. Abnormal lingular and lower lobe bronchi (adenopathy). (*A* and *B*) On the left, there is lobulation of the hilum. With contrast infusion, the enlarged nodes (N) and the pulmonary artery can be distinguished. On the right, the posterior wall of the bronchus intermedius is thickened. Lymph nodes are also visible in the right hilum.

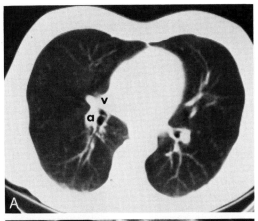

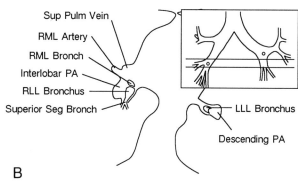

B

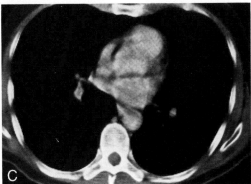

FIGURE 5–16. Normal right middle lobe bronchus level. (*A, B,* and *C*) The middle lobe bronchus arises anteriorly and extends anteriorly and laterally at an angle of about 45 degrees. Because it is also angled caudally, only a short segment of its lumen is visible. The superior segmental bronchus of the lower lobe arises posterolaterally. The superior pulmonary veins (v) lie anterior and medial to the bronchus, while the oval descending (interlobar) branch of the right pulmonary artery (a) lies beside and behind it. The appearance of the right hilum at this level is quite similar to that of the left hilum at the levels of the left upper lobe and lingular bronchi. On the left, the left lower lobe bronchus and pulmonary artery are similar in size.

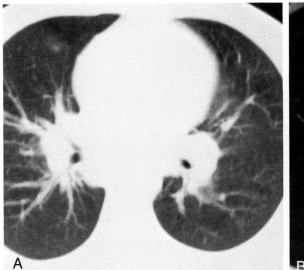

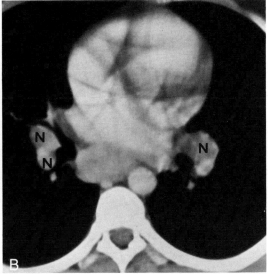

FIGURE 5–17. Abnormal right middle lobe bronchus level (adenopathy). (*A* and *B*) There is lobulation of the right hilum, and adenopathy is visible on mediastinal window scans. On the left, the hilum is enlarged relative to the bronchus, and adenopathy is clearly visible on mediastinal windows anterior to the bronchus.

lobe bronchus arises anteriorly and extends anteriorly, laterally, and inferiorly at angles of about 30 to 45 degrees (Fig. 5–16). Because of its obliquity, only a short segment of its lumen is visible at each level on CT, and this appearance should not be misinterpreted as bronchial obstruction. Often the superior segmental bronchus of the lower lobe arises posterolaterally at this level (Fig. 5–16).

At the level of the origin of the middle lobe bronchus, the superior pulmonary veins lie anterior and medial to the bronchus, as they do on the left, while the descending (interlobar) branch of the right pulmonary artery lies beside and behind it (Fig. 5–16). Because of this separation of artery and veins, the lateral hilum at this level (representing the artery) is oval in shape, without prominent lobulations. Any lobulation of significant size suggests hilar adenopathy (Figs. 5–17, 5–18). Contrast injection would be confirmatory.

Lower Lobe Bronchi (Basal Segments)

At this level, the hila are relatively symmetric, and comparing one side to the other can be helpful.

The main lower lobe bronchial trunk on each side (Fig. 5–16), which

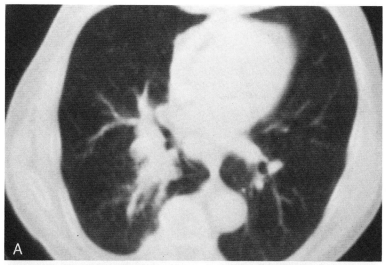
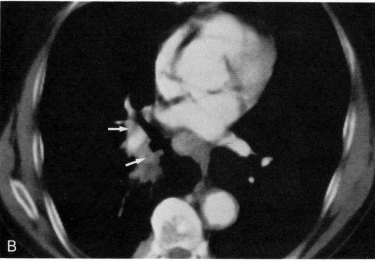

FIGURE 5–18. Right hilar carcinoma. *(A)* At a lung window setting, the right hilum is enlarged and lobulated. *(B)* With contrast infusion, the descending pulmonary artery is distinguishable from adenopathy (arrows).

eventually gives rise to the basal segmental bronchi, branches in a variable fashion. It is common for the lower lobe bronchial trunk on the right to divide into two basal bronchial branches or trunks, at a level above the origins of the basal segmental bronchi.

The basal segmental branches of the lower lobe bronchi also vary in appearance, depending on their courses (Fig. 5–19). On the right, the four segmental branches (medial, anterior, lateral, and posterior) are sometimes visible; on the left, there are three basal segments (anteromedial, lateral, and posterior). However, even on good quality scans it is not unusual for one or more segmental bronchi to be invisible with 1-cm collimation. With thin collimation, the segments are seen much better.

The segmental bronchi are accompanied by pulmonary artery branches that are somewhat larger than the bronchi (Fig. 5–19). At this level, the inferior pulmonary veins pass behind and medial to the bronchi to enter the left atrium. Hilar masses or lymph node enlargement can be diagnosed on the basis of contour abnormalities or asymmetries between the hila. Soft tissue densities which seem too large to be the pulmonary artery or vein branches should be regarded with suspicion (Figs. 5–20, 5–21).

Bronchial Abnormalities

The excellent contrast and spatial resolution of CT allow for good assessment of bronchial lesions, and CT is often performed to guide bronchoscopy in

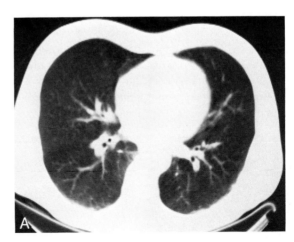

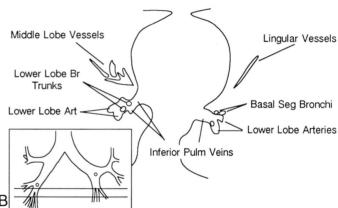

FIGURE 5–19. Normal lower lobe bronchi (basal segments). (*A* and *B*) On the right, the right lower lobe bronchus has bifurcated. On the left, three branches are seen. The inferior pulmonary veins are posterior and medial, and pulmonary artery branches accompany the bronchi.

Middle Lobe Vessels

Lingular Vessels

Lower Lobe Br Trunks

Lower Lobe Art

Basal Seg Bronchi

Lower Lobe Arteries

Inferior Pulm Veins

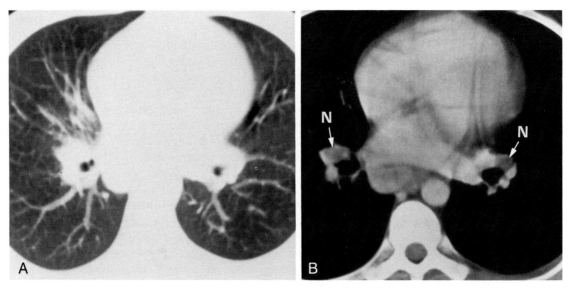

FIGURE 5–20. Abnormal lower lobe bronchi level (adenopathy). (*A* and *B*) The hila are enlarged bilaterally, and nodes (N) are visible at mediastinal window settings in the patient with sarcoidosis illustrated at higher levels.

patients who have a suspected hilar or bronchial abnormality. Bronchial wall thickening, the presence of an endobronchial mass, and narrowing of the bronchial lumen are accurate indicators of bronchial pathology. However, it must be kept in mind that bronchial abnormalities, which are primarily mucosal, can be missed using CT, because of their small size or minimal thickness. Also, volume averaging at the upper or lower edges of a bronchus can mimic the presence of bronchial obstruction. It is always a good idea to obtain additional views (preferably with thin collimation) of a questionable bronchial lesion, before making a definite diagnosis.

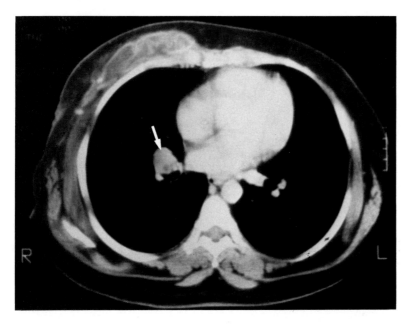

FIGURE 5–21. Right hilar adenopathy from lung cancer. At the level of the origins of lower lobe basal segments, the right hilum is enlarged, and adenopathy (arrow) is visible.

Bronchial wall thickening is most easily assessed on CT in regions where the hilar bronchi lie adjacent to lung—the posterior walls of the right main and both upper lobe bronchi, and the posterior wall of the bronchus intermedius. Smooth bronchial wall thickening can be due to inflammation or tumor infiltration (Figs. 5–8, 5–9), while a localized or lobulated thickening usually indicates tumor or lymph node enlargement (Figs. 5–11, 5–22).

Bronchial narrowing and endobronchial lesions, which may be extremely difficult to detect on plain radiographs, can be reliably diagnosed on CT (Figs. 5–23, 5–24). However, it may be difficult to distinguish endobronchial tumor from compression by an exobronchial mass (Fig. 5–25). Abrupt changes in bronchial caliber on CT usually indicate circumferential tumor infiltration or an endobronchial mass (Figs. 5–24, 5–26), but it is important to look at adjacent scans to confirm that the apparent bronchial narrowing does not reflect an oblique bronchial course, with the bronchus leaving the plane of scan (as with the right middle lobe bronchus).

Generally speaking, scans viewed with a lung window setting are best for identifying normal bronchi and detecting bronchial abnormalities, but often overestimate the degree of bronchial narrowing (Figs. 5–24, 5–25). Thus, a narrowed but patent bronchus may appear obstructed with this window setting, when 1-cm collimation is used. Also, a normal bronchus, slightly out of the plane of scan and being volume-averaged with adjacent soft tissue, can appear narrowed on lung window scans. Mediastinal window settings more accurately assess bronchial lumen diameter in the presence of an abnormality, but somewhat overestimate luminal size. If a bronchial lesion is suspected, both window settings should be used.

Differential Diagnosis of Hilar and Bronchial Abnormalities

Bronchogenic Carcinoma

The most common cause of hilar mass or lymph node enlargement is bronchogenic carcinoma. In patients with tumors arising centrally (usually squamous cell carcinoma), bronchial abnormalities (narrowing, obstruction) visible on CT are common, and the hilar mass can appear irregular because of local infiltration of the lung parenchyma. In such patients, an endobronchial lesion is commonly seen at bronchoscopy, correlating with the CT abnormality. If the bronchial abnormality is within 2 cm of the carina, resection may be difficult or impossible (Fig. 5–27); bronchoscopy rather that CT, however, is most accurate for making this determination.

When the carcinoma arises within the peripheral lung, and the hila are abnormal because of node metastases, the hilar mass or masses may be smoother and more sharply defined than when the hilar mass is primary. However, this distinction is not always easily made. Patients with a central mass and bronchial obstruction often show peripheral parenchymal abnormalities. In patients with hilar node metastases, a bronchial abnormality seen at CT usually reflects external compression by the enlarged hilar nodes, but bronchial invasion may also be present. Hilar node metastases are present at surgery in 15 to 40% of patients with lung cancer.

It is important to keep in mind that, in patients with bronchogenic carcinoma, enlarged hilar nodes visible on CT may not be due to node metastasis.

Text continued on page 82

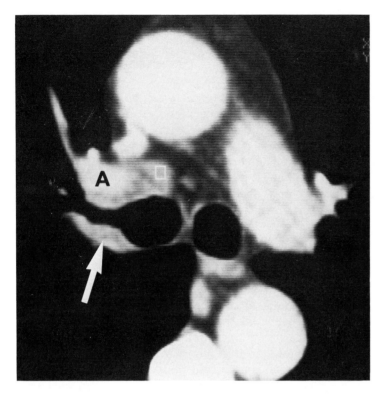

FIGURE 5–22. Bronchogenic carcinoma, right upper lobe bronchus. There is irregular thickening (arrow) of the posterior wall of the right upper lobe bronchus, with narrowing of its lumen, as a result of a carcinoma arising from its posterior wall. The truncus anterior (A) is opacified, as are pulmonary veins.

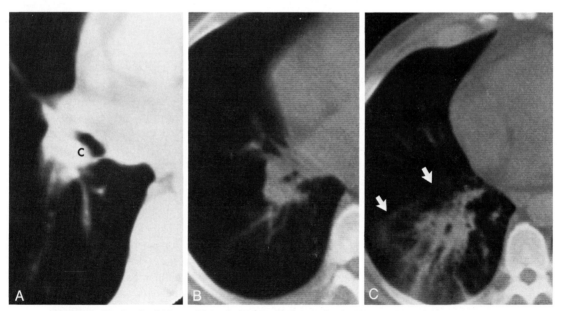

FIGURE 5–23. Carcinoid bronchial adenoma with hyperplastic hilar nodes. *(A)* In a patient with recurrent right lower lobe pneumonias, an endobronchial carcinoid tumor (c) is narrowing the bronchus intermedius. It appears focal and endobronchial, rather than infiltrative, because there are acute angles where it contacts the bronchus. *(B)* At a lower level, there is enlargement and lobulation of the right hilum, indicating adenopathy. *(C)* Patchy right lower lobe consolidation is present inferiorly. The major fissure (arrows) is displaced posteriorly, indicating lower lobe volume loss. At surgery, the hilar nodes were hyperplastic, resulting from the pneumonia. (Reproduced with permission. Webb WR, Gamsu G, Birnberg FA: CT appearance of bronchial carcinoid with recurrent pneumonia and hyperplastic hilar lymphadenopathy. J Comput Assist Tomogr, 7(4):707–709, 1983.)

FIGURE 5–24. Bronchogenic carcinoma, with right upper lobe bronchus obstruction. *(A)* With a lung window setting, there is thickening of the posterior wall of the right main bronchus (arrow), and the right upper lobe bronchus is invisible. This suggests narrowing or obstruction of the right upper lobe bronchus. The right hilum is enlarged. A poorly defined carcinoma is visible in the posterior lung. *(B)* At a mediastinal window setting, the upper lobe bronchus is obstructed (arrow) by an endobronchial mass, and a lateral hilar mass is visible. (Reproduced from Webb WR. Radiol Clin North Am, 21:723–739, 1983.)

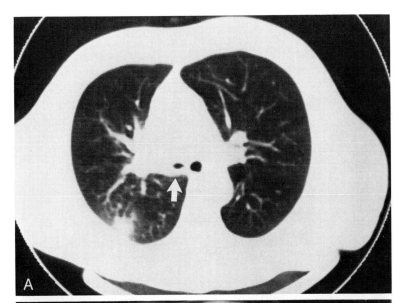

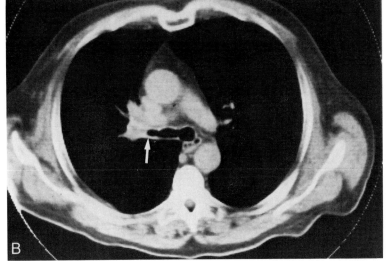

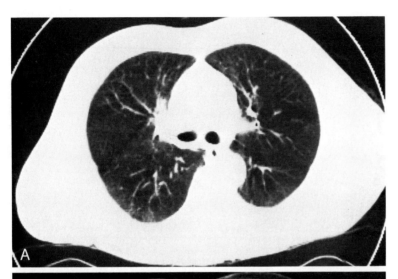

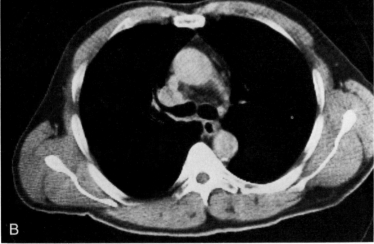

FIGURE 5–25. Lung cancer with right upper lobe bronchial compression. *(A)* With a lung window setting, as in Figure 5–24, there is thickening of the posterior wall of the right main bronchus, and the right upper lobe bronchus is not clearly seen. *(B)* With a mediastinal window setting, the right upper lobe segmental bronchi are visible but narrowed. Mass anterior to the upper lobe bronchus is also visible. The posterior wall of the upper lobe bronchus is thickened. (Reproduced with permission. From Webb WR, Gamsu G, Speckman JM: Computed tomography of the pulmonary hilum in patients with bronchogenic carcinoma. J Comput Assist Tomogr, 7:219–225, 1983.)

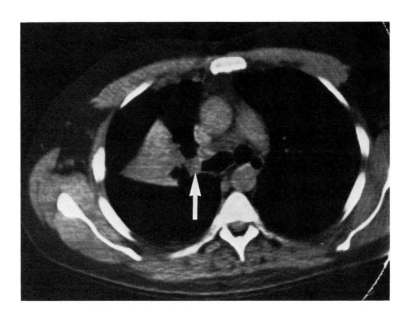

FIGURE 5–26. Endobronchial metastasis. In a patient with thyroid carcinoma, an endobronchial metastasis appears as a focal endobronchial mass (arrow) obstructing the right upper lobe bronchus. There is associated right upper lobe consolidation. (Reproduced from Webb WR. Radiol Clin North Am, 21:723–739, 1983.)

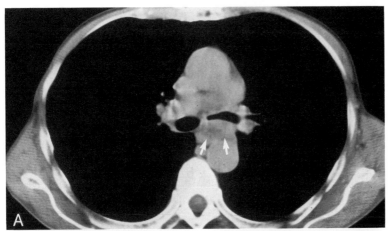

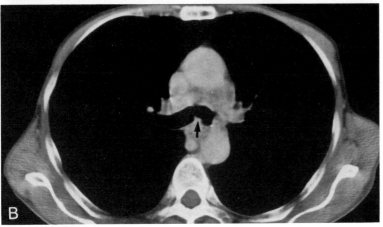

FIGURE 5–27. Bronchogenic carcinoma, left main bronchus. *(A)* Infiltrating tumor is narrowing the left main bronchus and producing a significant mass posterior to the bronchus (arrows). This appearance is typical of bronchogenic carcinoma. *(B)* There is thickening of the posterior carina (arrow), suggesting infiltration by tumor. This was confirmed at bronchoscopy, making this tumor unresectable.

Hyperplastic nodal enlargement often occurs in lung cancer patients, particularly when there is bronchial obstruction and distal pneumonia or atelectasis is present. Conversely, a normal-sized hilar node can harbor microscopic metastases.

Other Primary Bronchial Tumors

Other primary bronchial tumors can produce a hilar mass. The most common of these is so-called bronchial adenoma, usually carcinoid cell type (Fig. 5–23). This malignant tumor arises from the main, lobar, or segmental bronchi in 80% of cases. It tends to be slow growing and locally invasive. A well-defined endobronchial mass is typical, but a large, exobronchial hilar mass is sometimes seen as well. Carcinoid tumors are very vascular and can enhance somewhat following contrast infusion. Calcification occasionally occurs.

Benign bronchial tumors, such as fibroma, chondroma, or lipoma, will usually appear focal and endobronchial on CT, rather than infiltrative, and do not commonly produce an exobronchial mass. Obstruction is the primary finding on CT. They are relatively rare.

Lymphoma

Hilar adenopathy is present in 25% of patients with Hodgkin's and 10% of patients with non-Hodgkin's lymphoma. Hilar involvement is usually asymmetric. Multiple nodes in the hilum or mediastinum are usually involved. Endobronchial lesions can also be seen, or bronchi may be compressed by enlarged nodes, but this is much less common than with lung cancer. There are no specific features of the hilar abnormality seen in patients with lymphoma which allow a definite diagnosis.

Metastases

Metastases to hilar lymph nodes from an extrathoracic primary tumor are not uncommon. Hilar node metastases may be unilateral or bilateral. Endobronchial metastases can also be seen (Fig. 5–26), without there being hilar node metastases; these may appear to be focal and endobronchial or infiltrative. Head and neck carcinomas, thyroid carcinoma, genitourinary tumors (particularly renal cell), melanoma, and breast carcinomas are most commonly responsible for hilar or endobronchial metastases.

Inflammatory Disease

Unilateral or bilateral hilar lymphadenopathy, and bronchial narrowing, can be seen in a number of infectious or inflammatory conditions. Primary tuberculosis usually causes unilateral hilar adenopathy. Fungal infections, most notably histoplasmosis and coccidioidomycosis, cause unilateral or bilateral adenopathy. Sarcoidosis causes bilateral and symmetric adenopathy in most patients (Fig. 5–8).

In patients with prior tuberculosis or histoplasmosis, calcified hilar nodes are commonly seen. Calcified nodes can erode into a bronchus, causing obstruction—so-called broncholithiasis. Because of its ability to diagnose bronchial lesions and detect calcification, CT can be very helpful in diagnosing this entity.

Mucus

Blobs of mucus may simulate one or more endobronchial lesions on CT (Fig. 5–28); if you suspect this diagnosis, for instance, if you see a focal bronchial

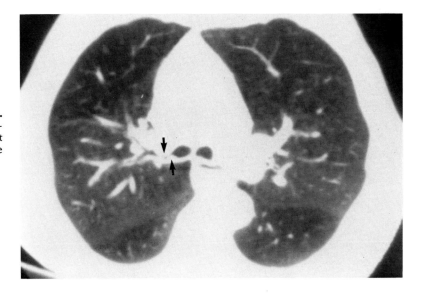

FIGURE 5–28. Bronchial mucus. Small collections of mucus (arrows) are visible within the right upper lobe bronchus. These cleared after coughing.

lesion when you don't expect one, obtain a repeat scan after having the patient cough. The abnormality will disappear. Large mucous plugs can also mimic hilar masses or be seen as a bronchial abnormality on CT.

Pulmonary Vascular Disease

CT is also useful in differentiating pulmonary vascular disease from hilar adenopathy. Pulmonary hypertension with dilatation of the pulmonary arteries is relatively common and can simulate a hilar mass on plain radiographs (Fig. 5–29). CT can accurately define the size of the pulmonary arteries in patients with arterial dilatation. Rarely, in patients with chronic pulmonary hypertension, pulmonary artery calcification can be seen as a result of atherosclerosis.

Encasement or compression of one of the main pulmonary arteries by tumor in patients with a bronchogenic carcinoma can be diagnosed with CT, and can be of value in assessing the extent of surgery required for resection. For example, tumor surrounding the left pulmonary artery generally indicates that

FIGURE 5–29. Pulmonary artery enlargement. Severe pulmonary hypertension has resulted in enlargement of the descending pulmonary arteries (A). The hila are smoothly enlarged, without lobulation, and the arteries maintain their normal oval shapes. There is some consolidation in the anterior right lung.

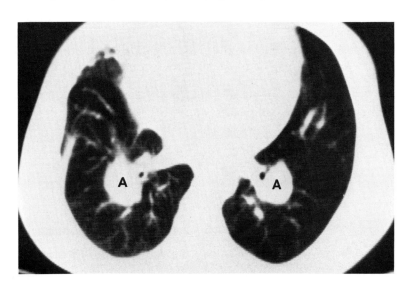

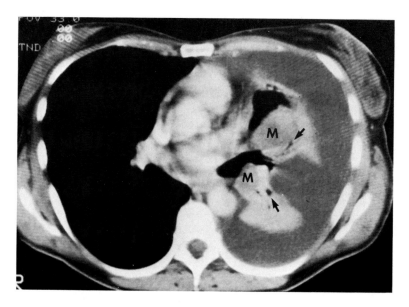

FIGURE 5–30. Hilar mass with atelectasis. In a patient with left hilar bronchogenic carcinoma, associated with collapse and pleural effusion, the hilar mass can be distinguished from collapsed lung following contrast infusion. The mass (M) appears less dense than opacified lung. Also, air-filled bronchi (arrows) delineate consolidated lung. There is also a large pleural effusion.

pneumonectomy rather than lobectomy will be required. However, one must be cautious; narrowing of the pulmonary artery can reflect compression rather than encasement. Adequate assessment requires the use of a bolus of intravenous contrast material.

Other than pulmonary artery dilatation because of pulmonary hypertension, or pulmonary artery involvement by tumor, pulmonary artery abnormalities are uncommon. Pulmonary artery aneurysms are rarely seen.

Mass Versus Atelectasis

In patients with a hilar mass and bronchial obstruction, collapse or consolidation of distal lung can obscure the margins of the mass, making it difficult to diagnose. On plain radiographs and conventional tomograms, the mass can sometimes be detected because of alterations in the shape of the collapsed or consolidated lobe or lobes (i.e., Golden's "S" sign). Similarly, alterations in the shape of a collapsed lobe can be seen on CT in the presence of a mass.

Also, in some patients, if a bolus of contrast is injected, and particularly if dynamic CT is performed, the collapsed lobe can be seen to enhance to a greater degree than the mass (Fig. 5–30). Of additional value in distinguishing mass and lung consolidation are air-filled bronchi, as seen on CT. These obviously indicate the presence of lung consolidation. In some patients, in the presence of total obstruction and complete lung collapse, low density, fluid-filled bronchi can be seen within the lung.

SUGGESTED READING

Naidich DP, Khouri NF, Scott WW Jr, et al.: Computed tomography of the pulmonary hila. 1. Normal anatomy. J Comput Assist Tomogr, 5:459–467, 1981.
Naidich DP, Khouri NF, Stitik FP, et al.: Computed tomography of the pulmonary hila. 2. Abnormal anatomy. J Comput Assist Tomogr, 5:468–475, 1981.
Webb WR, Glazer GM, Gamsu G: Computed tomography of the normal pulmonary hilum. J Comput Assist Tomogr, 5:476–484, 1981.
Webb WR, Glazer GM, Gamsu G: Computed tomography of the abnormal pulmonary hilum. J Comput Assist Tomogr, 5:485–490, 1981.
Webb WR, Gamsu G, Speckman JM: Computed tomography of the pulmonary hilum in patients with bronchogenic carcinoma. J Comput Assist Tomogr, 7:219–225, 1983.

6

Lung Disease

On CT, normal lung varies in appearance depending on the window settings used. With the lung window settings normally employed, the lungs appear very dark, but not as black as the air visible in the trachea or bronchi. This slight difference in attenuation between parenchyma and air should be sought in choosing the best window settings. If the lungs are viewed with too high a window mean value, they will appear too black, and information may be lost (soft tissue structures can be difficult to see, and areas of lucency within lung, such as bullae, may be missed). The lungs, after all, are not simply bags of air, and they should not appear to be. If too low a window mean value is used, the size of soft tissue structures in the lung (vessels or lung nodules) will be overestimated.

NORMAL ANATOMY

Intrapulmonary Fissures and Lobar Anatomy

Major Fissures

Because they are thin and oblique relative to the plane of the scan, the normal major fissures are not usually visible on CT obtained with 1-cm collimation. However, the position of each major fissure can be inferred from the position of the relatively avascular plane of lung 2 to 3 cm thick (representing the lung on each side of the fissure), which contains no large vessels (Fig. 6–1). In 10 to 20% of patients the major fissures are demonstrated on CT scans with 1-cm collimation as a thin line, although low window levels and narrow window widths may be required to see them. Sometimes, a ground-glass band of density is seen in the middle of the avascular area that surrounds the major fissure, reflecting volume averaging of the fissure itself. On thin-collimation scans, the major fissures are almost always recognizable as thin white lines.

Within the lower thorax, the major fissures angle anterolaterally, contacting the anterior third of the hemidiaphragms. They separate lower lobes posteriorly from upper lobe on the left, and middle and upper lobes on the right. In the upper thorax, the major fissures angle posterolaterally. Above the aortic arch, they contact the posterior chest wall and are usually no longer visible (only the upper lobe is seen at this level).

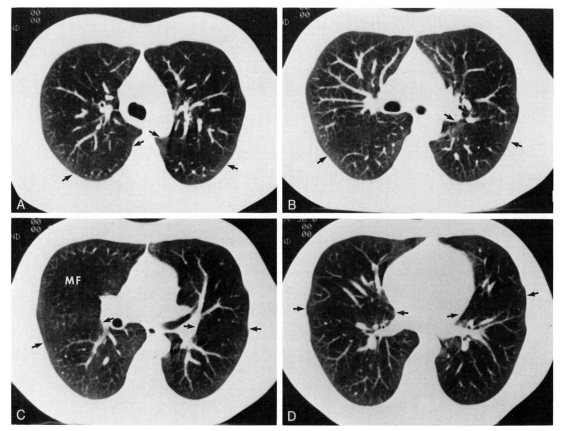

FIGURE 6–1. Normal fissures. *(A)* At the level of the aortic arch, an avascular band (arrows) within the posterior lungs marks the locations of the major fissures. They angle posterolaterally. *(B)* Several centimeters lower, the major fissures (arrows) are more anteriorly positioned. The upper lobes are anterior to the fissures. *(C)* The major fissures (arrows) remain visible. The location of the minor fissure (MF) is indicated by the rounded region, which contains no large vessels. *(D)* Near the diaphragm, the major fissures angle anterolaterally (arrows). The middle lobe is located anterior to the right major fissure.

Minor Fissure

The minor fissure is usually invisible, but its approximate location can be determined from the position of the avascular area, between the right upper lobe vessels above and the middle lobe vessels below, which lies roughly in the plane of scan (Fig. 6–1C). This avascular plane is visible in more than half of patients. On high-resolution CT (HRCT), the minor fissure can be seen as a white line of varying sharpness and thickness, depending on its orientation. Because the minor fissure often angles caudally or is concave caudally, it can be seen in two locations or can appear ring-shaped in the plane of the scan (Fig. 6–2), with the middle lobe between the fissure lines or in the center of the ring, and the upper lobe anterior to the most anterior part of the fissure.

Accessory Fissures

In patients with an azygos lobe, the four layers of the mesoazygos, or azygos fissure, are invariably visible above the level of the anomalously located azygos vein. The azygos fissure is C-shaped and convex laterally, beginning anteriorly at the right brachiocephalic vein and ending posteriorly at the right anterolateral surface of the vertebral body (see Fig. 3–10). Other accessory

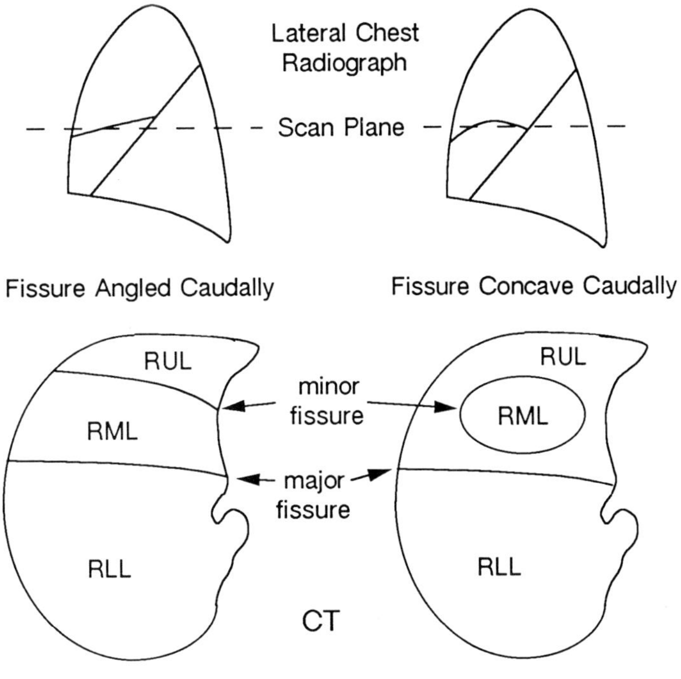

Lateral Chest
Radiograph

– Scan Plane –

Fissure Angled Caudally   Fissure Concave Caudally

FIGURE 6–2. Possible appearances of minor fissure. Depending on the orientation of the minor fissure, its appearance and the relationships of the lobes of the right lung can vary. If the minor fissure angles downward, both the middle and upper lobes can be seen on a single scan. If the minor fissure is concave caudally, it may appear ring-shaped. (RLL = right lower lobe; RML = right middle lobe; RUL = right upper lobe.)

RUL

RML

minor
fissure

RUL

RML

major
fissure

RLL

RLL

CT

fissures, most commonly the inferior accessory fissure, are occasionally seen on CT. They are not generally of significance in diagnosis.

MULTIPLE LUNG NODULES

Soon after it was introduced, CT was recognized as being much more sensitive than plain radiographs or conventional tomography in detecting lung nodules. Nodules as small as a few millimeters can be easily detected using CT, even with 1-cm collimation (Fig. 6–3). CT rapidly became routine for evaluating suspected pulmonary metastases.

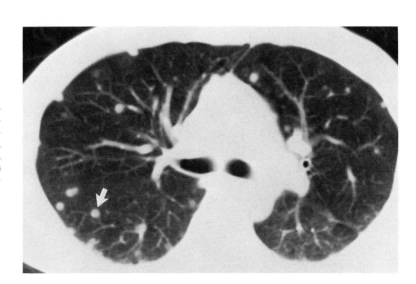

FIGURE 6–3. Multiple metastases. Multiple, small, well-defined nodules represent metastases from a renal cell carcinoma. Their peripheral location is typical. A few of these nodules (arrow) appear to be related to a pulmonary vessel.

Nodules can usually be distinguished from vessels seen in cross section by their size (if they are larger than the normal vessels in the same region). Also, nodules are usually visible on only one or two adjacent scans, while longitudinally oriented vessels can be followed on a number of adjacent scans, and can be traced to their point of origin, or can be seen to branch. Contrast injection is not usually of value in making this distinction, except for large central nodules in contiguity with the hilar vessels, because vascular opacification cannot be clearly seen at lung window settings.

Pulmonary nodules can occur in any part of the lung. However, pulmonary metastases resulting from tumor embolization have a predilection for the peripheral lung (Fig. 6–3). They are commonly visible in a subpleural location. However, normal subpleural lymphoid aggregates or granulomas, a few millimeters in diameter, can mimic this appearance. In a patient with suspected metastases, this may be problematic if no other, or larger, nodules are visible. Since these small peripheral densities are too small to biopsy percutaneously, follow-up CT (at 1 to 2 months) is often used. Metastases will increase in size.

The same rationale is used when small (2- to 3-mm) intraparenchymal nodules are seen. These small nodules can simply represent granulomas, and follow-up scans are often obtained to evaluate their significance.

In obtaining follow-up CT to assess a small lung nodule for change in size, it is important to obtain scans at exactly the same levels, and with the same window settings as in the original study. A small nodule can be missed if the patient breathes differently for two supposedly contiguous scans. (The nodule may fall at a level between the two "adjacent" scans, or can appear to be smaller if it is slightly out of the scan plane.) Identifying the pattern of branching vessels within the lung, in the region of the nodule, is an easy way of knowing exactly what level you are viewing. If the same vessels are visible on both the original and follow-up scans, and the nodule looks different, then the nodule *is* different. If a different branching pattern is visible, an apparent difference in nodule size may not be real. If follow-up scans are viewed at different window settings from the original study, a nodule may appear to be a different size. As stated above, low window mean settings make a nodule appear larger.

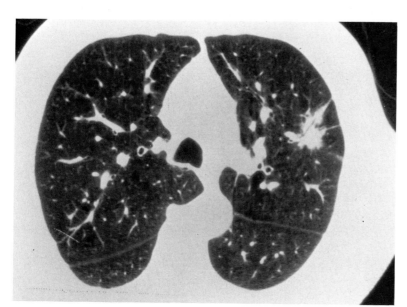

FIGURE 6–4. Spiculated carcinoma. High-resolution CT scan in a patient with an upper lobe nodule shows a spiculated mass that would be very suspicious for carcinoma. Note that the nodule contains an air bronchogram. An adenocarcinoma was found at surgery. Note the sharp definition of the major fissures with HRCT. (Reproduced with permission. From Webb WR: Radiographic evaluation of the solitary nodule. Am J Roentgenol, 154:701–708, 1990.)

Pulmonary metastases are typically round and well-defined (Fig. 6–3). Some metastases with surrounding hemorrhage can be ill-defined. Cavitation and calcification can be seen with some metastatic tumors. It has also been suggested that pulmonary metastases may be seen to have a connection with a pulmonary artery branch, reflecting their embolic nature (Fig. 6–3). However, this finding can be present with other causes of pulmonary nodules as well.

THE SOLITARY PULMONARY NODULE AND LUNG CANCER

It is not uncommon for a solitary nodule or focal lung mass to be visible on chest radiographs, and CT is often used in evaluating solitary nodules. CT is of value in confirming the presence of a parenchymal lesion suspected on plain films, determining the morphology of the nodule or mass, and detecting the presence of calcium (nodule densitometry).

Morphologic Characteristics of Some Solitary Nodules

In addition to conventional CT (contiguous 1-cm collimation), thin-slice, high-resolution CT scans can be quite valuable in delineating the morphology of pulmonary parenchymal lesions. I commonly obtain several contiguous high-resolution scans through the area of suspected abnormality in a patient with a lung nodule, mass, or focal pulmonary abnormality.

Lung Cancer

On CT, as on plain films, lung cancers can have a variety of appearances. Several findings, however, should suggest malignancy. One is poor definition of the edge of the lesion. Another common appearance on CT is spiculation of the margin of the nodule or mass (corona radiata or corona maligna), usually because of surrounding fibrosis (Fig. 6–4). This spiculated appearance is particularly common with adenocarcinomas. Lobulation also suggests the diagnosis of carcinoma, but may be seen with other lesions as well, particularly hamartomas.

Other "Nodules"

A few types of lung lesions which appear nodular on chest radiographs have morphologic characteristics visible on CT which are typical enough to allow a specific diagnosis to be made. These include vascular lesions (arteriovenous fistula and venous varix), focal consolidation or atelectasis, pleural masses, mucous plugs (Fig. 6–13), and rounded atelectasis (Fig. 6–21).

Arteriovenous Fistula

On CT, pulmonary arteriovenous (AV) fistulas take one of two forms: A single dilated vascular sac, visible as a smooth, sharply defined, round or oval

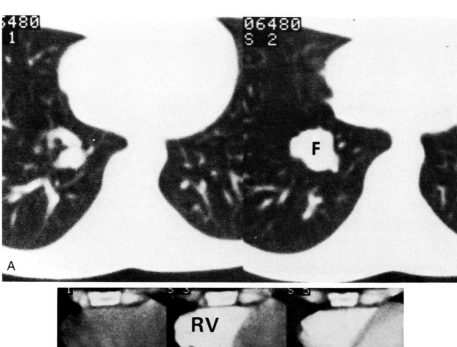

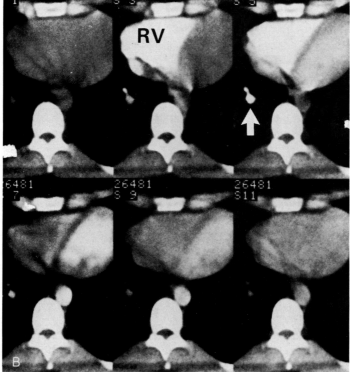

FIGURE 6–5. Arteriovenous fistula. *(A)* Two adjacent scans show a lobulated mass representing the fistula (F), and its large feeding vessels. *(B)* Following contrast injection, the fistula and its feeding vessels opacify rapidly (arrow), at the same time as the right ventricle (RV), and the contrast then washes out rapidly. (Reproduced with permission. From Godwin JD, Webb WR: Dynamic computed tomography in the evaluation of vascular lung lesions. Radiology, 138:629–635, 1981.)

nodule (most common); or a tangle of dilated tortuous vessels seen as a lobulated serpiginous mass. In each type, the feeding pulmonary artery branch and draining pulmonary vein are dilated and should be clearly seen on CT (Fig. 6–5). In most cases, the fistula will be subpleural in location. These findings should be sufficient to make a specific diagnosis.

Following the bolus injection of contrast, an AV fistula shows rapid opacification, followed by rapid washout of the contrast (Fig. 6–5). As would be expected, opacification occurs synchronous with, or just after, opacification of the right ventricle. Some solid tumors will also opacify after contrast injection, but this will not occur as rapidly as it will with an AV fistula, and the rapid washout of contrast will not be seen in patients with a solid tumor.

Venous Varix

In patients with elevated left atrial pressure, often as a result of mitral stenosis, central pulmonary vein branches can dilate, particularly on the right, simulating a lung nodule on plain radiographs. With CT this can be seen to correspond to the inferior pulmonary vein branch in most cases, and the dilated segment of vein opacifies after contrast infusion.

Focal Consolidation, Atelectasis, Scarring, and Granulomas

Focal consolidation can sometimes be diagnosed using CT in patients with a suspected nodule or mass. An area of focal consolidation typically appears ill-defined and may respect segmental or lobar boundaries or contain air bronchograms. Such focal consolidations can reflect pneumonia, atelectasis, or other inflammatory diseases. Infarcts can also result in focal consolidation, which may appear wedge-shaped and abut a pleural surface (producing the CT equivalent of a "Hampton hump"). It is important to remember, however, that some carcinomas, particularly adenocarcinomas and bronchioloalveolar cell carcinomas, can produce the appearance of consolidation on CT and can contain air bronchograms (Fig. 6–4).

Areas of scarring or atelectasis can sometimes mimic a solitary nodule on chest radiographs. Such areas are sometimes seen to be linear or geometric in shape (i.e., triangular) on CT, rather than nodular (round).

Inflammatory lesions, although seeming to represent a single nodule on plain film, may appear multifocal on CT, with several abnormal areas or "satellite" nodules being seen in the same region. This appearance suggests granulomatous disease (Fig. 6–6) and is less likely with carcinoma.

Pleural (Fissural) Lesions

Occasionally a pleural abnormality located in a fissure (for example, a plaque, loculated effusion, or benign mesothelioma) may be misinterpreted as a lung nodule (see Fig. 7–16). Looking for the fissures on CT, and obtaining thin-section scans, will usually allow you to avoid this mistake. Correlating the CT with the chest radiographs can also be of value.

CT Detection of Nodule Calcification

CT can be used to detect calcification in lung nodules, indicating that the nodule is benign. CT has largely replaced conventional tomography for the detection of nodule calcification, because of its greater sensitivity and because

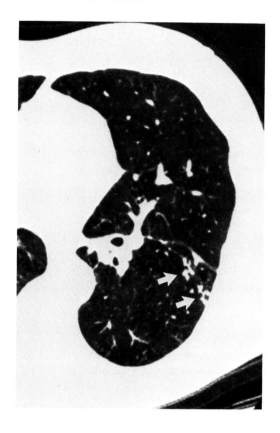

FIGURE 6–6. Small nodules representing atypical mycobacteria. High-resolution CT (HRCT) scan in a patient with an ill-defined 1-cm nodule visible on chest radiographs. On HRCT, the "nodule" is seen to consist of a number of smaller, well-defined nodular densities (arrows), which suggest a granulomatous process. (Reproduced with permission. From Webb WR: Radiographic evaluation of the solitary nodule. Am J Roentgenol, 154:701–708, 1990.)

it is more useful for detecting other abnormalities (i.e., mediastinal lymph node enlargement) in patients who have nodules.

Calcification of lung nodules can sometimes be seen using CT with conventional technique (1-cm collimation). However, thin section (1 to 2 mm) technique should be performed when using CT for this purpose. Calcium, easily diagnosable on thin section CT, is sometimes invisible when 1-cm collimation is used. Mediastinal window settings are best for detection of calcification.

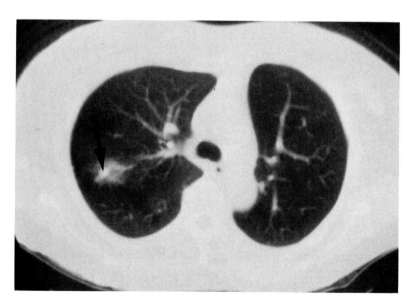

FIGURE 6–7. Eccentric calcification. CT scan in a patient with a right upper lobe nodule shows eccentric calcification (arrow). At surgery, this represented a carcinoma engulfing a granuloma. (Reproduced with permission. From Webb WR: Radiographic evaluation of the solitary nodule. Am J Roentgenol, 154:701–708, 1990.)

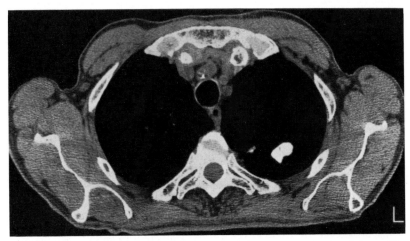

FIGURE 6–8. Diffuse calcification of a granuloma. On HRCT scan, an apical nodule is diffusely and densely calcified.

One should keep in mind that lung carcinomas can sometimes contain calcium, either as a result of calcification of the tumor or because the carcinoma has engulfed a preexisting granuloma (Fig. 6–7). Thus, when using CT to detect "benign" calcification, you must be sure that the calcification is "benign" in appearance; that is, it must be 1) diffuse (Fig. 6–8) or 2) central within the nodule and of significant size, criteria we are used to using when interpreting plain radiographs.

Also, unless it is diffusely calcified (Fig. 6–8), you should not call a calcified nodule greater than 2 cm in diameter benign; such large lesions have a significant chance of being malignant, even if some calcification is visible. Spiculated nodules also have a greater likelihood of being malignant than nodules which are smooth or lobulated. Generally, they should not be called benign, even if calcification is visible.

CT Nodule Densitometry

The technique of CT nodule densitometry was first reported in 1980. Although it remains somewhat controversial, it is gaining in acceptance and popularity. In understanding its use, it will be helpful to review some history.

Siegelman first suggested that nodule calcification invisible using plain radiographs or tomograms could be detected by measuring the CT number density of nodules on scans performed with thin collimation. In his initial report, 91 solitary nodules, which were apparently uncalcified, were studied using this technique. Averaging the highest CT numbers for each nodule, all 45 primary malignant lung tumors and 13 metastatic nodules were found to have a representative value of less than 164 H, while 20 of 33 benign nodules were identified as such by finding a representative CT number of over 164 H. Thus, approximately two-thirds of the benign nodules could be called benign by using nodule densitometry.

The controversy began when other investigators had difficulty replicating Siegelman's results, largely, it turned out, because of differences between the individual scanners and the reconstruction algorithms which were being used. In general, most benign nodules were found to have representative CT values much less than the 164 H cutoff which had been reported. However, other authors confirmed the potential utility of this technique, and Siegelman has subsequently confirmed his results in a larger series.

Further study of individual scanners, scanner geometry, and reconstruction algorithms emphasized the rather considerable variation in nodule density measurements obtained with different scanners, for nodules of different sizes or in different locations, and in patients of different size and with different chest wall thickness. These variations made the use of absolute CT number criteria, applicable to one machine, difficult or impossible to use with another. It was a difficult problem.

One approach to solving this problem was the development of an anthropomorphic phantom for use with chest CT (Fig. 6–9). This phantom can simulate the shape, dimensions, and density of thoracic structures in most patients. Cylinders of various diameters, made of plastic to correspond to the density of a calcified nodule (164 to 264 H) on Siegelman's scanner, serve as the reference density for simulating solitary pulmonary nodules.

When using this phantom, after a patient with a solitary nodule is scanned using thin collimation, the phantom is put together to simulate the same slice

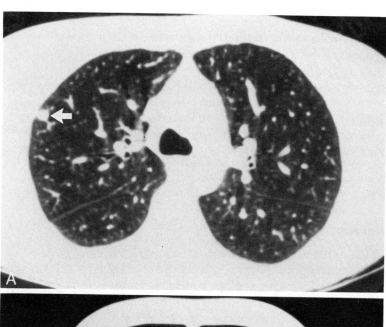

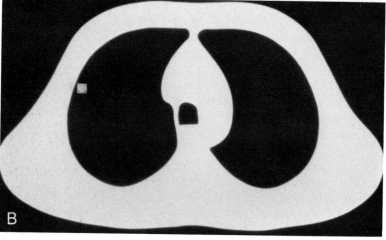

FIGURE 6–9. CT densitometry using a nodule phantom. *(A)* Thin-collimated CT scan in a patient with a small right lung nodule (arrow). *(B)* The CT phantom has been constructed to simulate the same slice level, nodule size, chest wall thickness, and nodule location, and the phantom has been scanned using identical technical factors.

CT NUMBERS

EXAM: 1799   STATION: 1

PRS: 1   PROSPECTIVE   IMAGE: 5

X\Y	126	127	128	129	130	131	132	133	134
283	-738	-640	-491	-401	-386	-347	-300	-370	-555
284	-648	-489	-294	-177	-126	-64	-24	-147	-430
285	-426	-269	-117	-35	18	82	94	-24	-319
286	-192	-81	5	38	87	141	118	2	-279
287	-118	-23	41	85	161	206	135	-25	-326
288	-187	-77	2	85	184	227	136	-88	-419
289	-354	-183	-55	52	146	186	72	-221	-554
290	-579	-396	-228	-103	3	42	-92	-405	-696
291	-737	-654	-538	-433	-337	-301	-375	-563	-751

C

FIGURE 6–9 *Continued (C)* CT numbers measured from the nodule include many pixels exceeding 100 H and some that exceed 200 H. *(D)* Numbers recorded from the phantom nodule are considerably lower. Thus, the nodule is calcified. (Reproduced with permission. From Webb WR: Radiographic evaluation of the solitary nodule. Am J Roentgenol, 154:701–708, 1990.)

CT NUMBERS

EXAM: 1799   STATION: 1

PRS: 1   PROSPECTIVE   IMAGE: 12

X\Y	117	118	119	120	121	122	123	124	125
202	-839	-618	-383	-241	-206	-283	-477	-742	-919
203	-627	-279	-61	12	30	-13	-146	-446	-782
204	-399	-64	32	36	38	27	-1	-196	-613
205	-265	13	35	33	31	19	23	-74	-482
206	-241	24	33	33	31	21	36	-52	-461
207	-339	-9	50	42	26	28	43	-113	-549
208	-533	-163	-2	34	37	26	-40	-316	-722
209	-765	-464	-226	-109	-86	-152	-323	-622	-890
210	-921	-799	-623	-499	-473	-562	-714	-880	-972

D

level, chest wall thickness, nodule location, and size. Then the phantom is scanned, using the identical CT technique as was used in scanning the patient, and the density of pixels in the patient's nodule and the phantom nodule are compared. If pixels in the lung nodule are denser than those in the phantom nodule, calcium is considered to be present (Fig. 6–9); if not, the nodule is considered to be uncalcified (or indeterminate) and potentially malignant. Thus, the phantom is assumed to provide a measurement of density independent of equipment-related or patient-related variations, and its use in CT nodule densitometry has been generally accepted.

It is recommended that in order to call a nodule benign, using this technique, dense pixels must be diffuse or central within the nodule, must account for 10% or more of its cross-sectional area, and must be visible on more than one scan—in other words, the calcification must be of significant size and characteristic of a benign lesion (diffuse or central). Also, as stated above, this technique should not be used in evaluating nodules which appear spiculated or are greater than 2 cm in size.

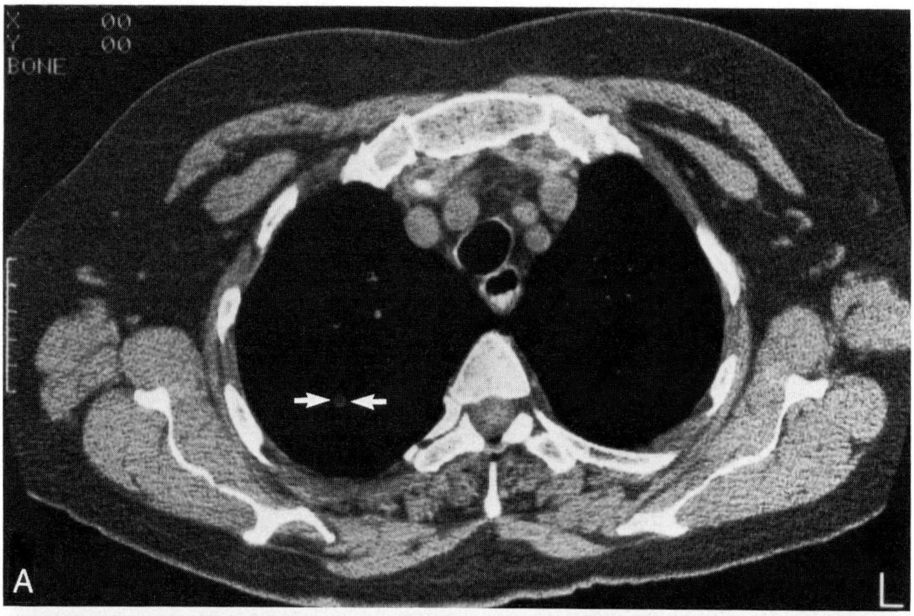

CT NUMBERS

EXAM 390 STATION 1

PRS 1 PROSPECTIVE IMAGE 7

Y \ X	187	188	189	190	191	192	193	194	195
291	-804	-633	-265	-52	-62	-128	-200	-394	-436
292	-644	-270	-137	-97	-117	-101	-43	-158	-290
293	-364	-110	-60	-90	-83	-131	-102	-94	-217
294	-380	-119	-118	-145	-116	-137	15	-36	-14
295	-294	-101	-59	-107	-63	-167	-173	-177	-179
296	-404	-70	-86	-111	-88	-87	-64	85	-49
297	-637	-319	-22	-50	-20	-53	-32	-159	-520
298	-760	-464	-151	-83	-72	-169	-123	-272	-722
299	-889	-844	-632	-336	-142	-235	-396	-728	-950

B

FIGURE 6–10. Hamartoma with fat density. *(A)* HRCT scan with mediastinal window settings in a patient with a small lung nodule detected on plain films. The nodule (arrows) is difficult to see and appears similar in density to subcutaneous fat. *(B)* CT numbers are mostly between −40 and −120 H. (Reproduced with permission. From Webb WR: Radiographic evaluation of the solitary nodule. Am J Roentgenol, 154:701–708, 1990.)

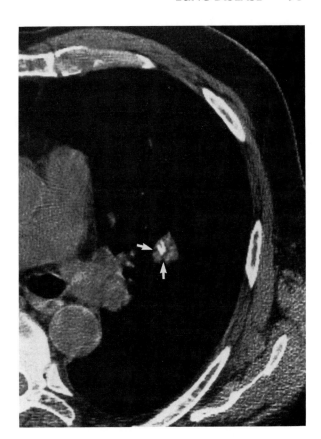

FIGURE 6–11. Hamartoma with fat and calcium.
HRCT scan shows dense calcification and areas of low
density (arrows) representing fat.

It should be noted, however, that the use of a phantom is not always
necessary in performing nodule densitometry. Some current scanners are better
densitometers, and less susceptible to variations in CT number measurement,
than the scanners which prompted the invention of this phantom. In our
institution we routinely perform nodule densitometry without using a nodule
phantom. We generally regard nodules with CT numbers of more than 200 to
be calcified. However, in deciding on what number threshold to use in calling a
nodule calcified, you can be as conservative as you wish. Nodules which show
visible calcification will generally have measured CT numbers of about 400 H
(Fig. 6–8).

Hamartomas

CT with thin collimation can also be valuable in diagnosing pulmonary
hamartomas. Using CT, about two-thirds of hamartomas can be correctly diagnosed because of visible fat (Fig. 6–10), either focal or diffuse (60%), fat and
focal calcification (30%) (Fig. 6–11), or diffuse calcification (10%). In order to
conclude that a nodule contains fat, however, CT numbers should range between
–40 H and –120 H.

Use of CT to Guide Biopsy of a Solitary
Nodule

If CT does not allow a specific diagnosis to be made in a patient with a
solitary nodule, and no calcification is visible, a biopsy may be considered

necessary for diagnosis. Depending on the clinical situation, and the beliefs of the patient's physician, several options are available. These include needle lung biopsy or bronchoscopy. To some degree, CT can be used to help make this choice.

Bronchoscopy is most accurate in diagnosing central masses which have an endobronchial component, while needle biopsy is best for peripheral lung lesions. If an endobronchial lesion is seen with CT, there is bronchial narrowing at the site of the nodule, or if a bronchus can be seen to pass through the mass lesion, bronchoscopy directed to the proper site is most appropriate. Also, in some patients, CT will show a bronchial lesion which is beyond the visibility of the bronchoscope, and thus it can guide the subsequent biopsy attempt (usually a brushing of the appropriate bronchus). If there is no evidence of an abnormal bronchus at CT, needle biopsy should probably be performed first.

Computed tomography can be helpful in planning a needle aspiration biopsy, even if CT is not used for the biopsy itself. First, CT can indicate the depth of the lesion, and the needle can be marked accordingly. This is of particular value if only single plane fluoroscopy is available for the biopsy procedure. Secondly, CT can help in planning the biopsy approach. If bullae lie in the path of the needle, or if the needle must cross a fissure to reach the lesion, the risk of pneumothorax is increased, and a different approach might be chosen.

CYSTIC AND CAVITARY LUNG DISEASE

This category includes a number of different kinds of diseases which have in common the presence of air-containing spaces, cysts, or cavities within the lung. Many can be distinguished by their CT or HRCT appearances.

Bronchiectasis and Bronchial Abnormalities

Conventional CT is of limited value in diagnosing bronchiectasis, because tubular or cylindrical bronchiectasis is easily missed using this technique. However, HRCT is more accurate than conventional CT and has replaced bronchography in many institutions. In patients with suspected bronchiectasis, HRCT scans are obtained at 1- or 2-cm intervals from the lung apices to bases, to show the extent of disease throughout both lungs.

In patients with bronchiectasis, the dilated and thick-walled bronchi are usually visible on several adjacent scans (Fig. 6–12). The smaller pulmonary artery branch, lying adjacent to the dilated, ring-shaped bronchus, gives their combined shadow the appearance of a signet ring. The "signet ring sign" (Fig. 6–12) is characteristic of this entity.

Mucous plugs (Fig. 6–13) associated with bronchiectasis, cystic fibrosis, allergic bronchopulmonary aspergillosis, bronchial obstruction, or congenital bronchial atresia can sometimes produce nodular densities which are difficult to diagnose on chest radiographs. On CT their relation to the bronchial tree, their often branching shape, and associated bronchiectasis can allow the correct diagnosis to be made.

In patients with bronchiolitis obliterans (Swyer-James syndrome), in addition to findings of bronchiectasis, areas of pulmonary hyperlucency can also be

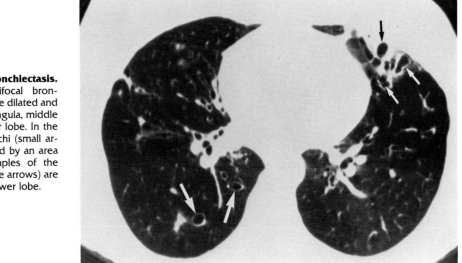

FIGURE 6–12. Bronchiectasis. HRCT shows multifocal bronchiectasis. Bronchi are dilated and thick walled in the lingula, middle lobe, and right lower lobe. In the lingula, dilated bronchi (small arrows) are surrounded by an area of atelectasis. Examples of the signet ring sign (large arrows) are visible in the right lower lobe.

seen on CT, probably as a result of decreased perfusion within areas of lung which are poorly ventilated.

Lung Abscess and Septic Embolism

A lung abscess can occur with a variety of bacterial, fungal, and parasitic infections. The hallmark of lung abscess is necrosis or cavitation within an area of pneumonia or dense consolidation, which can appear quite irregular (Fig. 6–14). Necrosis can sometimes be seen on CT if contrast is injected, even if the lesion does not contain air; the necrosis appears as a focal area of low density (it remains unopacified) within the consolidation. Cavitation is said to be present if air is visible within the lesion, and often CT is obtained to confirm this diagnosis when the plain radiograph is suggestive. CT can also be helpful in distinguishing

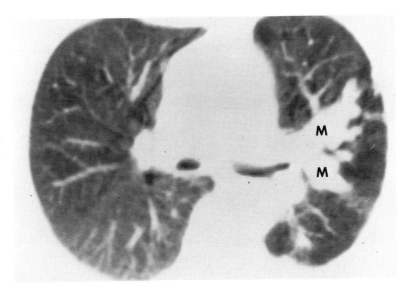

FIGURE 6–13. Mucous plug. The presence of a large mucous plug (M) can be diagnosed because of its typically tubular or branching appearance.

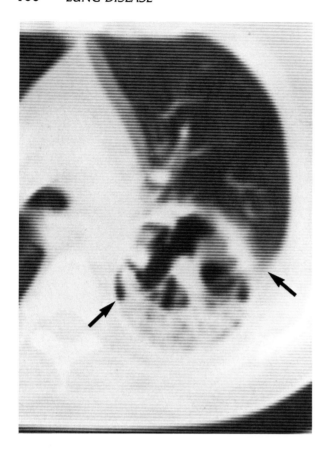

FIGURE 6–14. Bacterial lung abscess. A large, poorly defined cavity with an irregular wall is visible. Septations or residual lung are present within the cavity. There are acute angles (arrows) where the abscess meets the chest wall. This finding is of value in distinguishing abscess and empyema.

a lung abscess from an empyema. The CT appearances of lung abscess and empyema will be contrasted in Chapter 7.

In immunosuppressed patients, CT can be helpful in detecting infectious lung diseases at an early stage, when the patient is symptomatic, but before the chest film suggests the diagnosis. The detection of cavitary nodules in this setting can be quite helpful.

In patients with septic embolism, cavitation of lung nodules is common. Sometimes the nodules or cavities can be seen to be peripheral and associated with small pulmonary artery branches, suggesting their embolic nature.

In patients with a preexisting cyst or cavity, a mycetoma or fungus ball can form as a result of saprophytic infection, usually by Aspergillus. On CT, a round or oval mass (the fungus ball) can be seen within the cavity, in a dependent location, and is typically mobile. Thickening of the cavity wall is common.

Neoplasms

Both primary lung carcinomas and metastases can cavitate. Typically a cavitary carcinoma has a thick, irregular, and nodular wall (see Fig. 5–9), but some metastatic tumors, particularly those of squamous cell origin, can be relatively thin walled.

Pulmonary parenchymal involvement is seen in 10% of patients with Hodgkin's disease at the time of presentation, as either direct extension from hilar nodes, or discrete mass-like lesions which may contain air bronchograms or cavitate. These may be peripheral and subpleural in location. Note that lung involvement does not usually occur in the absence of radiographically demonstrable mediastinal (and usually ipsilateral hilar) adenopathy in previously untreated patients.

CONGENITAL LESIONS

Bronchogenic Cyst

The appearance of mediastinal bronchogenic cysts has been described. Pulmonary parenchymal cysts can appear to be solid, or if infected, can contain air. When fluid-filled, pulmonary bronchogenic cysts are typically well defined, round or oval, and can appear to be of fluid or soft-tissue density, depending on the nature of their contents. When a cyst contains air, outlining its wall, the wall typically appears very thin, although there may be consolidation of surrounding lung because of infection.

Sequestration

Pulmonary sequestrations can appear cystic or solid on CT. From 70 to 90% are located posteromedially on the left; all have anomalous systemic arterial supply from the thoracic or abdominal aorta. There is no pulmonary artery supply to the lesion.

An intralobar sequestration typically contains air, but is quite variable in appearance. On CT, it can appear cystic or multicystic (sometimes with air-fluid levels); it can appear to represent hyperlucent lung (with no recognizable wall); it can appear to represent consolidated and collapsed lung; or it may show a combination of these findings (Fig. 6–15). Extralobar sequestration, which is usually diagnosed in infants or children, produces a solid mass. A few cases of sequestration have been reported in which the feeding systemic artery was

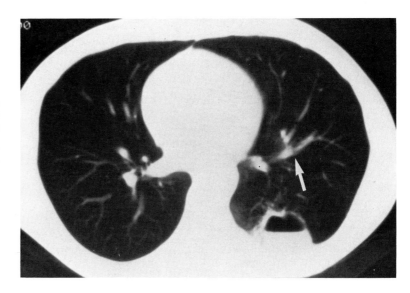

FIGURE 6–15. Sequestration. An intralobar sequestration presents with an air- and fluid-filled cyst in the left lower lobe. A bronchogenic cyst would have a similar appearance. Note that pulmonary vessels and bronchi (arrow) are displaced anteriorly by the sequestration.

visible on contrast-enhanced CT, but this requires a large vessel, a large bolus, and a fair amount of luck.

Hypogenetic Lung Syndrome

This rare anomaly, almost always occurring on the right side, is characterized by (1) hypoplasia of the lung with abnormal segmental or lobar anatomy, (2) hypoplasia of the pulmonary artery, (3) anomalous pulmonary venous return, usually to the inferior vena cava, and (4) anomalous systemic arterial supply to a portion of the hypoplastic lung, usually the lower lobe. Although these four features often coexist, the hypogenetic lung syndrome shows a considerable amount of variation in the degree to which each feature is expressed.

On CT, the hypoplastic lung is recognizable because of dextrocardia and mediastinal shift to the right side (Fig. 6–16). The hypoplastic lung may also show abnormal bronchial anatomy, deficient bronchial divisions, or mirror-image bronchial or pulmonary artery branching. When the anomalous (scimitar) vein is present, it is clearly visible on CT. Hypoplasia of the pulmonary artery is usually recognizable by the decreased size of vessels within the hypoplastic lung.

PARENCHYMAL LUNG DISEASE

Consolidative Lung Disease and Atelectasis

CT is not generally used to diagnose patients with pulmonary consolidation (air-space disease) visible on chest radiographs, because in most cases the diagnosis of such diseases is clinical. In some cases, however, CT may be done to look for associated findings such as pleural abnormalities, bronchial obstruction or associated mass, adenopathy, or cavitation.

In some patients with a mass suspected on the basis of plain radiographs, CT may show that the lesion represents a consolidative process, such as a

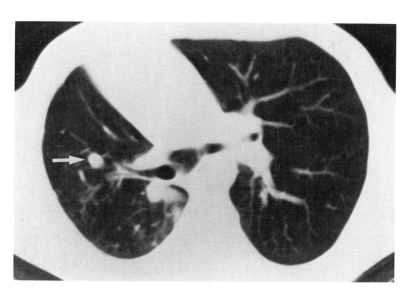

FIGURE 6–16. Hypogenetic lung syndrome. The right lung is reduced in volume, and the mediastinum is shifted toward the right. The scimitar vein (arrow) is visible within the right lung.

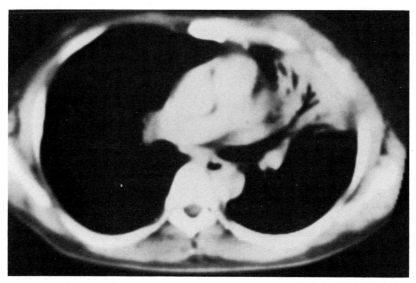

FIGURE 6–17. Actinomycosis pneumonia. There is dense consolidation of the lingula with air bronchograms. Thickening of soft tissues of the adjacent chest wall indicates chest wall involvement.

pneumonia. The CT findings of air space consolidation are similar to those usually seen on plain radiographs, with obscuration of pulmonary vessels and visible air-filled bronchi (air bronchograms) being the most characteristic findings (Fig. 6–17). Patchy consolidation (Fig. 6–18) or air-space nodules (or "acinar" nodules), measuring approximately 0.5 to 1 cm in diameter, can also be seen on CT in patients with air-space diseases, usually on the edges of confluent areas of consolidation; these are characteristic of endobronchial spread of tuberculosis, but can be seen with other infections, various causes of pulmonary edema or hemorrhage, or with alveolar cell carcinoma and lymphoma. Also, consolidation may have a lobar or segmental distribution.

Atelectasis: Types and Patterns

Atelectasis most commonly occurs because of bronchial obstruction (obstructive atelectasis) (Fig. 5–23), pleural effusion, or other pleural processes which allow the lung to collapse (passive atelectasis) (Figs. 5–30, 7–4), or lung fibrosis (cicatrization atelectasis). These can have different appearances. General signs of volume loss on CT are the same as those we use on chest radiographs.

FIGURE 6–18. Patchy consolidation from pneumonia. Small nodular densities on the edges of larger areas of consolidation represent so-called air-space nodules.

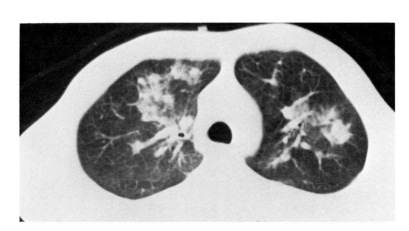

RIGHT UPPER
LOBE COLLAPSE

LEFT UPPER
LOBE COLLAPSE

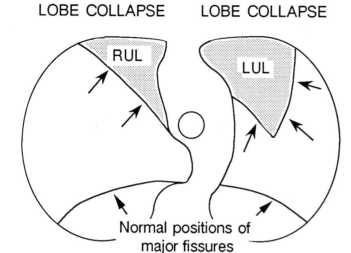

FIGURE 6–19. Typical patterns of upper lobe collapse.

Mediastinal shift (particularly anteriorly) and displacement of fissures are well seen on CT.

Obstructive Atelectasis

This often occurs because of a central endobronchial lesion, and thus, the bronchi should be examined closely. For the most part, the CT findings of obstructive atelectasis are what would be expected from our experience with plain films. Typically, the affected lobe is partially or completely consolidated. Air bronchograms may be visible, but typically they aren't. Low density fluid or mucus (low density relative to opacified lung) within obstructed bronchi can sometimes be seen as well. The air- or fluid-filled bronchi can be dilated in the presence of atelectasis, simulating bronchiectasis.

On CT, atelectasis can be diagnosed when displacement of fissures is seen. As on plain films, typical patterns of collapse can be identified (Figs. 6–19, 6–20).

Right Upper Lobe Collapse. The major fissure rotates anteriorly and

RIGHT MIDDLE
LOBE COLLAPSE

LEFT LOWER
LOBE COLLAPSE

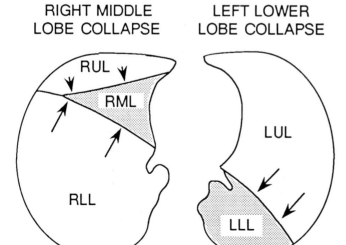

FIGURE 6–20. Typical patterns of middle and lower lobe collapse.

medially as the upper lobe progressively flattens against the mediastinum (Fig. 6–19). The fissure can be bowed anteriorly. In the presence of a hilar mass, an appearance similar to "Golden's S sign," as seen on plain radiographs, is visible.

Left Upper Lobe Collapse. As on the right, the major fissure rotates anteromedially. However, above the hilum, the superior segment of the lower lobe may displace part of the upper lobe away from the mediastinum, giving the posterior margin of the collapsed lobe a "V" shape (Fig. 6–19). A similar appearance is sometimes seen on the right.

Middle Lobe Collapse. As the middle lobe loses volume, the minor fissure, which normally is difficult to see because it lies in the plane of scan, rotates downward and medially and becomes visible on CT. The collapsed lobe assumes a triangular shape, with one side of the triangle abutting the mediastinum (Fig. 6–20). The upper lobe can be seen anterolaterally, bordering the collapsed lobe, with the lower lobe bordering it posterolaterally. These aerated lobes usually separate the collapsed middle lobe from the lateral chest wall.

Lower Lobe Collapse. On either side, the major fissure rotates posteromedially (Fig. 6–20). The collapsed lobe contacts the posterior mediastinum and maintains contact with the medial diaphragm below.

Passive Atelectasis

In the presence of pleural effusion, lung tends to retract or collapse toward the hilum, and fluid entering the fissures allows the lobes to separate (Figs. 5–30, 7–4). With the injection of contrast material, the lung opacifies and is clearly distinguishable from surrounding fluid. Air bronchograms may be seen within the collapsed lobes.

A very interesting form of passive atelectasis is so-called rounded atelectasis. This entity reflects focal, collapsed, and often folded lung. It almost always occurs in association with pleural disease, and is commonly seen in patients with asbestos related pleural thickening. However, at the time the diagnosis is made, the pleural disease may be largely resolved.

Rounded atelectasis occurs most commonly in the posterior lung, in the paravertebral regions, and may be bilateral. Bending or bowing of adjacent bronchi and arteries towards the area of atelectasis, because of volume loss or folding of lung, is characteristic (Fig. 6–21). This appearance has been likened to a "comet tail." Air bronchograms within the mass can sometimes be seen. In the presence of pleural disease, and these typical findings, the diagnosis can usually be suggested. If there is no evidence of pleural disease, either thickening, effusion, or plaques, you should be cautious in making the diagnosis of round atelectasis, and biopsy may be warranted.

Cicatrization Atelectasis

This occurs in the presence of pulmonary fibrosis and may be associated with tuberculosis, radiation, or chronic bronchiectasis. In this condition, there is no evidence of bronchial obstruction. Rather, air bronchograms and bronchial dilatation (bronchiectasis) are usually visible within the area of collapse. The volume loss is often severe.

Interstitial Lung Disease

Conventional and high-resolution CT can be used to evaluate diffuse interstitial lung diseases. We prefer HRCT because it provides much better resolution of lung anatomy and pathology.

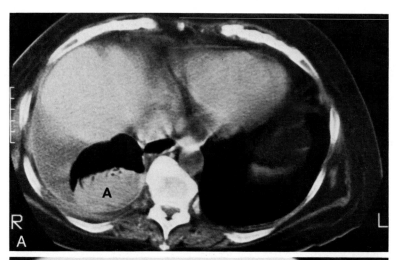

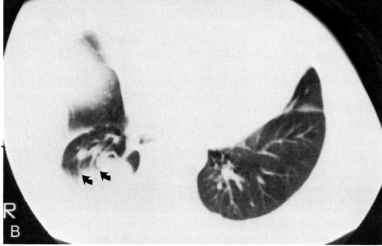

FIGURE 6–21. Rounded atelectasis. *(A)* Adjacent to an area of pleural thickening and effusion, the atelectatic lung (A) shows air bronchograms curving into its edge. *(B)* At a lung window setting, the curved vessels and bronchi (arrows) entering the atelectatic lung are visible, and there is posterior displacement of the major fissure, indicating volume loss.

Generally, HRCT is used in four ways in this setting: (1) to detect lung disease in patients with symptoms of respiratory distress or abnormal pulmonary function tests who have normal chest radiographs (approximately 10% of patients with interstitial disease have normal chest radiographs); (2) to characterize lung disease as to its pathologic nature (e.g., is there honeycombing?), and perhaps to make a specific diagnosis; (3) to localize areas of abnormality in patients who are going to have a lung biopsy; and (4) to follow patients who are being treated for a known disease.

As stated in the first chapter, most patients scanned with HRCT in our institution have scans performed at 4-cm intervals from the lung apices to bases (usually five or six levels), both supine and prone, at full inspiration.

In considering the use of HRCT for the diagnosis of diffuse lung disease, it is necessary to review the HRCT anatomy of the secondary pulmonary lobule. The lung is a lobular organ, and HRCT can show many features of the secondary pulmonary lobule in both normals and abnormals. Also, many lung diseases produce characteristic findings at the lobular level.

HRCT Findings in Normals

Secondary pulmonary lobules are polygonal, measuring approximately 2 to 3 cm in diameter. They are marginated by interlobular septa, which contain

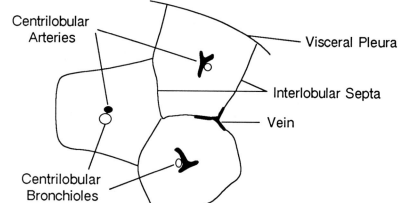

FIGURE 6–22. Normal pulmonary lobules.

veins and lymphatics (Fig. 6–22). In the center of the lobule are pulmonary artery and bronchiolar branches. On high-resolution CT, normal interlobular septa are sometimes visible as very thin, straight lines of uniform thickness which are 1 to 2 cm in length and contact the pleural surface, but usually, well-defined septa are not visible in normals (Fig. 6–4). Branching vessels seen in relation to the septa represent veins. A linear, branching, or dot-like density seen within the secondary lobule, or within a centimeter of the pleural surface, represents the intralobular artery branch. The centrilobular bronchiole is not normally visible. The visible artery in the center of the lobule is not seen to extend to the pleural surface in the absence of atelectasis.

HRCT Findings in Abnormals

On high-resolution CT, interstitial lung diseases produce some characteristic alterations in the appearances of lobular structures and some specific alterations in lobular anatomy.

Interstitial Thickening. Thickening of the interlobular septa can be seen in patients with a variety of interstitial lung diseases (Fig. 6–23). Within the central lung, the thickened septa can outline an entire lobule (1 to 3 cm in diameter), which appears hexagonal or polygonal in shape, and commonly contains a visible, central arterial branch. Within the peripheral lung, thickened septa (1 to 2 cm in length) can be seen extending to the pleural surface. Thickening of longer septa, several centimeters in length, which marginate more than one lobule, can also be seen. Often, thickened septa within the peripheral lung are associated with some overlying pleural (or subpleural) thickening, or fissural thickening. Interstitial thickening can make the edges of vessels and bronchi, or the pleural surfaces, appear irregular or serrated, throughout the lung.

Pulmonary Fibrosis, Honeycombing, and Architectural Distortion. Fibrosis associated with areas of lung destruction and the disorganization of lung architecture (honeycombing) results in a cystic appearance on HRCT which is characteristic (Fig. 6–24). Honeycombing produces cystic spaces several millimeters to several centimeters in diameter, which are often peripheral in location and are characterized by thick, clearly definable walls. Honeycombing is often associated with septal and pleural thickening, which are usually irregular. Also, intralobular bronchioles may be visible on HRCT in patients with honeycombing because of a combination of bronchiolectasis and thickening of the peribron-

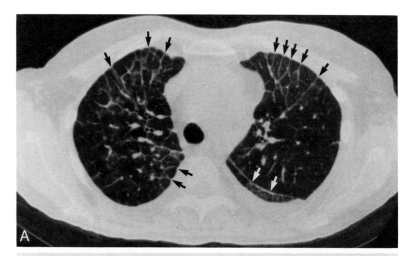

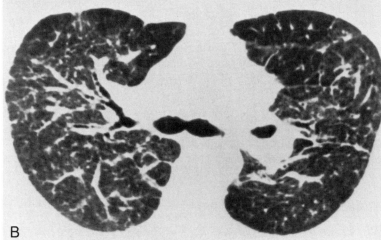

FIGURE 6–23. Thickening of the interlobular septa. *(A)* In a patient with lymphangitic spread of carcinoma, HRCT scan shows evidence of septal thickening (black arrows) characteristic of this disease. Apparent thickening of the left major fissure (white arrows) represents subpleural interstitial thickening. Notice that the pleural surface appears irregular where it is contacted by the thick septa. *(B)* In a patient with sarcoidosis and pulmonary fibrosis, irregular septal thickening is visible throughout the lung. The edges of the vessels and bronchi appear quite irregular.

FIGURE 6–24. Pulmonary fibrosis and honeycombing. In a patient with idiopathic pulmonary fibrosis and honeycombing, HRCT scan shows characteristic small, thick walled cysts (honeycomb cysts), most evident peripherally. Bronchi within the central lung are dilated as a result of traction bronchiectasis.

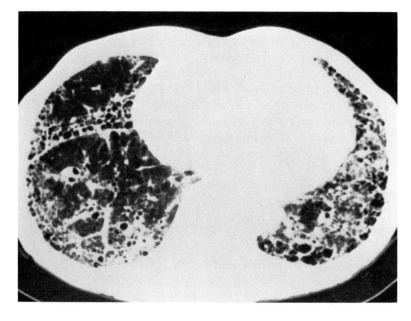

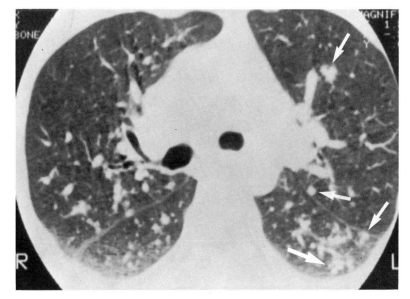

FIGURE 6–25. Interstitial nodules (sarcoidosis). HRCT scan in a patient with biopsy-proven sarcoidosis shows several large and small nodules (arrows), representing granulomas or groups of granulomas. Some are seen in relation to the pleura or vessels. Metastatic tumor would be included in the differential diagnosis of these nodules.

chiolar interstitium. In patients with septal thickening, the presence of honeycombing can help distinguish fibrosis from other causes of septal thickening (i.e., lymphangitic spread). Traction bronchiectasis is another finding in patients with fibrosis. Conglomerate masses of fibrous tissue can be seen in the upper lobes of patients with sarcoidosis or silicosis.

Nodules. Small or miliary nodules, a few millimeters to 1 cm in diameter, can be detected on HRCT in patients with granulomatous diseases such as sarcoidosis (Fig. 6–25), and in patients with metastatic tumor and silicosis. Interstitial nodules are usually well defined and can sometimes be seen in relation to the interlobular septa.

Bronchial Abnormalities. As indicated above, HRCT is useful in diagnosing large bronchial abnormalities, such as bronchiectasis. It can also be used to diagnose small bronchiolar abnormalities involving the peripheral lung, such as occur in early cystic fibrosis (Fig. 6–26). Since small bronchioles are centrilobular,

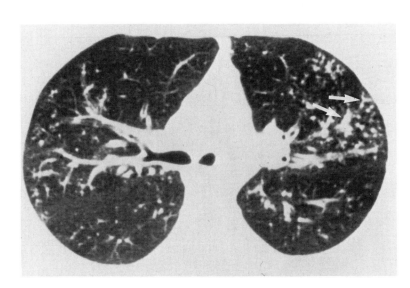

FIGURE 6–26. Cystic fibrosis. HRCT scan in a young girl with cystic fibrosis shows branching bronchi and bronchioles (arrows), which are filled with mucus or pus. Central bronchi are abnormally thick walled.

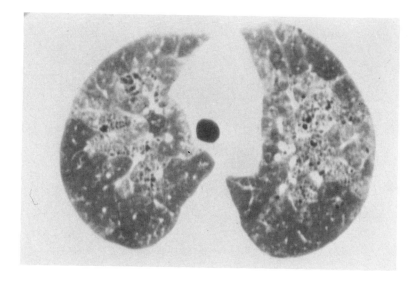

FIGURE 6–27. "Ground-glass" density. In a patient with central honeycombing, a hazy, geographic increase in lung density is visible. Active disease (desquamative interstitial pneumonitis) was present at biopsy.

bronchial or peribronchial inflammation typically results in centrilobular abnormalities. In patients with early cystic fibrosis, mucous plugs can be seen within very small peripheral bronchi or bronchioles.

Ground-Glass Density. In some patients with minimal interstitial disease, alveolitis, alveolar wall thickening, or minimal air-space consolidation, a hazy increase in lung density can be observed on HRCT, which typically has a patchy distribution (Fig. 6–27). It is differentiated from true consolidation in that it does not obscure pulmonary vessels. In some patients, this appearance correlates with "activity" of the interstitial process on biopsy (alveolar wall thickening, alveolar filling, or desquamation of alveolar lining cells). This appearance is nonspecific and can be seen with a variety of diseases (pneumonia, edema,

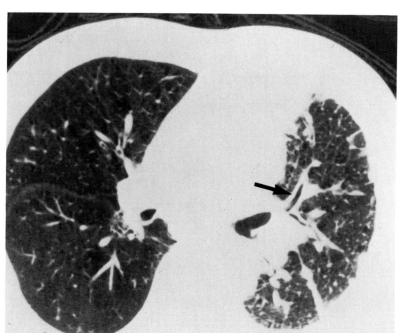

FIGURE 6–28. Lymphangitic spread of carcinoma. In addition to septal thickening and nodularity of the fissure, there is peribronchial cuffing centrally (arrow).

desquamative interstitial pneumonitis, bronchiolitis obliterans with organizing pneumonia, alveolar proteinosis, etc.) but, in most patients, the disease is treatable and the diagnosis should be pursued.

HRCT Appearances in Specific Diseases

Lymphangitic Spread of Carcinoma. Smooth septal thickening, seen on HRCT, is characteristic of pulmonary lymphangitic spread of carcinoma, and this is often the predominant finding (Fig. 6–23A). Some nodularity of the septa, presumably reflecting tumor nodules, may also be seen, but is not common. Thickening of the peribronchial and perivascular interstitium within the central (parahilar) lung results in peribronchial cuffing (Fig. 6–28). In a patient with the appropriate history, the HRCT appearance of lymphangitic spread is diagnostic. Often, the plain radiograph will be normal or equivocal in this setting. Pulmonary edema can produce similar findings.

Idiopathic Pulmonary Fibrosis. Patients with pulmonary fibrosis frequently show irregular septal thickening (Fig. 6–23B), as contrasted with the smooth septal thickening seen with edema or lymphangitic spread of carcinoma. Depending on the severity of the disease, honeycombing and traction bronchiectasis are commonly visible (Fig. 6–24). Honeycombing is most severe in the peripheral lung in many patients with this disease, a finding which can be helpful in differential diagnosis. However, this distribution can be seen with other processes as well. Ground-glass density (Fig. 6–27) can indicate the presence of active disease.

Sarcoidosis. The most frequent findings are interstitial nodules, 3 mm to 1 cm in diameter, seen on HRCT as either subpleural nodules, nodular thickening of the peribronchoarterial (parahilar) interstitium, or nodular or irregular thickening of interlobular septa (Figs. 6–23B, 6–25). Septal thickening, architectural distortion, honeycombing, and central conglomerate masses with crowded, ectatic bronchi are findings indicative of the fibrosis seen in longstanding disease. Patchy areas of increased ground-glass density have been shown to correlate with increased uptake on gallium scans and may be indicative of an active alveolitis.

Eosinophilic Granuloma of the Lung. On HRCT, thin-walled cystic lesions are seen in a majority of patients. Other findings include small nodules (< 5mm in diameter), larger cavitating nodules, areas of ground-glass density, and honeycombing.

Lymphangioleiomyomatosis. HRCT demonstrates thin-walled cysts diffusely throughout the lungs, with normal intervening lung tissue seen in less severely involved areas. Interlobular septal thickening is generally absent or of mild severity. When seen in a patient with a characteristic history (a female with dyspnea, spontaneous pneumothorax, and chylous pleural effusions), the findings are diagnostic.

Emphysema

On conventional CT, emphysema can be diagnosed if areas of low attenuation are visible; a paucity of vessels or draping of vessels around bullae may also be seen. However, emphysema is most accurately detected and diagnosed using HRCT. On HRCT, emphysema results in focal areas of very low density which can be easily contrasted with surrounding normal lung parenchyma if sufficiently low window means (< −600 H) are used. Emphysema is distin-

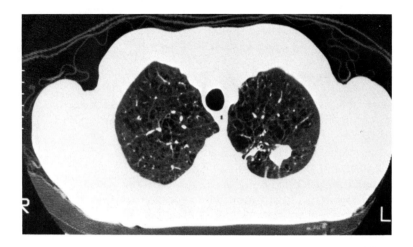

FIGURE 6–29. Emphysema. On HRCT scan, cystic low-density areas do not have visible walls, except where marginated by interlobular septa. This is the same patient with left apical nodule as shown in Figure 6–8.

guishable from honeycombing in that the cystic areas lack visible walls (Fig. 6–29).

Emphysema may be classified as centrilobular, panlobular, paraseptal, and bullous. To some extent these can be differentiated on HRCT.

Centrilobular emphysema is most common, is usually associated with smoking, and is typically worse in the apices (Fig. 6–29). Sometimes it appears "centrilobular" on HRCT. Panlobular emphysema may be more extensive than centrilobular disease, or may be related to other causes such as alpha$_1$-antitrypsin deficiency, being worse at the lung bases.

Paraseptal emphysema is also common (Fig. 6–30). It is usually focal emphysema, involving peripheral lung adjacent to the chest wall and mediastinum. Emphysematous spaces several centimeters in diameter are typical, and their walls are easily seen. This form of emphysema may or may not be associated with more diffuse disease.

Bullous emphysema can produce large areas of bullous destruction, particularly in young men. Bullae can contain fluid as well as air; often this reflects infection.

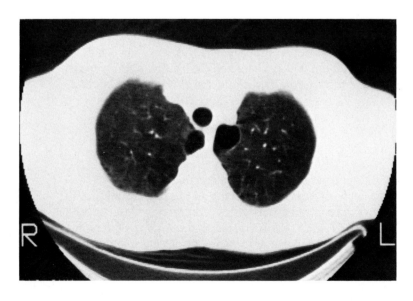

FIGURE 6–30. Paraseptal emphysema. The emphysematous areas are larger and have more easily seen walls. A paramediastinal location is typical.

SUGGESTED READING

Khouri NF, Meziane MA, Zerhouni EA, et al.: The solitary pulmonary nodule. Assessment, diagnosis, and management. Chest, 91:128, 1987.

Osborne D, Vock P, Godwin JD, Silverman PM: CT identification of bronchopulmonary segments: 50 normal subjects. Am J Roentgenol, 142:47–52, 1984.

Proto AV, Ball JB: Computed tomography of the major and minor fissures. Am J Roentgenol, 140:439–448, 1983.

Siegelman SS, Khouri NF, Leo FP, et al.: Solitary pulmonary nodules: CT assessment. Radiology, 160:307–312, 1986.

Webb WR: High-resolution CT of the lung parenchyma. Radiol Clin North Am, 27:1085–1097, 1989.

Webb WR: CT of the solitary pulmonary nodule. Am J Roentgenol, 154:701–708. 1990.

7

Pleura, Chest Wall, and Diaphragm

Computed tomography (CT) plays an important role in the diagnosis of pleural and chest wall abnormalities. The cross-sectional format and excellent density resolution of CT often provide anatomic information that cannot be obtained using conventional radiographic techniques.

TECHNICAL CONSIDERATIONS

In general, the pleura and chest wall are well evaluated using standard thoracic CT techniques. In most instances, however, because patients are positioned with their arms raised over the head for chest CT, the anatomy of the chest wall musculature and axilla which is depicted is somewhat different from that portrayed in most anatomy textbooks. Occasionally, in patients with suspected chest wall disease, it may be helpful to scan the patient with arms down (at his or her sides), in order to avoid this distortion.

One must keep in mind that the diaphragm and posterior pleural space extend well below the lung bases, and scans inferior to the diaphragmatic domes must be obtained to evaluate these structures completely. Scanning with the patient in the prone position may be of assistance in evaluating pleural diseases; free pleural effusions shift to the dependent portion of the pleural space when the patient is moved from the supine position to the prone or decubitus position, whereas loculated effusions or fibrosis shows little or no change. Also, the movement of an effusion helps reveal underlying pulmonary parenchymal or pleural lesions that are otherwise obscured.

Mediastinal window settings are most suitable for evaluating the soft tissues of the chest wall, pleura, and diaphragm. However, lung window settings or extended window settings allow more accurate estimation of the size, contour, and appearance of pleural lesions at their interface with adjacent lung. Appropriate window settings must be used to evaluate bony lesions of the chest wall. High-resolution CT (HRCT) techniques can demonstrate the anatomy of the lung-pleura-chest wall interface better than can conventional CT. CT following contrast infusion is helpful in showing pleural thickening, and in allowing its differentiation from pleural fluid.

Occasionally, multiplanar reconstruction of images can clarify the relationship of chest wall or pleural processes to the lung or mediastinal structures.

PLEURA

Anatomy

Because of the oblique orientation of the lateral ribs, usually only a short segment of each rib is visible on a single CT scan; each progressively more anterior rib represents the one arising at a higher thoracic level (Fig. 7–1). For example, at any given level, the fourth rib lies anterior to the fifth, and the fifth lies anterior to the sixth. At the level of the lung apex, the first rib can be identified by its anterior position and by its articulation with the manubrium immediately below the level of the clavicle.

In some patients, a bony spur projects inferiorly from the undersurface of the first rib at its junction with the manubrium. In cross section, this bony spur can appear to be surrounded by lung and can mimic a lung nodule. This appearance is usually bilateral and symmetric, providing a clue as to its true nature.

Costal Pleura

On conventional CT or HRCT, a 1- to 2-mm thick stripe of density is commonly seen in the intercostal spaces, between the visible rib segments (Fig. 7–1). This stripe represents the combined thicknesses of the two pleural layers, endothoracic fascia, and innermost intercostal muscle (primarily intercostal muscle). The visceral and parietal pleura themselves are not normally visible on CT, but in the presence of pleural thickening or effusion, a stripe of density is visible passing internal to the ribs, and sometimes separated from the rib or innermost

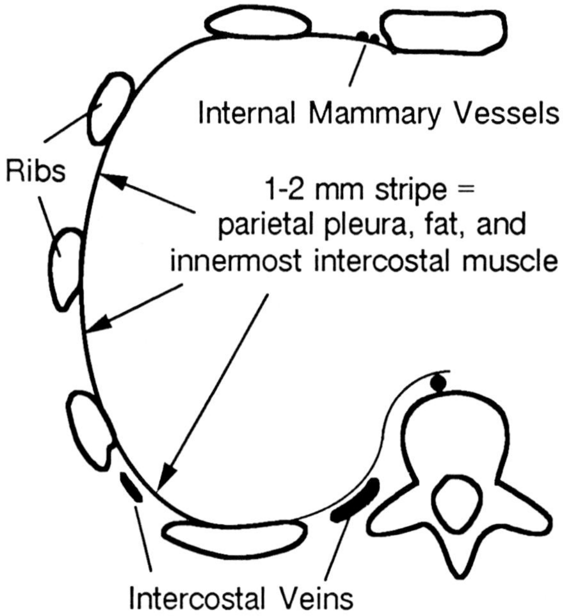

Internal Mammary Vessels

Ribs

1-2 mm stripe =
parietal pleura, fat, and
innermost intercostal muscle

Intercostal Veins

FIGURE 7–1. Normal pleura. A 1- to 2-mm line of density at the pleural surface primarily represents the innermost intercostal muscle, combined with the density of the two pleural layers and the endothoracic fascia. In the paravertebral region, this stripe is much thinner or invisible.

intercostal muscle by a layer of extrapleural fat. In the paravertebral regions, the innermost intercostal muscle is absent, and a much thinner line (or no line at all) is visible at the pleural surface, adjacent to paravertebral fat.

Intrapulmonary Fissures

These have been described previously (see Fig. 6–1). Normal collections of fat extending into the inferior aspects of the major fissures at the diaphragmatic surface can simulate fissural pleural thickening or effusion. These will be low in density at mediastinal window settings.

Inferior Pulmonary Ligament

On each side, below the level of the pulmonary hilum, the parietal and visceral pleural layers join, forming a fold that extends inferiorly along the mediastinal surface of the lung and ends at the level of the diaphragm. This fold, the inferior pulmonary ligament, anchors the lower lobe. On CT images viewed at lung window settings, it appears as a small triangular density 1 cm or less in size with its apex pointing laterally into the lung and its base against the mediastinum. On each side, it usually lies adjacent to the esophagus (Fig. 7–2). Pleural effusion or pneumothoraces can be limited and marginated by the inferior pulmonary ligament.

A very similar density can be seen on the right, lateral to the inferior vena cava (and thus anterior to the inferior pulmonary ligament), extending inferiorly to the diaphragm, and then laterally for several centimeters along the diaphragmatic surface (Fig. 7–2). This represents the right phrenic nerve and its pleural reflection. A similar density can be seen on the left as well. Its only significance is that it is commonly seen and is just as commonly confusing.

Pleural Abnormalities

Pleural thickening or fluid is visible on CT as a water or soft tissue density, often crescentic or lenticular in shape, internal to a rib (Fig. 7–3).

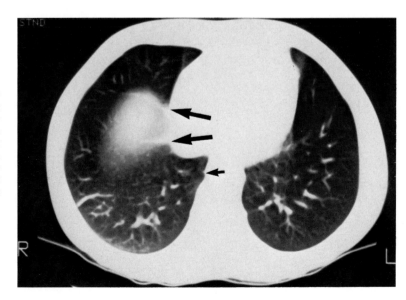

FIGURE 7–2. Inferior pulmonary ligament and right phrenic nerve. A small triangular density (small arrow) adjacent to the esophagus represents the right inferior pulmonary ligament. Longer linear densities near the surface of the right diaphragm (large arrows) represent the phrenic nerves.

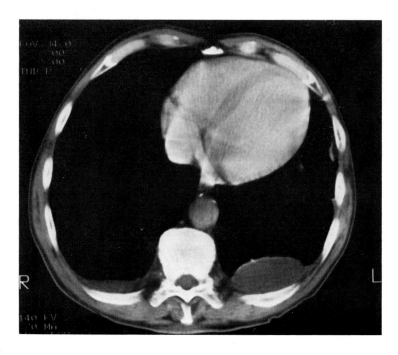

FIGURE 7–3. Pleural fluid. A crescent-shaped fluid collection on the right is internal to the visible rib segment. On the left, the fluid collection is lenticular in shape, but tapers laterally. These appearances are typical of pleural abnormalities.

Thickened pleura can often be distinguished from pleural fluid after contrast infusion; the thickened pleura will often enhance. The presence of pleural thickening, with or without effusion, suggests pleural inflammation or infection, or neoplastic involvement of the pleura. The presence of effusion without visible pleural thickening suggests the presence of a transudative effusion (Fig. 7–4), such as might occur with congestive heart failure. However, in some cases, this appearance can be seen early in the course of infection or in patients with metastatic tumor.

Normal extrapleural fat pads, a few millimeters thick, can sometimes be seen internal to a rib, particularly in the lower posterolateral thorax, and may not always be distinguishable from pleural thickening or fluid. However, the normal fat pads will often be symmetric, while pleural abnormalities generally aren't. In some patients, pleural thickening or effusion can be seen to be separated from

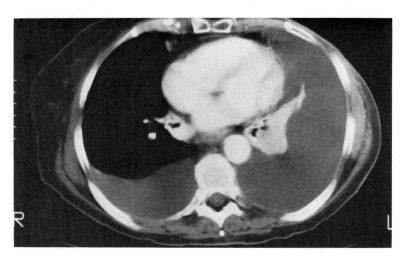

FIGURE 7–4. Pleural effusions. Large bilateral effusions appear lower in density than the contrast enhanced left lower lobe and heart. There is no evidence of pleural thickening; the thin line seen at the pleural surface represents the 1- to 2-mm stripe normally seen, which does not pass internal to the ribs. This appearance is typical of a transudative effusion.

intercostal muscle by these normal fat pads. The visibility of these fat pads is considerably improved on HRCT.

Pleural Fluid Collections

Small pleural effusions can be difficult to distinguish from pleural thickening. The diagnosis of free pleural fluid requires a change in patient position from supine to decubitus or prone. Large effusions often extend into the major fissures, displacing the lower lobes medially and posteriorly.

The visceral pleura covers the surface of the lung, and its inferior extent is defined by the inferior extent of lung in the costophrenic angles. The parietal pleura is contiguous with the chest wall and diaphragm and extends well below the level of the lung bases, in the costophrenic angles. Thus, pleural fluid collections in the costophrenic angles can be seen below the lung base and can mimic collections of fluid in the peritoneal cavity.

The parallel curvilinear configuration of the pleural and peritoneal cavities at the level of the perihepatic and perisplenic recesses allows fluid in either cavity to appear as an arcuate or semilunar density displacing liver or spleen away from the adjacent chest wall. The relationship of the fluid collection to the ipsilateral diaphragmatic crus (see below) helps to determine its location. Pleural fluid collections in the posterior costophrenic angle lie posterior to the diaphragm and cause lateral displacement of the crus. Peritoneal fluid collections are anterior to the diaphragm.

Pleural fluid can also be distinguished from ascites by the clarity of the interface of the fluid with the liver and spleen (Fig. 7–5). With pleural fluid the interface is hazy whereas with ascites it is sharp. In patients with both pleural and peritoneal fluid, the diaphragm often can be seen as a uniform, curvilinear structure of muscle density with relatively low-density fluid both anteriorly and posteriorly, or medially and laterally (Fig. 7–5). Fluid seen posterior to the liver is within the pleural space (Fig. 7–11); the peritoneal space does not extend into this region (this is the "bare area" of the liver).

A large pleural effusion will allow the lower lobe to float anteriorly and lose volume. The posterior edge of the lower lobe, when surrounded by fluid

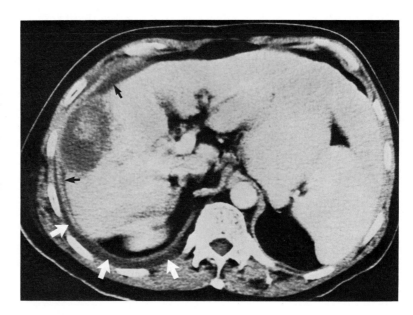

FIGURE 7–5. Pleural effusion and ascites. In a patient with a liver abscess, there are both pleural effusion and ascites. Effusion (white arrows) is posterior to the diaphragm. Ascites (small black arrows) is medial to the diaphragm and shows a sharp interface with the liver. Note that the diaphragm is visible as a white stripe with fluid on each side. No ascites is visible posterior to the liver.

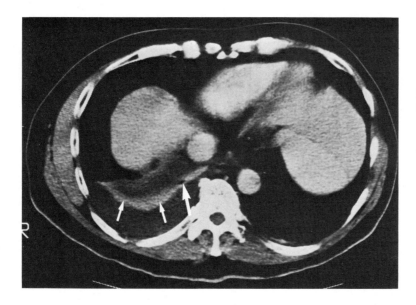

FIGURE 7–6. Subpulmonic effusion with a "pseudodiaphragm." In a patient with a large right pleural effusion, the collapsed posterior lower lobe (arrows) simulates the diaphragm. However, an air bronchogram (large arrow) within this density, and contiguity with the lower lobe at more cephalad levels, indicate its true nature.

both anteriorly and posteriorly, can appear to represent the diaphragm (a "pseudodiaphragm"), with pleural fluid posteriorly and ascites anteriorly (Fig. 7–6). Sequential scans at more cephalad levels, however, generally will allow the correct interpretation to be made. Typically the arcuate density of the atelectatic lower lobe becomes thicker superiorly, is contiguous with the remainder of the lower lobe, and often contains air bronchograms.

Many effusions appear to be near to water in density. CT numbers cannot be used reliably to predict the specific gravity of the fluid or its cause. Acute or subacute hemothorax can sometimes be inhomogeneous in density with some areas—particularly dependent regions—having a CT attenuation value greater than that of water.

Fissural Fluid

A focal or loculated collection of pleural fluid in a major or minor fissure can have a confusing appearance on CT images and can be misinterpreted as

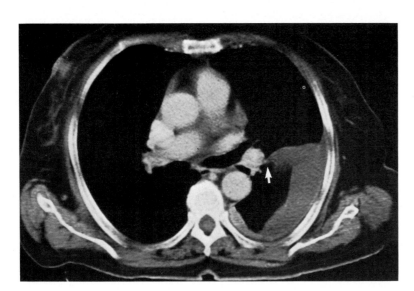

FIGURE 7–7. Fluid in a fissure. In this patient, fluid extends into the left major fissure. The fluid tapers medially (arrow), forming a "beak."

representing a parenchymal mass. However, careful analysis of contiguous images usually will confirm the relationship of the mass to the plane of the fissure. If the abnormality also is of fluid density, the diagnosis becomes more likely. The edges of the fluid collection may be seen to taper, conforming to the fissure, forming a "beak" (Fig. 7–7). Correlation of CT scans with the plain radiographs can help, particularly for fluid localized in the minor fissure.

Parapneumonic Effusions

Pleural fluid can accumulate in patients with pneumonia, even when the pleural space is uninfected. This is termed a parapneumonic effusion, and probably results from increased permeability of the visceral pleura. Distinguishing pleural effusion from adjacent consolidated lung may be difficult unless contrast material is injected, resulting in opacification of the lung. The pleural fluid remains low in density while the consolidated lung increases in density.

Empyema and Its Differentiation from Lung Abscess

With conventional radiographic techniques, empyemas may be difficult or impossible to differentiate from peripheral lung abscesses abutting the chest wall. This distinction can be an important one to make because empyemas are usually treated by tube thoracostomy and systemic antibiotics, whereas most lung abscesses only require antibiotics and postural drainage.

Typically, on CT, an empyema has a regular shape and is round, elliptical, or lenticular in cross section (Figs. 7–8, 7–9). The outer edge of the lesion is sharply demarcated from adjacent lung. When a bronchopleural fistula is present and air is contained within the empyema cavity, or when air is introduced into the empyema at thoracentesis, its inner margin usually appears smooth and its wall is of uniform thickness. Lung abscesses, on the other hand, are irregularly shaped and often contain multiple loculated collections of air and fluid (see Figs. 6–14, 7–8, 7–10). Their inner surfaces often are irregular and ragged, and their outer edges may be poorly defined because of adjacent pulmonary parenchymal consolidation.

At their point of contact with the chest wall, empyemas can show acute or obtuse angles (Figs. 7–8, 7–9), while abscesses typically have acute angles (see Fig. 6–14). Empyemas also will compress and displace lung and vessels, acting like a space-occupying mass, while lung abscesses destroy lung without

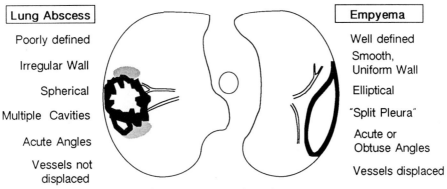

FIGURE 7–8. Empyema versus lung abscess.

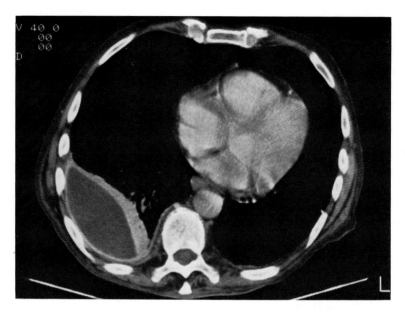

FIGURE 7–9. Empyema. An empyema is lenticular in shape and well defined. After contrast injection, the thickened visceral and parietal pleura and the "split pleura" sign are visible.

displacing it (usually). In some cases, empyema cavities, unlike lung abscess cavities, can change shape when the patient moves from the supine to the prone or decubitus position.

When an abscess or empyema does not contain air and appears to be of homogeneous density on plain radiographs, contrast-enhanced CT scans can demonstrate the wall of the lesion and provide a clue as to its fluid-filled nature. The walls of both empyemas and abscesses may be enhanced with contrast infusion, while their fluid contents are not. The walls of an empyema represent the visceral and parietal pleural surfaces, split apart by the fluid collection; with contrast infusion, this "split pleura" appearance is commonly visible, and the thickened, split pleural layers usually appear smooth and of uniform thickness (Figs. 7–8, 7–9).

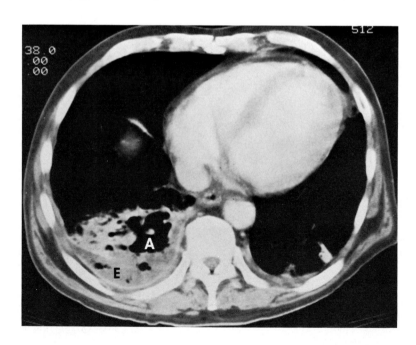

FIGURE 7–10. Lung abscess with empyema and bronchopleural fistula. The cavitary, air-filled lung abscess (A) is irregular in shape and is associated with consolidation of the adjacent lung. An empyema (E) marginated by thickened pleura is also seen. Air within the pleural collection indicates a bronchopleural fistula.

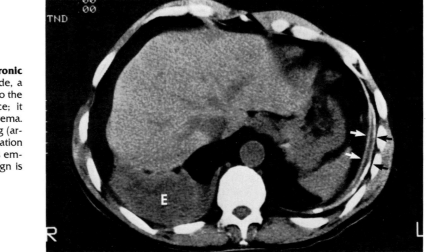

FIGURE 7–11. Acute and chronic empyemas. On the right side, a fluid collection (E) posterior to the liver is in the pleural space; it represents an acute empyema. On the left, pleural thickening (arrows) with areas of calcification reflects a healed tuberculous empyema. The "split pleura" sign is present.

Organizing Empyema

In patients with chronic empyema, especially when it is tuberculous in origin, ingrowth of fibroblasts can result in pleural fibrosis and the development of chronic pleural thickening (Fig. 7–11). CT may show a thickened pleural peel, which can cause lung restriction and decreased lung volume. Frequently, a thickened layer of extrapleural fat is also visible separating the parietal pleura and the ribs (this layer is considerably thicker than the fat pads, which can be seen normally). Calcification, which typically is focal in its early stages (Fig. 7–11), may become extensive (Fig. 7–12).

Dense pleural thickening, even with calcification, does not indicate that the pleural disease is inactive. Loculated fluid collections resulting from active infection (Figs. 7–12) may be seen on CT within the thickened pleura.

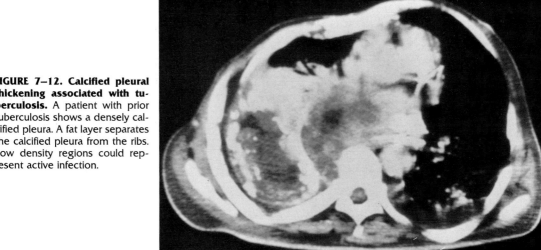

FIGURE 7–12. Calcified pleural thickening associated with tuberculosis. A patient with prior tuberculosis shows a densely calcified pleura. A fat layer separates the calcified pleura from the ribs. Low density regions could represent active infection.

Thoracostomy Tubes

Infected pleural fluid collections often become loculated, and can be difficult to drain. CT is sometimes indicated to evaluate thoracostomy tube position when the tube is functioning poorly. Malpositioned chest tubes can lie within a fissure, within a loculated fluid collection (while other collections remain undrained), or outside the empyema.

Asbestos-Related Pleural Disease

Asbestos-related pleural thickening has a typical appearance on CT. Early pleural thickening is discontinuous; pleura plaques (focal areas of thick pleura) are visible adjacent to the inner surfaces of ribs or vertebral bodies, and the intervening pleura is normal (Fig. 7–13). The pleural disease is typically bilateral. Calcification is common. Diffuse pleural thickening, which is probably the result of prior asbestos-related benign pleural effusion, can also be seen (Fig. 7–14). In patients with asbestos-related pleural disease, the pleural thickening, plaques, or calcification typically involves the parietal pleura, but this is difficult to recognize on CT unless the presence of pleural fluid separates the visceral and parietal pleural layers.

The diaphragmatic pleura is commonly involved in patients with asbestos-related pleural disease. However, the diaphragm lies roughly in the plane of the scan, and the detection of uncalcified pleural plaques on the diaphragmatic surface can be difficult. In some patients, diaphragmatic pleural plaques are visible deep in the posterior costophrenic angle, below the lung base; in this location, the pleural disease can be localized to the parietal pleura, because only parietal pleura is present. Pleural plaques along the mediastinum have been considered unusual in patients with asbestos-related pleural disease but are

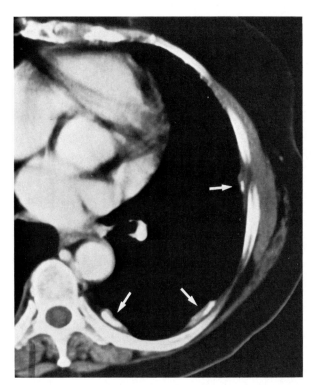

FIGURE 7–13. Asbestos-related pleural plaques. Typical calcified pleural plaques (arrows) are visible. They are often internal to ribs.

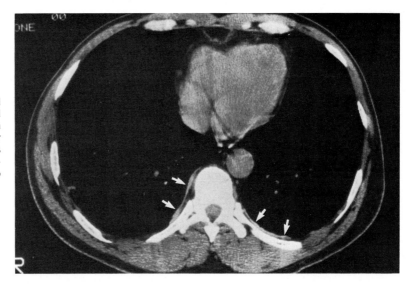

FIGURE 7–14. Asbestos-related pleural thickening. Linear pleural thickening (arrows) can be seen with asbestos exposure or other causes of pleural disease such as rheumatoid arthritis. The thickened pleura is visible internal to the ribs.

visible on CT scans in about 40% of patients. Paravertebral pleural thickening is also common. Although it is unusual, pleural thickening can involve a fissure and can result in a localized intrapulmonary pleural plaque. This may simulate a lung nodule on CT unless the plane of the fissure is identified.

Malignant Mesothelioma

Diffuse mesothelioma is a highly malignant, progressive neoplasm with an extremely poor prognosis. It is characterized morphologically by gross and nodular pleural thickening. However, hemorrhagic pleural effusion is often present and may obscure the underlying pleural thickening, which in early cases can be minimal. Malignant mesothelioma spreads most commonly by local infiltration of the pleura. In most patients, malignant mesothelioma is related to asbestos exposure, and although it is rare in the general population, the incidence in asbestos workers is 5 to 7%.

In patients with malignant mesothelioma, CT can expedite the initial diagnosis and define the extent of tumor. Usually, irregular or nodular pleural thickening is visible, which may surround the lung (Fig. 7–15). Often, it is most pronounced within the inferior thorax. Pleural fluid collections which are commonly associated can be difficult to distinguish from mesothelioma. However, CT scans with the patient in the prone or decubitus position can help to distinguish the underlying mesothelioma or pleural thickening from free fluid. Also, enhancement of the tumor after infusion of contrast medium also can help differentiate it from adjacent fluid collections.

Although pleural mesothelioma is visible most frequently along the lateral chest wall, mediastinal pleural thickening or concentric pleural thickening is seen with extensive disease (Fig. 7–15). The abnormal hemithorax can appear contracted and fixed, with little change in size during inspiration. Thickening of the fissures, particularly the lower part of the major fissures, can reflect tumor infiltration of the fissures or associated pleural effusion. Malignant mesothelioma typically spreads by local invasion, involving the mediastinum and sometimes the chest wall, but hematogenous pulmonary metastases and distant metastases do occur.

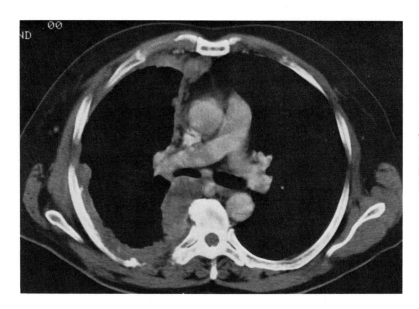

FIGURE 7–15. Malignant mesothelioma. There is circumferential nodular pleural thickening involving the right hemithorax. The right lung is reduced in volume compared to the left.

Benign Mesothelioma

Benign or localized mesothelioma (pleural fibroma) is an uncommon tumor, usually detected incidentally on chest radiographs. However, it can be associated with hypoglycemia and hypertrophic pulmonary osteoarthropathy. It usually arises from the visceral pleura and therefore can be within a fissure (Fig. 7–16) but more commonly involves the costal pleural surface. CT shows solitary, smooth, sharply defined, often large lesions contacting a pleural surface. It can be difficult to localize a fissural lesion to the fissure on CT without thin collimation.

Usually a benign mesothelioma will appear homogeneous on CT, but necrosis can result in a multicystic appearance with or without contrast infusion. Although it is generally believed that pleural abnormalities result in obtuse angles at the point of contact of the lesion and chest wall, benign mesotheliomas

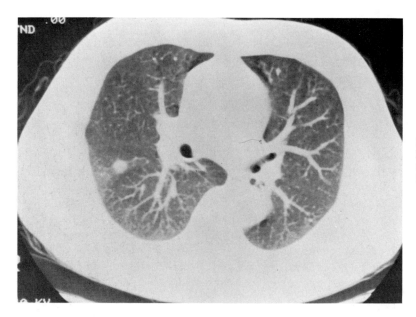

FIGURE 7–16. Benign mesothelioma. A nodular density represents a benign mesothelioma in the minor fissure.

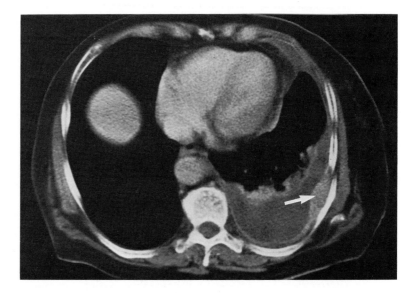

FIGURE 7–17. Pleural metastasis. There is pleural thickening evident after contrast infusion. An enhancing pleural mass (arrow) and pleural effusion are visible.

typically show acute angles with slightly tapered pleural thickening adjacent to the mass. This thickening may reflect a small amount of fluid accumulating in the pleural space at the point where the visceral and parietal pleural surfaces are separated by the mass. A similar "beak" or "thorn" sign often is visible on plain radiographs in patients with a benign fissural mesothelioma.

Metastases

In patients with intrathoracic or extrathoracic tumors, metastases to the pleura can cause nodular pleural thickening and pleural effusion. Usually, pleural effusion masks the underlying pleural mass or masses on plain radiographs, but occasionally they can be seen using CT. In particular, in patients with a malignant thymoma which has metastasized to the pleura, pleural effusion is often absent and the pleural metastases can be visible. They usually are discrete and form obtuse angles at their junctions with the chest wall.

With contrast infusion, pleural metastases, regardless of their origin, will often increase in density on CT relative to the adjacent effusion and thus become visible (Fig. 7–17). In many cases of pleural metastasis, nodular pleural thickening indistinguishable from that in patients with malignant mesothelioma is found

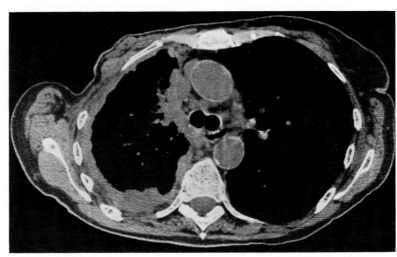

FIGURE 7–18. Pleural metastasis. Diffuse nodular pleural thickening simulates mesothelioma.

(Fig. 7–18), and extension into the fissures can also be seen. Uncommonly, malignant pleural effusion is unassociated with detectable pleural thickening.

Lymphoma

Pleural effusions are found in 15% of patients with Hodgkin's disease, and usually reflect lymphatic or venous destruction rather than pleural involvement, because they tend to resolve following local mediastinal or hilar radiation. Pericardial effusions, on the other hand, present in 5%, usually indicate direct involvement of the pericardium.

CHEST WALL

Chest Wall Abnormalities

Intrathoracic Lesions with Secondary Chest Wall Involvement

Several pulmonary infections can involve the chest wall by direct extension. These include actinomycosis (see Fig. 6–17), nocardiosis, and tuberculosis. If the chest wall disease is associated with adjacent pulmonary consolidation rather than a mass, differentiation from neoplasm may be possible.

Direct invasion of the chest wall by a peripheral bronchogenic carcinoma is common. Similarly, Hodgkin's disease can involve structures of the chest wall by direct invasion from the mediastinum or lung in a small percentage of cases. Malignant mesothelioma is a less common tumor that also can invade the chest wall.

The CT diagnosis of chest wall invasion can be difficult. A variety of CT findings can indicate chest wall invasion. These include the presence of obtuse angles at the point of contact between tumor and pleura, increased density of extrapleural fat, soft tissue mass, and rib destruction. Only rib destruction and significant chest wall mass have proved to be reasonably accurate indicators, and they reflect gross disease.

Diagnosing chest wall invasion when a tumor simply abuts the pleura should be avoided. Tumors adjacent to the pleura—even when associated with local pleural thickening, pleural effusion, or other findings which seem to suggest chest wall invasion—may not be invasive. In a patient with bronchogenic carcinoma, pleural effusion can occur for a variety of reasons, including obstructive pneumonia, and lymphatic or pulmonary venous obstruction by tumor. Only those patients with demonstration of tumor cells in the pleural fluid are considered unresectable. Reliable findings of chest wall invasion include bone destruction and a discrete extrapleural mass (Fig. 7–19). Such lesions are readily accessible to biopsy guided by CT.

Superior Sulcus (Pancoast) Tumors

Invasive tumors arising in the superior pulmonary sulcus produce the characteristic clinical findings of Horner's syndrome and shoulder and arm pain; this presentation is termed Pancoast's syndrome. In the past, tumors of the superior sulcus carried a very poor prognosis, but combined therapy with radiation followed by resection of the upper lobe, chest wall, and adjacent

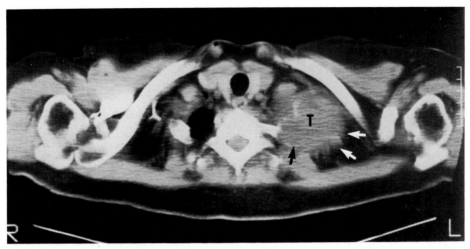

FIGURE 7–19. Pancoast tumor. A patient with a superior sulcus tumor (T) shows rib destruction (black arrow) and invasion of fat by tumor (white arrows).

structures has resulted in 5-year survival rates of 30%. In patients being considered for this combined therapy, CT scans can provide information on the anatomic extent of tumor spread that is useful in planning both the radiation therapy and the surgical approach to the tumor.

Extension of tumor posteriorly or laterally at the lung apex involves primarily the chest wall and nerves (Fig. 7–19). Although chest wall invasion does not prevent resection, extensive chest wall and bone involvement makes surgical treatment difficult, and the prognosis for patients with extensive chest wall disease is poor. Invasion of tumor posteromedially will involve the ribs or vertebral bodies. This occurs in one-third to one-half of cases and can usually be seen on CT scans. Anterior and medial extension of tumor can involve the esophagus, trachea, and brachiocephalic vessels. Invasion of these structures or the vertebral body precludes resection.

AXILLARY SPACE

Anatomy

As usually defined, the axilla is bordered by the fascial coverings of the following muscles: the pectoralis major and pectoralis minor anteriorly; the latissimus dorsi, teres major, and subscapularis posteriorly; the chest wall and serratus anterior medially; and the coracobrachialis and biceps laterally. However, when patients are scanned with their arms above their heads, the axilla is open laterally (see Fig. 2–1).

The axilla contains the axillary artery and vein, branches of the brachial plexus, some branches of the intercostal nerves, and a large number of lymph nodes, all surrounded by fat. The axillary vessels and the brachial plexus extend laterally, near the apex of the axilla, close to the pectoralis minor muscle. In general, the axillary vein lies below and anterior to the axillary artery, whereas the brachial plexus is largely above and posterior to the artery. Although these vessels usually can be seen on CT images, in many normal persons it is impossible to distinguish artery and vein within the axilla.

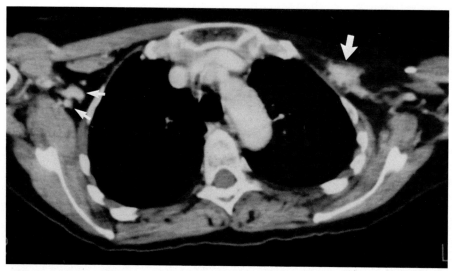

FIGURE 7–20. Axillary mass in a patient with recurrent breast cancer after radical mastectomy.
This patient has been scanned with arms down. The right axilla is normal, with vessels (small arrows) accounting for most of the visible soft tissue. On the left, the pectoralis muscles have been removed. A mass (large arrow) is visible in relation to axillary vessels. (Reproduced with permission. From Shea WJ Jr., deGeer G, Webb WR: Chest wall after mastectomy. Radiology, 162:162-164, 1987.)

Lymphadenopathy or Mass

Axillary lymph nodes, usually up to 1 cm but occasionally 1.5 cm in diameter, can be seen in normal subjects. Lymph nodes larger than 2 cm in diameter are generally considered pathologic (see Fig. 4–1). Axillary lymphadenopathy is seen most frequently in patients with lymphoma or metastatic carcinoma. Lymph node masses are detected most easily by observing both axillae for asymmetry. Enlarged lymph nodes high within the axilla lie beneath the pectoral muscles and may not be palpable, but these nodes can be detected by CT. Axillary masses in relation to nerves of the brachial plexus can also be demonstrated using CT (Fig. 7–20).

BREAST

Soft tissues of the breasts are seen on CT scans of women patients in the supine position. Localized breast masses occasionally are visible, but their CT appearance is usually nonspecific. Breast masses detected incidentally on CT images generally should be evaluated by physical examination and conventional mammography.

Breast Carcinoma

CT has not become an established technique for the routine evaluation of patients with breast cancer. However, CT can aid the planning of radiation therapy by providing an accurate measurement of chest wall thickness and by detecting internal mammary lymph node metastases.

Mastectomy

In women who have had a mastectomy, characteristic alterations in chest wall anatomy are seen, depending on the surgical procedure performed.

CT is sometimes used to evaluate suspected local tumor recurrence and to guide needle biopsy.

A radical mastectomy consists of complete removal of the breast tissue and pectoralis major and pectoralis minor muscles and extensive axillary lymph node dissection (Fig. 7–20). On CT, although most of the pectoralis muscles are absent, residual pectoralis major muscle is sometimes seen at its sternal or costal attachment. This should not be misinterpreted as recurrent tumor.

A typical modified radical mastectomy consists of removal of the breast and pectoralis minor muscle and an axillary lymph node dissection. The precise techniques for this procedure can vary among surgeons, and a discussion with the surgeon concerning the procedure performed is advisable before interpreting the CT scans. In patients who have undergone a modified radical mastectomy, the amount of pectoralis minor muscle remaining is variable. Without careful clinical correlation, it is sometimes difficult to distinguish postsurgical changes from tumor recurrence. This is a particular problem when the patient has difficulty elevating both arms symmetrically for the CT examination. With the arms raised, asymmetry of the pectoralis muscles is accentuated, and the scans are often very difficult to interpret. It is therefore best to obtain scans with the patient's arms at her sides.

A simple mastectomy consists of removal of only breast tissue; the underlying musculature remains intact. Residual breast tissue will remain when segmental or partial mastectomy is performed.

DIAPHRAGM

Anatomy

Because of the transaxial plane of CT, the central portion of the diaphragm does not appear as a distinct structure, and its position can only be inferred by the position of the lung base above, and upper abdominal organs below. However, as the more peripheral portions of the diaphragm extend caudally toward their sternal and costal attachments, the anterior, posterior, and lateral portions of the diaphragm become visible adjacent to retroperitoneal fat (Fig. 7–21). Where the diaphragm is contiguous with the liver or spleen, it cannot usually be delineated by CT unless thin collimation CT is used and a subdiaphragmatic fat layer is present.

The right and left diaphragmatic crura are tendinous structures that arise inferiorly from the anterior surfaces of the upper lumbar vertebral bodies and intervening disks, and are continuous with the anterior longitudinal ligament of the spine. The crura ascend anterior to the spine, on each side of the aorta, and then pass medially and anteriorly, joining the muscular diaphragm anterior to the aorta, to form the aortic hiatus (Fig. 7–21). The right crus, which is larger and longer than the left, arises from the first three lumbar vertebral levels; the left crus arises from the first two lumbar segments.

The diaphragmatic crura can be mistaken for enlarged lymph nodes or masses because of their rounded appearance; para-aortic lymph nodes can

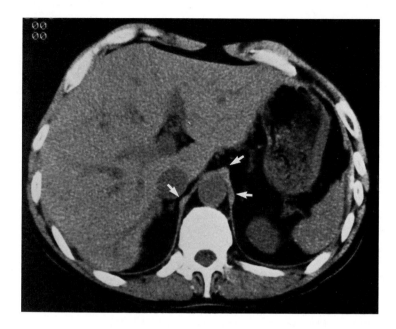

FIGURE 7–21. Normal diaphragm. The diaphragm is outlined by retroperitoneal fat. Where it contacts the liver and spleen, it is not usually visible as a discrete structure. The diaphragmatic crura can appear lumpy (arrows). Here they pass anterior to the aorta to form the aortic hiatus.

indeed be seen in a similar position. However, on contiguous CT scans, the crura merge gradually with the diaphragm at more cephalad levels. The diameter of the crura also will vary with lung volume, increasing in thickness at full inspiration compared with expiration.

Openings in the Diaphragm

The diaphragm is perforated by several openings that allow structures to pass from the thorax to the abdomen. The aortic hiatus is posterior; it is bounded posteriorly by the vertebral body and anteriorly by the crura (Fig. 7–21). Through it pass the aorta, the azygos and hemiazygos veins, the thoracic duct, intercostal arteries, and splanchnic nerves. The esophageal hiatus is situated more anteriorly, in the muscular portion of the diaphragm. Through it pass the esophagus, the vagus nerves, and small blood vessels. The foramen of the inferior vena cava pierces the fibrous central tendon of the diaphragm anterior to and to the right of the esophageal hiatus.

Of these three structures, the aortic hiatus is defined most readily. On CT scans, the esophageal foramen is visible as an opening at the junction of the esophagus and stomach. The foramen of the inferior vena cava must be inferred from the position of the inferior vena cava. The foramina of Morgagni and of Bochdalek are not visible on CT scans in normal individuals.

Diaphragmatic Abnormalities

Hernias

Abdominal or retroperitoneal contents can herniate into the chest through congenital or acquired areas of weakness in the diaphragm or through traumatic diaphragmatic ruptures. Hernias of the stomach through the esophageal hiatus are the most common.

Hernias through the foramen of Bochdalek were thought to be uncommon in adults; however, CT has shown that small Bochdalek defects may occur in as many as 5% of normals. This is the most common type of diaphragmatic hernia

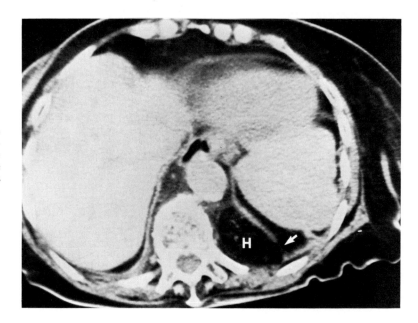

FIGURE 7–22. Bochdalek hernia. In this patient, the hernia (H) consists of a collection of retroperitoneal fat. A small defect in the diaphragm (arrow) is visible at this level.

in infants. Most are left-sided, and although often they are located in the posterolateral diaphragm, they can occur anywhere along the posterior costodiaphragmatic margin (Fig. 7–22). Bochdalek hernias in adults usually contain retroperitoneal fat or kidney.

Parasternal hernias through the foramen of Morgagni are relatively rare. Most Morgagni's hernias occur on the right and, in contrast to Bochdalek hernias, usually contain an extension of the peritoneal sac. Their contents can include omentum, liver, or bowel. The presence of bowel anterior to the heart can suggest the presence of a hernia, but this is not usually the case.

Diaphragmatic rupture can result from penetrating or nonpenetrating trauma to the abdomen or thorax. In nearly all cases, the left hemidiaphragm is affected, with ruptures of the central or posterior diaphragm being the most frequent. Omentum, stomach, small or large intestine, spleen, or kidney may all herniate through the diaphragmatic rent.

Diaphragmatic Eventration

Local eventration of the right hemidiaphragm and superior displacement of the liver can be confused radiographically with a peripheral pulmonary or pleural mass. CT scans after infusion of contrast medium can demonstrate opacification of normal intrahepatic vessels in the apparent mass, allowing its identification. In addition, scans reformatted in the coronal plane can show that the "mass" has the same density as liver.

SUGGESTED READING

Hulnick DH, Naidich DP, McCauley D: Pleural tuberculosis evaluated by computed tomography. Radiology, 149:759–765, 1983.

Im J–G, Webb WR, Rosen A, et al.: Costal pleura: Appearances at high–resolution CT. Radiology, 171: 125–131, 1989.

Mirvis S, Dutcher JP, Haneyt PJ, et al.: CT of malignant pleural mesothelioma. Am J Roentgenol, 140:665–670, 1983.

Rabinowitz JG, Efremidis SC, CohenB, et al.: A comparative study of mesothelioma and asbestosis using computed tomography and conventional chest radiography. Radiology, 144:453–460, 1982.

Stark DD, Federle MP, Goodman PC, et al.: Differentiating lung abscess and empyema. Radiology and computed tomography. Am J Roentgenol, 141:163–167, 1983.

THE ABDOMEN AND PELVIS

2

8

Introduction to CT of the Abdomen and Pelvis

While magnetic resonance imaging (MRI) has replaced computed tomography as the imaging method of first choice for most indications in the central nervous system, computed tomography remains a primary imaging modality in the abdomen. With the rapid scan times of most modern CT scanners, motion artifact is usually minimal. Efficacious use of contrast agents allows accurate differentiation of bowel from other structures in the abdomen. Computed tomography is as comprehensive as MRI, but remains more available and cheaper than MRI.

Evaluation of the abdomen by CT requires greater patient preparation, attention to technique, and individualization than CT evaluation of any other area of the body. The best quality studies are produced when the radiologist is present to evaluate the patient clinically, assess the nature of the imaging problem, and tailor the study to optimize the information the examination provides.

APPROACH

When a patient presents for an abdominal CT scan, the radiologist should assess the clinical problem to be evaluated by taking a brief patient history and reviewing all pertinent previous imaging studies. Medical history of importance to CT examination includes the current indication for the study, contrast allergies, cardiac and renal impairments, past abdominal surgeries, radiation therapy, etc. In some cases, such as when there is a question of an abdominal mass, a brief physical examination is helpful. Previous imaging studies are reviewed to ensure that all previous abnormalities and questionable findings are appropriately reevaluated.

Decisions to be made to individualize the examination include

1. Contrast: intravenous, oral, rectal, vaginal
2. Area scanned: anatomic landmarks
3. Scan parameters: slice thickness and spacing
4. Technique: dynamic sequence, scan times, reconstruction matrix

The radiologist should review the scan before the patient leaves the CT suite to ensure a superior quality study. Any questionable areas should be reevaluated as needed.

GASTROINTESTINAL CONTRAST

Nearly all CT scans of the abdomen require the administration of intraluminal contrast agents to opacify the gastrointestinal tract. The usual agents are radiopaque, consisting of dilute concentrations of barium or iodinated agents. Concentrations of 1 to 3% are optimal for CT, as compared to the 30 to 60% solutions used for fluoroscopy studies. Barium mixtures and water-soluble iodinated agents are equally effective. A number of commercial preparations are available specifically for CT.

We routinely use dilutions of 3 ml of 60% iodinated oral contrast agent in every 100 ml of water. Our standard bowel preparation for CT includes a clear liquid diet beginning at midnight before the CT exam. The patient ingests only oral contrast agents for the last 4 hours before the examination. Oral contrast is given in four doses of 400 ml each at 10:00 pm the night before, at 2 hours before the exam, at 30 minutes before the exam, and immediately before the exam. This dosage regimen will usually opacify the entire bowel, including the colon and rectum. Opacification of the upper gastrointestinal tract can be attained rapidly by giving 200 ml doses of oral contrast agents every 10 minutes for 30 to 40 minutes before the CT examination. The same dilution of water-soluble contrast can be given as an enema to rapidly opacify the colon. A basic rule of abdominal CT is that no one can receive "too much" oral contrast. Air provides both excellent contrast and bowel distention when used for CT of the gastrointestinal tract. The colon can be insufflated by placement of a Miller air tip enema tube such as that routinely used for double contrast barium enemas. The stomach and duodenum can be distended by use of effervescent granules which release carbon dioxide on contact with fluid in the stomach.

INTRAVENOUS CONTRAST

Intravenous contrast agents improve the quality of abdominal CT by opacifying blood vessels and increasing the density of vascular abdominal organs. When properly used, intravenous contrast improves the detection of most pathologic processes. Intravenous infusion by controlled mechanical injection provides more reliable contrast effect than drip infusion by gravity. For most abdominal CT scans we use a 150 ml dose of 60% iodinated agent, given at 2.5 ml per second for 20 seconds, followed by 1 ml per second for 100 seconds. We begin scanning 40 seconds after initiation of contrast infusion to allow circulation of contrast into the abdominal vessels.

OTHER CONTRAST APPLICATIONS

When scanning the female pelvis, particularly when evaluating for pathology of the female organs, we ask the patient to place a tampon in her vagina. The tampon appears as a cylinder of air density on CT, allowing positive identification of the vagina.

Sterile iodinated contrast can be injected into indwelling catheters, drainage tubes, sinus tracts, etc., to evaluate extent of disease. Dilution of contrast to a 1 to 3% concentration is needed to avoid streak artifact on CT.

SCAN PARAMETERS AND TECHNIQUE

Slice thickness of 8 to 10 mm is sufficient for most applications of abdominal CT. When volume averaging is a problem, such as with small renal or pancreatic lesions, 5-mm-thick slices are used. Thinner slices are seldom useful because anatomic misregistration due to variations in breath holding is a bigger problem than volume averaging. Most scans are performed using contiguous slices (10 mm thick at 10-mm intervals). However, survey examinations may be performed at longer intervals (10-mm-thick slices at 15- to 20-mm intervals) to save radiation dose and time with minimal loss of information.

Scan times of 1 to 2 seconds should always be used to diminish motion artifact from peristalsis and pulsating blood vessels. The time between individual slices (interscan delay) should be kept to a minimum to ensure scanning during maximum opacification by intravenous contrast agents. Image reconstruction is usually performed using a 512x512 or 320x320 pixel matrix. To decrease reconstruction time during biopsy procedures, a 256x256 matrix will usually suffice.

IMAGE PHOTOGRAPHY

Each CT image of the abdomen contains much more information than can be displayed by any one window width and level setting. Routine "soft tissue" windows (window width = 400 H, window level = 30 to 50 H) define most abdominal anatomy. However, the liver should always also be inspected using narrow "liver windows" (window width = 150 H, window level = 70 to 80 H) to increase contrast within the liver and improve detection of subtle lesions. The lung bases are included on scans through the upper abdomen and should be inspected using "lung windows" (window width = 2000 H, window level = − 500 H). Lastly, inspection of the bones using "bone windows" (window width = 2000 H, window level = 600 H) may yield important clues to pathologic findings within the abdomen.

9

Liver

ANATOMY

The vascular anatomy of the liver defines the surgical approach to hepatic resection. Resectability of hepatic lesions can be determined by CT only if hepatic vascular anatomy is clearly understood. A knowledge of three dimensional hepatic anatomy is essential to correlate lesion location with various hepatic imaging methods. Previous concepts of hepatic lobar anatomy can be ignored in favor of current anatomic considerations that relate directly to surgical resection of hepatic lesions. A key concept to remember is that the hepatic veins run in the interlobar and *inter*segmental fissures, while the portal veins, hepatic arteries, and bile ducts course together within the *intra*segmental parenchyma. Portal veins and hepatic arteries supply the parenchyma of the segments through which they course. Hepatic veins drain both segments bordering the fissures which the veins help define.

Hepatic vascular territories divide the liver into three lobes and four segments (Fig. 9–1). The right and left lobes are separated by the major lobar fissure. This fissure is defined by the middle hepatic vein in the cranial third of the liver and by a line drawn from the center of the inferior vena cava through the gallbladder fossa to the liver edge in the lower portion of the liver. The right hepatic lobe is divided into anterior and posterior segments by the right intersegmental fissure. This fissure is defined by the course of the right hepatic vein in the cranial aspect of the liver and by a line drawn midway between the anterior and posterior branches of the right portal vein in the caudal aspect of the liver. The left hepatic lobe is divided into medial and lateral segments by the left intersegmental fissure marked by the left hepatic vein in the cranial aspect of the liver and by the prominent fissure of the ligamentum venosum and falciform ligament in the caudal aspect of the liver. The medial segment was formerly called the "quadrate lobe."

Lesions confined to the right or left lobe can be surgically removed by right or left hepatic lobectomy carried up to but not including the middle hepatic vein. Lateral segmentectomy of the left lobe and technically more difficult posterior segmentectomy of the right lobe can be performed for lesions confined to the corresponding segments. Extended right lobectomy, which includes removal of the medial segment of the left lobe, can be performed if the volume of hepatic parenchyma in the remaining lateral segment of the left lobe is sufficient to sustain life. Accurate localization of lesions on CT and other imaging methods is critical to surgical planning.

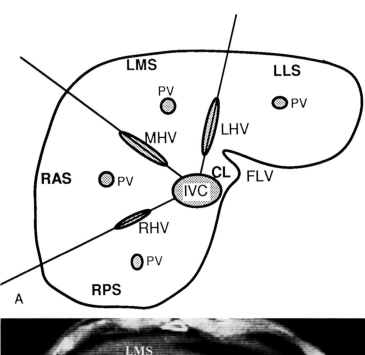

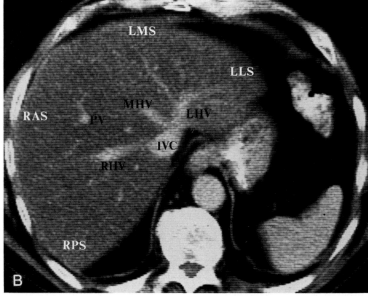

FIGURE 9–1. Hepatic segmental anatomy. Diagram *A* and CT image *B* demonstrate the hepatic venous anatomy, which provides landmarks for the fissures dividing the liver into lobes and segments. The hepatic and portal veins are prominent in *B* because the liver has diffuse fatty infiltration that lowers the CT attenuation of the liver parenchyma. (RPS, RAS = posterior and anterior segments of the right lobe; LMS, LLS = medial and lateral segments of the left lobe; CL = caudate lobe; RHV, MHV, LHV = right, middle, and left hepatic veins; PV = portal veins; IVC = inferior vena cava; FLV = fissure of the ligamentum venosum.)

The caudate lobe is separated from the rest of the liver by the fissure of the ligamentum venosum anteriorly and the inferior vena cava posterolaterally. It is supplied by branches of both right and left hepatic arteries and portal veins, and drains venous blood directly into the inferior vena cava by multiple small veins. The papillary process of the caudate lobe extends toward the lesser sac and may appear separate from the rest of the caudate lobe, simulating a mass or enlarged lymph node.

Several fissures and ligaments deserve special mention either because they are particularly prominent or because they define important perihepatic spaces. The falciform ligament consists of two closely applied layers of peritoneum extending from the umbilicus to the diaphragm in a parasagittal plane. The caudal free end of the falciform ligament contains the ligamentum teres, which is the obliterated umbilical vein remnant. The reflections of the falciform ligament separate over the posterior dome of the liver to form the coronary ligaments, which define the "bare area" of the liver not covered by peritoneum. The coronary ligaments reflect between liver and diaphragm and prevent ascites or other intraperitoneal fluid from covering the "bare area" of the liver. The absence of fluid over the "bare area" is an important sign in the differentiation of ascites from pleural effusion on CT. The remainder of the falciform ligament and ligamentum teres continues into the liver to form a prominent fat-filled fissure often mistaken for the main interlobar fissure. In actuality, the fissure of the ligamentum teres and falciform ligament defines the left intersegmental fissure dividing medial and lateral segments of the left lobe.

The fissure of the ligamentum venosum contains the remnant of the ductus venosus, which in fetal life carried oxygenated blood from the umbilical vein to the inferior vena cava. The fissure is commonly fat-filled and prominent on CT, separating the caudate lobe and the left lobe.

The lesser omentum suspends the lesser curve of the stomach and the duodenal bulb from the inferior surface of the liver, attaching within the fissure of the ligamentum venosum. The lesser omentum is subdivided into the gastro-hepatic ligament and the hepatoduodenal ligament. The gastrohepatic ligament contains cardinal veins, which serve as an important sign of portal hypertension when they become dilated. The free rightward end of the hepatoduodenal ligament carries the portal vein, hepatic artery, and common bile duct between the porta hepatis and the duodenum. The hepatoduodenal ligament provides the anterior border of the foramen of Winslow opening into the lesser sac.

TECHNIQUE

Optimal detection of liver mass lesions by CT requires scanning both before and after intravenous contrast administration. While intravenous contrast will generally improve visualization of liver masses, on some occasions the mass will become isodense with the liver parenchyma and will escape detection if only contrast-enhanced scans are performed.

Our standard technique is to obtain baseline liver scans before contrast, and then repeat the entire scan of the liver after contrast. Both studies are done using 10-mm-thick slices at contiguous 10 mm intervals through the entire liver. Intravenous contrast is administered by power injector at 2.5 ml per second for 20 seconds, followed by 1.0 ml per second for 100 seconds for a total dose of 150 ml of 60 percent contrast agent. Scanning is begun 20 seconds following initiation of contrast injection. We use scan times of 2 to 3 seconds with 6-second interscan delay for table movement. Using this technique the entire liver can generally be scanned within the first 2 to 3 minutes of contrast injection to ensure maximal enhancement.

To characterize the enhancement pattern of a liver mass, we use a dynamic CT protocol with scanning at a single anatomic level. A single slice level through the midportion of the mass is selected. Contrast is given by power injector in a 100 ml dose at 2.5 ml per second. Six scans per minute are obtained for the first 2 minutes, then three scans per minute for the next 5 minutes, and final scans are obtained at 12, 17, and 23 minutes post injection. This protocol is most commonly used for CT characterization of suspected cavernous hemangioma.

DIFFUSE LIVER DISEASE

Fatty Liver

Fatty infiltration of the liver is one of the most common abnormalities diagnosed by liver CT. Fatty infiltration is a nonspecific response of hepatocytes to a variety of insults, including alcoholism, cirrhosis, obesity, diabetes, chemotherapy, steroid therapy, hyperalimentation, and malnutrition. Fatty infiltration lowers the CT attenuation of the liver parenchyma, causing hepatic vessels to stand out in relief (Fig. 9–1B). The normal CT attenuation of the liver is equal to or greater than that of the normal spleen, both before and after intravenous contrast administration. Fatty infiltration makes involved portions of the liver appear more lucent than the splenic parenchyma. Three patterns of fatty infiltration are seen on CT:

1. *Diffuse.* The entire liver is uniformly reduced in density. Vessels stand out in prominent relief especially following contrast administration, but run their normal course through the liver without displacement by mass effect (Fig. 9 – 1B). The liver is usually enlarged and enhances minimally. This pattern is the most common and easiest to recognize.

2. *Focal.* A geographic or fan-shaped portion of the liver is fatty-replaced while the remainder of the liver remains of normal density. The low density may extend to the liver surface but no bulge in contour is seen (Fig. 9–2). Vessels run their normal course through the area of involvement.

3. *Multifocal.* Patchy areas of decreased attenuation are scattered through the liver. Tumors may be simulated by the islands of fatty infiltration or by focal sparing, which leaves islands of normal parenchyma surrounded by fatty infiltration.

Focal fatty infiltration can be differentiated from hepatoma, metastases, and other tumors by the following signs (Fig. 9–2):

1. Angulated geometric margins (non-spherical shape)
2. Interdigitating margins with slender fingers of normal or fatty tissue

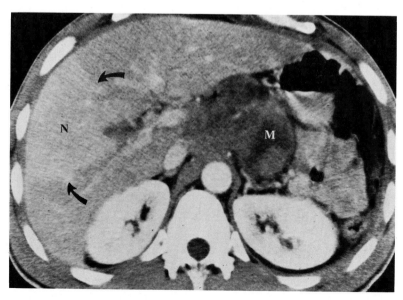

FIGURE 9–2. Focal fatty liver. This geographic pattern of fatty infiltration developed within 2 weeks of the placement of this patient with lymphoma on chemotherapy. The higher density wedge-shaped area (N) is normal liver parenchyma that has been spared the process of fatty infiltration. Note the sharp straight margins of demarcation (arrows) between normal high density and fatty low density areas of the liver. M is a mass of adenopathy due to lymphoma.

3. Absence of mass effect or vessel displacement

4. Rapid change over time. Fatty changes can be seen within 3 weeks following the insult and can resolve within 6 days after removing the insult.

Further confirmation of fatty replacement can be provided by other imaging tests. Ultrasound will show the area of fatty infiltration as a corresponding area of increased echogenicity. Technetium sulphur colloid liver scans will show normal activity in the area of involvement since the reticuloendothelial cells are not displaced. Xenon scintigraphy will show uptake in the area of involvement since xenon is fat avid. Percutaneous biopsy is an option in difficult cases.

Cirrhosis

Cirrhosis is a chronic diffuse liver disease characterized by progressive destruction of hepatocytes and distortion of hepatic architecture with extensive collagen deposition. The common forms of cirrhosis are Laënnec's due to alcoholism, postnecrotic due to various types of hepatitis and toxic injury to the liver, and biliary due to chronic intrahepatic cholestasis. Patients with cirrhosis may show the following findings (Fig. 9–3):

1. Fatty infiltration with hepatomegaly is characteristic of early cirrhosis

2. Non – uniform attenuation due to chronic fatty infiltration and irregular fibrosis

3. Irregular lobulated hepatic contour due to areas of atrophy and nodular regeneration

4. Intrahepatic regenerating nodules

5. Atrophy of the right lobe with hypertrophy of the left and caudate lobes is common in alcoholic cirrhosis

6. Decreased liver volume when cirrhosis is chronic

7. Increased size and prominence of the intrahepatic fissure due to shrunken liver parenchyma

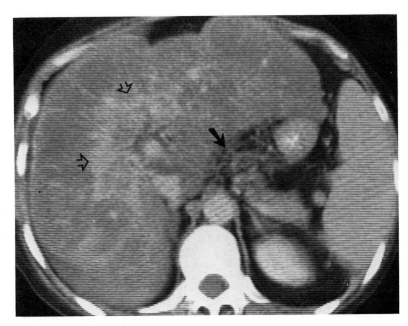

FIGURE 9–3. Cirrhosis. CT image of the liver demonstrates signs of advanced cirrhosis. The periphery of the liver is lower in density than that of the spleen, indicating fatty replacement of the liver. The higher density areas centrally (open arrows) are due to extensive scarring and collagen deposition. The contour of the liver is lobulated and the left lobe is enlarged. A tangle of collateral vessels (closed arrow) in the gastrohepatic ligament indicates the presence of portal hypertension.

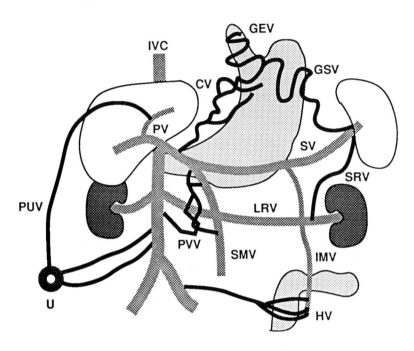

FIGURE 9–4. Portosystemic collaterals. Schematic representation of portosystemic venous collaterals that may be seen in portal hypertension. (IVC = inferior vena cava; PV = portal veins; SV = splenic vein; SMV = superior mesenteric vein; IMV = inferior mesenteric vein; LRV = left renal vein; HV = hemorrhoidal veins; PVV = paravertebral veins; SRV = splenorenal veins; GSV = gastrosplenic veins; GEV = gastroesophageal varices; CV = cardinal veins (in gastrohepatic ligament); PUV = paraumbilical vein; U = umbilicus.

8. Signs of portal hypertension
9. Ascites.

Patients with cirrhosis are at high risk of developing portal hypertension and hepatocellular carcinoma. Each CT scan in patients with cirrhosis must be carefully analyzed for signs of these conditions.

Portal Hypertension

Portal hypertension results from progressive fibrosis of the hepatic vascular bed with development of portosystemic collaterals and eventually hepatofugal flow (that is away from, instead of into, the liver). Portal hypertension causes

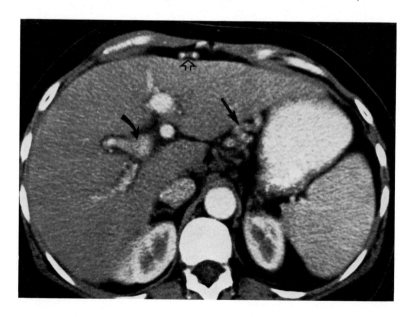

FIGURE 9–5. Portal hypertension. CT signs of portal hypertension are demonstrated in this slice through the porta hepatis. The portal vein (curved arrow) is enlarged, measuring 15 mm. Dilated and tortuous cardinal veins (arrow) are seen in the gastrohepatic ligament. The paraumbilical vein (open arrow) is patent and enlarged. Visualization of a patent paraumbilical vein is the most specific CT sign of portal hypertension.

major morbidity in the cirrhotic patient because of the risk of hepatic encephalopathy and variceal hemorrhage. Portal hypertension can be diagnosed on CT by the presence of the following:

1. Portosystemic collaterals (Figs. 9–4 and 9–5)
2. Increased size of the portal venous system (larger than 1.1 to 1.3 cm)
3. Portal vein thrombosis seen as an enlarged low density portal vein that fails to enhance (Fig. 9–7)
4. Splenomegaly due to splenic congestion
5. Ascites.

The enlarged collateral vessels characteristic of portal hypertension may be subtle and easily missed. You see what you look for!

FOCAL LIVER MASSES

Solid Liver Masses

A primary goal of liver imaging is to differentiate significant liver masses from insignificant ones. Clinically significant liver masses include metastases, hepatoma, and hepatic adenoma. Cavernous hemangioma, hepatic cyst, and focal nodular hyperplasia are clinically insignificant focal liver masses that must be discriminated.

Metastases. Metastases are the most common malignant tumor in the liver. Liver metastases can originate from almost any primary malignancy, but most arise from the gastrointestinal tract, especially the colon. Usually metastases are multiple, but the greatest problems in differentiation occur when they are solitary. A wide spectrum of CT appearances (Fig. 9–6) is possible, including

1. Well-defined, low density solid mass (most common)
2. High density solid mass, especially when the liver is fatty-replaced

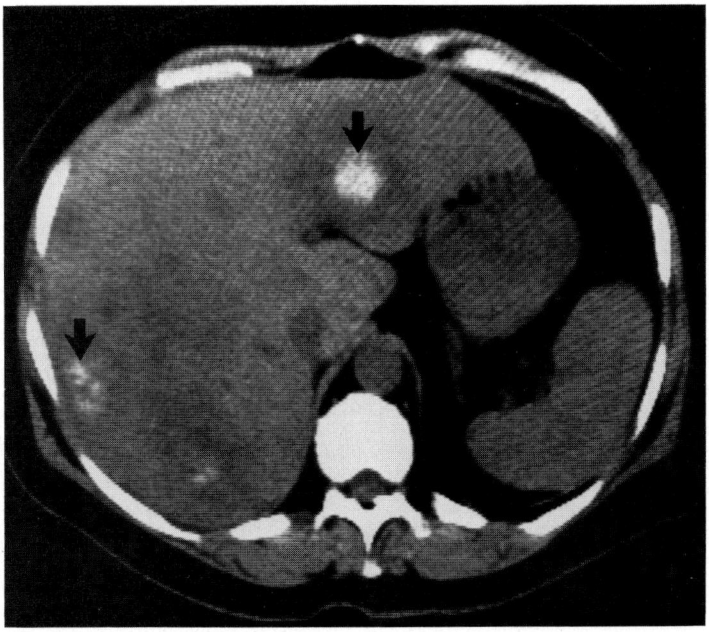

FIGURE 9–6. Liver metastases. Metastatic deposits from mucinous adenocarcinoma of the colon cause multiple focal mass densities in the liver, some of which are calcified (arrows). Calcified metastases are characteristic of mucinous carcinomas and necrotic tumors.

3. Cystic/necrotic mass, especially when the primary tumor is mucinous colon or ovarian carcinoma, lung, melanoma, or carcinoid tumor

4. Partially calcified mass, especially when the metastatic deposit is necrotic.

In summary, metastases can look like almost every other lesion in the liver, and must always be considered a possibility.

Hepatoma. Hepatocellular carcinoma is the most common primary hepatic malignancy. Eighty percent of hepatomas arise in cirrhotic livers. Elevated serum alpha-fetoprotein is a common clinical clue to the diagnosis. Three patterns of tumor growth are seen: solitary tumor (50%), diffuse infiltrative tumor (30%) (Fig. 9–7), and multinodular tumor (20%). On CT most are low density on unenhanced scans and enhance prominently during the arterial phase on dynamic contrast injection. Areas of tumor necrosis are common, and calcification is present in 25%. Tumor invasion of hepatic and portal veins (Fig. 9–7) is frequent. Fatty metamorphosis within hepatomas is common histologically and has been reported on CT.

Hepatic Adenoma. Hepatic adenomas are rare but much talked about benign tumors. They are significant lesions because of the risk of major hemorrhage associated with their presence. Hepatic adenomas are composed entirely of hepatocytes and are completely devoid of bile ducts and Kupffer cells. Areas of hemorrhage and necrosis are nearly always present within the tumor. Most patients present with an abdominal mass, gastrointestinal complaints, or hemoperitoneum due to tumor rupture. Oral contraceptives are a risk factor, both for tumor growth and rupture. Surgical removal is recommended. The imaging findings are

1. Hypodense heterogeneous mass on unenhanced CT
2. Hemorrhage within the tumor common
3. Marked heterogeneity on enhanced CT with areas of increased, normal, and decreased density within the tumor

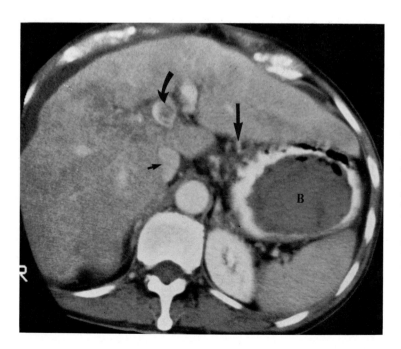

FIGURE 9–7. Hepatocellular carcinoma. A diffusely infiltrating hepatoma causes subtle low density in the right lobe, with mass effect on vascular structures. Note the subtle indentation of the inferior vena cava (small arrow). The tumor occupies the entire right lobe of the liver. Tumor thrombus causes a low density center (curved arrow) in the portal vein. Enlarged collateral vessels between liver and stomach (large arrow) indicate the presence of accompanying portal hypertension. The patient also has ascites and a bezoar (B) in his stomach.

4. Absent radionuclide uptake within the tumor on technetium-99m labelled sulfur colloid liver scan

5. Multiple tumors in 30%.

Focal Nodular Hyperplasia. In contrast to hepatic adenoma, focal nodular hyperplasia contains all the histologic elements of normal liver including Kupffer cells. Fibrous bands and stellate fibrous scars are common, but hemorrhage and necrosis are rare. Most patients are asymptomatic and the tumor is discovered incidentally. No treatment is indicated. The imaging findings are

1. Hypodense homogeneous mass on unenhanced CT scan
2. Hyperdense or isodense mass on enhanced CT scan
3. Normal radionuclide uptake within the tumor in 40 to 70% on technetium-99m labelled sulfur colloid liver scan
4. Multiple tumors in 7%.

Cavernous Hemangioma. Cavernous hemangiomas are the second most common focal mass lesion in the liver, exceeded in frequency only by metastases. They are the most common benign liver neoplasms, found in up to 7% of patients on autopsy series. They are often discovered incidentally during hepatic imaging by ultrasound or computed tomography. They may be found at any age and are more common in women. While most are solitary, 10% of the affected patients have multiple lesions easily mistaken for metastases. The tumors consist of large, thin-walled, blood-filled vascular spaces lined by epithelium and separated by fibrous septa. Blood flow through the complex vascular spaces is very slow, resulting in characteristic prolonged retention of contrast agents on CT. The majority of lesions are less than 5 cm in size, are asymptomatic, and pose no threat to the patient. Larger *giant cavernous hemangiomas* may cause symptoms by pressure effect, hemorrhage, or arteriovenous shunting. The imaging findings are (Fig. 9–8)

1. Well-defined hypodense mass of the same density as other blood-filled spaces, such as the portal vein on unenhanced CT scans, are observed
2. Nodule-like areas of enhancement develop from the periphery when contrast is given as a rapid bolus
3. Areas of enhancement become confluent and the entire lesion may gradually become isodense or hyperdense relative to the liver parenchyma
4. Contrast enhancement usually persists within the lesion for 20 to 30 minutes following contrast injection
5. Large lesions have discrete areas of fibrosis and occasionally calcification which remain hypodense throughout the period of enhancement.

When these classic findings are observed, the CT examination can be considered diagnostic of cavernous hemangioma with a high degree of confidence.

Cystic Liver Masses

Simple Hepatic Cyst. Simple hepatic cysts are believed to be congenital and due to maldevelopment of bile ducts. They are usually solitary, but may be multiple, especially in patients with adult polycystic disease. Simple hepatic cysts appear on CT as round, fluid density masses with sharply defined, smooth, thin walls (Fig. 9–9). They have no internal structure and show no enhancement with

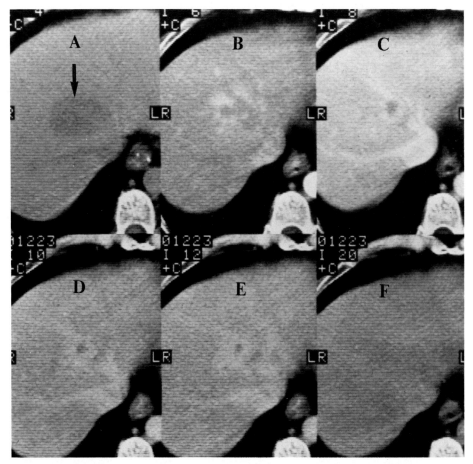

FIGURE 9–8. Cavernous hemangioma. A series of timed sequential images follows a bolus of contrast through a liver mass and demonstrates the characteristic findings of a cavernous hemangioma (arrow). *A,* obtained prior to contrast administration, shows a well-defined hypodense mass. *B to E,* obtained 30 seconds, 1 minute, 2 minutes, and 5 minutes, respectively, following a bolus of intravenous contrast, demonstrate the characteristic enhancement of the lesion from periphery to center. *F,* obtained 10 minutes after contrast injection, shows that the lesion has become isodense and undetectable.

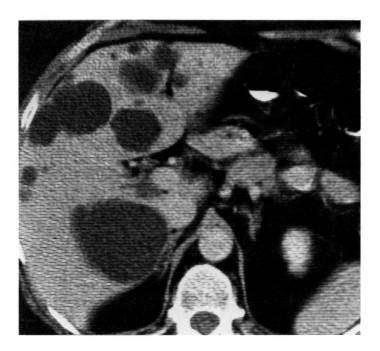

FIGURE 9–9. Multiple simple hepatic cysts. Multiple simple hepatic cysts have uniform low internal density and sharp margins with the surrounding hepatic parenchyma. No cyst walls are evident. The lesions do not enhance with intravenous contrast administration.

contrast administration. Lesions with this appearance in asymptomatic patients may be confidently diagnosed as simple hepatic cysts.

The following diseases must be considered in symptomatic patients and when the cystic hepatic lesion is not characteristic of simple hepatic cyst:

Pyogenic abscess. This is usually solitary but often multiloculated with thickened enhancing walls (Fig. 9–10). When multiple, lesions are often grouped and consist of multiple microabscesses. Gas is present within the lesion in 20% of cases. Patients are usually septic and are often jaundiced. Fine needle aspiration is indicated for bacterial culture. Catheter or surgical drainage is needed.

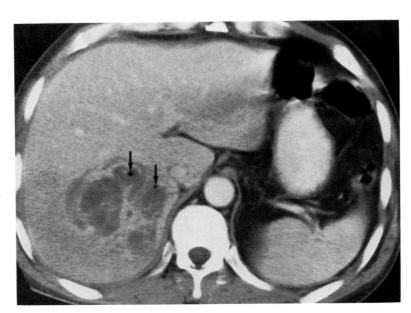

FIGURE 9–10. Pyogenic liver abscess. A liver abscess containing *Escherichia coli* has multiple irregular septations and contains a few bubbles of air (arrows). Because of the multiple loculations, this abscess did not respond to percutaneously placed catheter drainage and required surgical debridement.

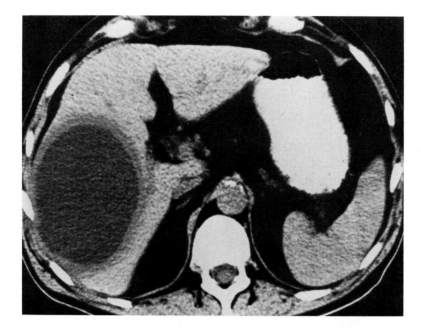

FIGURE 9–11. Amebic abscess.
A 50-year-old American living in Thailand returned to the United States with this mass in his liver. While the internal density is homogeneously low, a distinct thick wall is present and was observed to enhance with intravenous contrast administration. Serologic titers were positive for amebiasis.

Amebic abscess. This is usually solitary with a well-defined, nodular, enhancing wall (Fig. 9–11). Appearance overlaps that of pyogenic abscess, but patients are generally not septic and have a history of travel to endemic areas. Diagnosis is made by clinical and radiographic findings and is confirmed by serology. Treatment is with metronidazole. Drainage is not needed.

Echinococcus Cyst. Infestation with the Echinococcus tapeworm results in the formation of single or multiple cystic masses. The cysts are usually well-defined and have calcification in their walls in 50%. Daughter cysts can be visualized with the parent cyst in 70%. The remainder may be difficult to differentiate from simple cysts. Surgery is the treatment of choice.

Cystic/Necrotic Liver Tumor. Necrotic, hemorrhagic, or primarily cystic

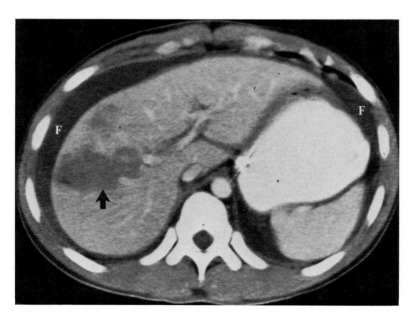

FIGURE 9–12. Liver laceration. A CT image of the liver in a 16-year-old boy injured in a motor vehicle accident demonstrates a low density band (arrow) through the liver. The low density band is due to hematoma within a laceration of the liver. Fluid (F) around the liver, spleen, and stomach is free blood within the peritoneal cavity. CT is excellent for quantitating the amount of hemoperitoneum, but the entire abdomen and pelvis must be surveyed.

tumors may mimic simple hepatic cysts. Most will have thickened walls, nodularity, internal debris, or show evidence of contrast enhancement. Metastases are most common and usually multiple. Biliary cystadenomas and cystadenocarcinomas are uncommon cystic tumors. Hepatocellular carcinoma may rarely be cystic.

LIVER TRAUMA

CT accurately depicts the extent of liver injury and quantitates the amount of hemoperitoneum following blunt abdominal trauma. Liver injuries may be classified as contusions or lacerations with variably sized intrahepatic and subcapsular hematomas. Hemoperitoneum associated with liver injury generally implies a laceration extending through the liver capsule with bleeding and/or bile leakage into the peritoneal cavity. Lacerations may be linear or stellate and are defined on CT by hematoma within the area of injury (Fig. 9–12). The hematoma may be isodense with unenhanced liver parenchyma. Visualization of the hematoma and the laceration is improved by intravenous contrast administration, which enhances liver parenchyma.

SUGGESTED READING

Alpern MB, Lawson TL, Foley WD, et al.: Focal hepatic masses and fatty infiltration detected by enhanced dynamic CT. Radiology, 158:45–49, 1986.

Baker MK, Wenker JC, Cockerill EM, et al.: Focal fatty infiltration of the liver: Diagnostic imaging. Radiographics, 5:923–939, 1985.

Balfe DM, Mauro MA, Koehler RE, et al.: Gastrohepatic ligament: Normal and pathologic CT anatomy. Radiology, 150:485–490, 1984.

Brant WE, Floyd JL, Jackson DE, et al.: The radiological evaluation of hepatic cavernous hemangioma. JAMA, 257:2471–2474, 1987.

Bree RL, Schwab RE, Glazer GM, et al.: The varied appearances of hepatic cavernous hemangiomas with sonography, computed tomography, magnetic resonance imaging, and scintigraphy. Radiographics, 7:1153–1175, 1987.

Harbin WP, Robert NJ, Ferrucci JT: Diagnosis of cirrhosis based on regional changes in hepatic morphology. Radiology, 135:273–283, 1980.

Mathieu D, Bruneton JN, Drouillard J, et al: Hepatic adenomas and focal nodular hyperplasia: Dynamic CT study. Radiology, 160:53–58, 1986.

Mukai JK, Stack CM, Turner DA, et al.: Imaging of surgically relevant hepatic vascular and segmental anatomy. Part 1. Normal anatomy. Am J Roentgenol, 149:287–292, 1987.

Mukai JK, Stack CM, Turner DA, et al.: Imaging of surgically relevant hepatic vascular and segmental anatomy. Part 2. Extent and resectability of hepatic neoplasms. Am J Roentgenol, 149:293–297, 1987.

Murphy BJ, Casillas, J., Ros PR, et al.: The CT appearance of cystic masses of the liver. Radiographics, 9:307–322, 1989.

Pagani JJ: Intrahepatic vascular territories shown by computed tomography (CT)—The value of CT in determining resectability of hepatic tumors. Radiology, 147:173–178, 1983.

Piekarski J, Goldberg HI, Royal SA, et al.: Difference between liver and spleen CT numbers in the normal adult: Its usefulness in predicting the presence of diffuse liver disease. Radiology, 137:727–729, 1980.

Rubenstein WA, Auh YH, Whalen JP, et al.: The perihepatic spaces: Computed tomographic and ultrasound imaging. Radiology, 149:231–239, 1983.

Sauerbrei EE, Lopez M: Pseudotumor of the quadrate lobe in hepatic sonography: A sign of generalized fatty infiltration. Am J Roentgenol, 147:923–927, 1986.

Sexton CC, Zeman RK: Correlation of computed tomography, sonography, and gross anatomy of the liver. Am J Roentgenol, 141:711–718, 1983.

Subramanyan BR, Balthazar EJ, Madamba MR, et al.: Sonography of portosystemic venous collaterals in portal hypertension. Radiology, 146:161–166, 1983.

Waller RM, Oliver TW, McCain AH, et al.: Computed tomography and sonography of hepatic cirrhosis and portal hypertension. Radiographics, 4:677–715, 1984.

Weinstein JB, Heiken JP, Lee JKT, et al.: High resolution CT of the porta hepatis and hepatoduodenal ligament. Radiographics, 6:55–74, 1986.

Welch TJ, Sheedy PF, Johnson CM, et al.: Radiographic characteristics of benign liver tumors: Focal nodular hyperplasia and hepatic adenoma. Radiographics, 5:673–682, 1985.

10

Biliary Tree and Gallbladder

BILIARY TREE

Anatomy

The bile ducts arise as biliary capillaries between hepatocytes. Interlobular bile ducts coalesce to form two main trunks from the right and left lobes of the liver. The common hepatic duct is formed in the porta hepatis by the junction of the main right and left bile ducts. The cystic duct runs posteriorly and inferiorly from the gallbladder neck to join the common hepatic duct and form the common bile duct. The common bile duct runs ventral to the portal vein and to the right of the hepatic artery, descending from the porta hepatis along the free right border of the hepatoduodenal ligament to behind the duodenal bulb. Its distal third turns directly caudally, descending in the groove between the descending duodenum and the head of the pancreas just ventral to the inferior vena cava. It tapers distally as it ends in the sphincter of Oddi, which protrudes into the duodenum as the ampulla of Vater. The common bile duct and the pancreatic duct share a common orifice in 60% of cases and have separate orifices in the other 40%. In any case, they are in such close proximity that tumors in the ampullary region will generally obstruct both ducts.

Normal size intrahepatic bile ducts are not usually visible on routine CT. The common hepatic duct is occasionally visualized in the porta hepatis, and the common bile duct is frequently seen descending adjacent to the descending duodenum. It is fair to use the generic term "common duct" to refer to both the common hepatic and the common bile ducts, since the cystic duct junction marking their anatomic partition is not routinely visualized on CT. The normal common duct does not exceed 7 mm in diameter when seen on CT. The portal triad in cross section has been likened to Mickey Mouse's head (Fig. 10–1), with Mickey's face representing the larger and more inferior portal vein, the right ear representing the common duct, and the left ear representing the hepatic artery. Dilatation of the bile duct is then seen as enlargement of Mickey's right ear. The bile ducts may be difficult to differentiate from blood vessels without intravenous contrast administration. Air or contrast agents from the gastrointestinal tract may reflux into the biliary tree owing to a number of causes (Table 10–1).

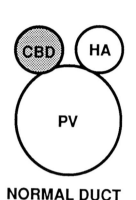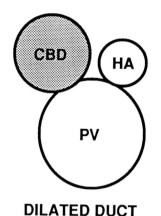

FIGURE 10–1. Anatomy of Portal Triad. Diagrammatic representation of the cross-sectional anatomy of the portal triad when the common bile duct is normal (left) and dilated (right). (PV = dorsally positioned portal vein; HA = hepatic artery; CBD = common bile duct.)

NORMAL DUCT   **DILATED DUCT**

Biliary Obstruction

CT is about 95% accurate in determining the presence, level, and cause of biliary obstruction. The major causes of biliary obstruction are gallstones, tumor, stricture, and pancreatitis. A rare but interesting cause of biliary obstruction is Mirizzi syndrome. A gallstone impacted in the cystic duct induces cholangitis or erodes into the common duct to cause obstructive jaundice.

CT diagnosis of biliary obstruction depends upon the demonstration of dilated bile ducts. The biliary tree dilates proximal to the point of obstruction, while bile ducts below the obstruction remain normal or are reduced in size. When cirrhosis, cholangitis, or periductal fibrosis prohibits dilatation of the bile ducts in obstructive jaundice, the CT will be falsely negative. The CT findings of biliary obstruction (Fig. 10–2) are

1. Multiple branching tubular, round, or oval low density structures representing dilated intrahepatic biliary ducts course toward the porta hepatis

2. Dilatation of the common duct in the porta hepatis seen as a tubular or oval fluid density structure greater than 7 mm diameter

3. Enlargement of Mickey's right ear (the common duct in the hepatoduodenal ligament) to greater than 7 mm diameter

4. Dilatation of the common duct in the pancreatic head seen as a round fluid density structure larger than 7 mm

5. Enlargement of the gallbladder to greater than 5 cm diameter, when the obstruction is distal to the cystic duct.

Clues to the cause of biliary obstruction (Fig. 10–3) include the following:

1. Abrupt termination of a dilated extrahepatic biliary duct is characteristic of a malignant process even in the absence of a visible mass. Common tumors causing biliary obstruction are pancreatic carcinoma, ampullary carcinoma, and cholangiocarcinoma. A mass is often visible on CT at the point of biliary obstruction.

TABLE 10–1. Gas in the Biliary Tree or Reflux of Contrast into the Biliary Tree

Post-Operative	***Perforated Ulcer***
Sphincterotomy	Choledochoduodenal fistula
Choledochoenterostomy	
	Carcinoma
Gallstone Fistula	Choledochoenteric fistula
Cholecystoduodenal fistula	

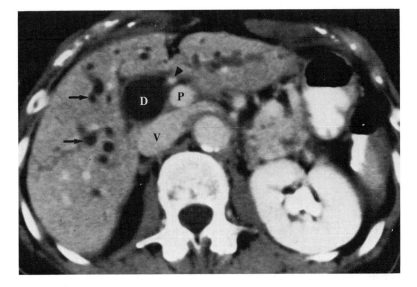

FIGURE 10–2. Dilated Bile Ducts. The greatly dilated common bile duct (D) is seen superior to the inferior vena cava (V) and to the right of the hepatic artery (arrowhead) and portal vein (P). Dilated intrahepatic bile ducts (arrows) are seen as low density branching tubular structures within the liver.

2. Gradual tapering of a dilated duct is seen most commonly with benign disease such as inflammatory stricture or pancreatitis. Calcifications in the pancreas are a clue to the presence of chronic pancreatitis.

3. Gallstones obstructing the bile ducts are seen as calcific or soft-tissue density structures within the bile duct surrounded by a crescent of fluid density bile. Some stones are isodense with bile and are not detectable by CT.

Cholangiocarcinoma

Cholangiocarcinoma is a slow growing primary carcinoma of the bile ducts. While it may arise anywhere in the biliary tree, it occurs most frequently in the common bile duct between the cystic duct and the ampulla of Vater. The tumor is frequently small at the time of discovery because it causes jaundice early in its course. Focal or generalized biliary dilatation leads to the point of tumor obstruction. The tumor itself may be isodense with surrounding parenchyma, or too small to see on CT. When visible, it is generally hypodense compared with liver parenchyma and infiltrates surrounding tissues.

Caroli's Disease

Caroli's disease is a rare congenital anomaly of the biliary tract characterized by saccular dilatation of the intrahepatic biliary tree, cholangitis, and gallstone formation in the absence of cirrhosis or portal hypertension. CT demonstrates nonuniform dilatation of the intrahepatic biliary tree with focal areas of tubular and saccular enlargement (Fig. 10–4).

Choledochal Cyst

Choledochal cyst is a congenital segmental dilatation of the common bile duct. Three major types have been described: (1) symmetric ectasia of the entire

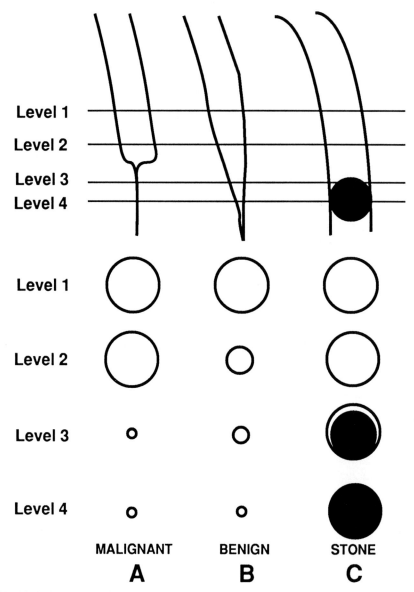

FIGURE 10–3. Clues to the Cause of Biliary Obstruction. Malignant tumors cause abrupt termination of the distal common bile duct as in *(A)*. Inflammatory strictures and pancreatitis cause progressive tapering of the distal common bile duct, as in *(B)*. Impacted gallstones *(C)* may be seen as rounded structures in the distal common bile duct. The CT density of gallstones varies from calcific density to fat density.

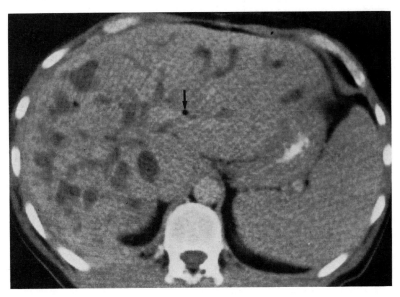

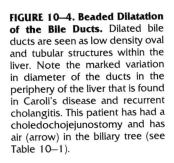

FIGURE 10–4. Beaded Dilatation of the Bile Ducts. Dilated bile ducts are seen as low density oval and tubular structures within the liver. Note the marked variation in diameter of the ducts in the periphery of the liver that is found in Caroli's disease and recurrent cholangitis. This patient has had a choledochojejunostomy and has air (arrow) in the biliary tree (see Table 10–1).

common duct (most common) (Fig. 10–5), (2) diverticulum of the common bile duct, and (3) localized fusiform dilatation of the distal common bile duct (choledochocele). On CT choledochal cyst appears as a well-defined, fluid-filled structure separate from the gallbladder and associated with dilatation of the intrahepatic biliary tree. Identification of bile ducts joining the cystic mass proves the diagnosis.

GALLBLADDER

Anatomy

The gallbladder lies in a fossa formed by the junction of the right and left lobes of the liver. While the position of the fundus is quite variable, the neck and body of the gallbladder are invariably related to the region of the porta hepatis and major interlobar fissure. The gallbladder is in close proximity to the duodenal bulb and hepatic flexure of the colon.

Ultrasound, not CT, is the primary imaging modality for the gallbladder. However, significant gallbladder pathology may be diagnosed by CT, especially when screening the acutely ill patient. Normal bile is of fluid density (0 to 20 H) on CT. The gallbladder wall enhances avidly with contrast administration.

Gallstones

While gallstones may be detected by CT, its sensitivity is much less than that of ultrasound or oral cholecystography. Gallstones vary in CT density from negative numbers indicating fat density (pure cholesterol stones) to high positive numbers of calcified stones (Fig. 10–6). Fissured stones may contain linear streaks of air. Some gallstones may not be seen on CT because they are isodense with bile, or because they are too small. Contrast in adjacent bowel loops may obscure or mimic gallstones.

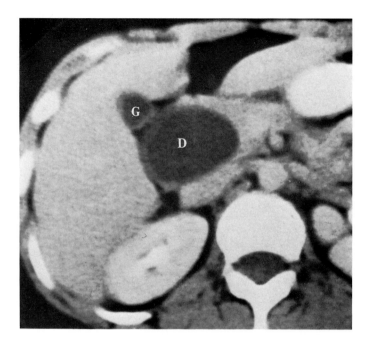

FIGURE 10–5. Choledochal Cyst. The common bile duct (D) is massively enlarged. The neck of the gallbladder (G) is seen adjacent to the dilated common bile duct.

Acute Cholecystitis

Acute cholecystitis is usually diagnosed clinically, or by ultrasound or radionuclide hepatobiliary scan. Cases are seen on CT usually because they are atypical or complicated. Gangrenous cholecystitis may lead to perforation, abscess, fistula, or peritonitis. Acalculous cholecystitis occurs most commonly in critically ill patients, especially following surgery, trauma, burns, or in patients on hyperalimentation. Emphysematous cholecystitis may produce deceptively mild symptoms but carries a high morbidity and mortality. The CT findings in acute cholecystitis (Fig. 10–7) are

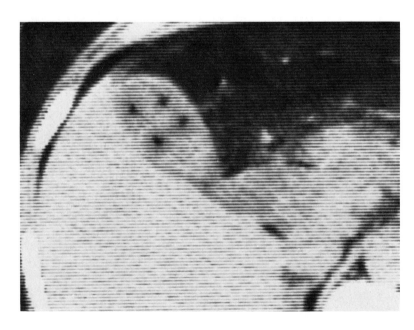

FIGURE 10–6. Gallstones. These gallstones are easily seen within the gallbladder because their high fat content makes them less dense than bile. Note the low density centers of pure cholesterol.

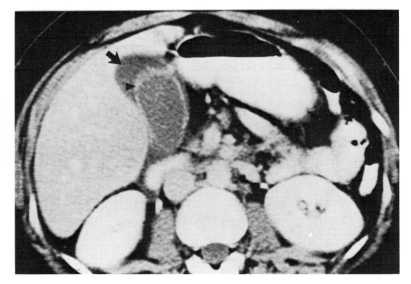

FIGURE 10–7. Acute Cholecystitis. The gallbladder wall (arrowhead) enhances brightly following intravenous contrast administration in this patient with acalculous cholecystitis. Note the pericholecystic fluid (arrow).

1. Gallstones in 95%
2. Distended gallbladder lumen > 5 cm
3. Thickening of the gallbladder wall > 3 mm
4. Halo of subserosal edema in the gallbladder wall
5. Pericholecystic fluid collection associated with perforation
6. Increase in bile density (20 H) due to biliary stasis, intraluminal pus, hemorrhage, or cellular debris
7. Air in the gallbladder wall (emphysematous cholecystitis).

Gallbladder Carcinoma

Primary carcinoma of the gallbladder is commonly misdiagnosed preoperatively. CT provides an excellent method of evaluation. Chronic cholelithiasis is the major risk factor for this tumor. Calcification of the gallbladder wall (porcelain gallbladder) is associated with a 10 to 25 percent incidence of developing carcinoma. CT findings in gallbladder carcinoma are

1. Intraluminal soft tissue mass
2. Focal or diffuse thickening of the gallbladder wall
3. Subhepatic mass replacing the gallbladder
4. Gallstones (80%)
5. Calcification of the gallbladder wall, particularly if interrupted
6. Extension of tumor into liver, subhepatic space, extrahepatic bile ducts, or adjacent bowel.

SUGGESTED READING

Barakos JA, Ralls PW, Lapin SA, et al.: Cholelithiasis: Evaluation with CT. Radiology, 162:415–418, 1987.
Baron RL: CT diagnosis of choledocholithiasis. Semin Ultrasound CT MR, 8:85–102, 1987.
Lane J, Buck JL, Zeman RK: Primary carcinoma of the gallbladder: A pictorial essay. Radiographics, 9:209–228, 1989.
May GR, James EM, Bender CE, et al.: Diagnosis and treatment of jaundice. Radiographics, 6:847–890, 1986.

11

Spleen

ANATOMY

The spleen occupies a relatively constant position in the left upper quadrant of the abdomen. It is a soft and pliable organ that conforms to the shape of adjacent structures. The diaphragmatic surface is smooth and convex, conforming to the dome of the diaphragm, while the visceral surface has concavities for the stomach, kidney, and colon. The splenic artery and vein course in close relationship with the pancreas to the splenic hilum, where each vessel divides into multiple branches.

The CT density of the normal spleen is always less than or equal to the CT density of the normal liver. Most splenic lesions are seen best on contrast-enhanced CT scans. The spleen enhances irregularly following bolus injection of contrast agents, forming transient pseudomasses due to variable rates of blood flow through its pulp (Fig. 11–1). Lobulations in the splenic contour may also be mistaken for masses, but can generally be identified on serial slices as part of the spleen.

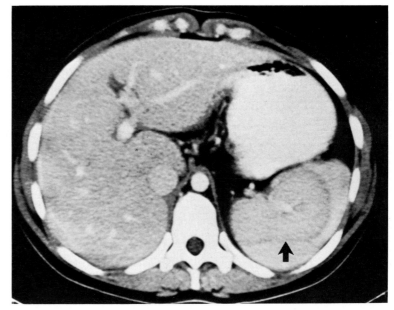

FIGURE 11–1. Splenic pseudomass. Inhomogeneous enhancement of the spleen produces a pseudomass (arrow) during the early stage of intravenous contrast administration using a power injector. Images obtained a few minutes later (not shown) demonstrated uniform density of the spleen.

Accessory spleens are present in 10 to 30% of individuals. These appear as round or oval masses up to 2 to 3 cm in diameter, most commonly located in the hilum of the spleen and around the tail of the pancreas. They have the same CT density as the spleen. Accessory spleens may hypertrophy following splenic resection. A radionuclide liver-spleen scan using technetium sulphur colloid can confirm a hypertrophied accessory spleen as functioning splenic tissue.

TECHNIQUE

The spleen is best examined using contiguous 10-mm-thick slices following intravenous injection of contrast agents. Unenhanced scans add little diagnostic information. When splenic pseudomasses due to early non-uniform contrast distribution (Fig. 11–1) are suspected, rescanning the spleen a few minutes later will usually demonstrate uniform enhancement.

SPLENOMEGALY

Spleen size varies with age, body habitus, and nutrition. Younger adults tend to have larger spleens than older adults. Judging spleen size is largely subjective. Size greater than 12 cm in the long axis and extension below the costal margin or substantially below the upper pole of the left kidney are signs of enlargement. The causes of splenomegaly are exhaustive but generally fall into myeloproliferative, infectious, congestive, and infiltrative categories. Most conditions affect CT density of the spleen minimally, so differentiation is based upon other CT findings or clinical evaluation.

LOW DENSITY LESIONS IN THE SPLEEN

Infarction

This classically appears as a wedge-shaped hypodense area. However, since infarcts are often multiple, of variable size, and frequently fuse with each other, the wedge shape is often lost. The key finding is extension of the low density area to the capsule of the spleen without causing mass effect (Fig. 11–2). The infarcted areas progressively atrophy, eventually resulting in notching of the splenic contour and occasionally calcification. Sickle cell and cardiac disease, lymphoma, and metastases are predisposing conditions to splenic infarction. Infarcts provide fertile soil for abscess formation.

Lymphoma

The spleen is the largest lymphoid organ in the body, so it is hardly surprising that involvement by lymphoma is common (Fig. 11–3). Lymphoma of the spleen may cause splenomegaly, a large solitary mass, or multiple focal

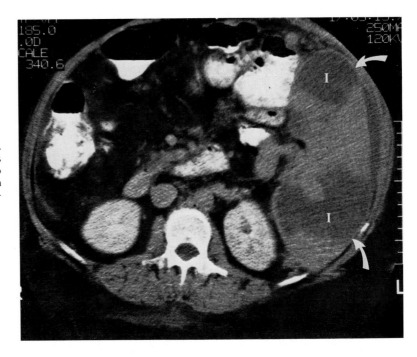

FIGURE 11–2. Splenic infarction. Splenic infarctions (I) are seen as low density areas extending to the splenic capsule (arrows) in this patient with massive splenomegaly.

nodules. However, lymphoma, especially Hodgkin's lymphoma, may involve the spleen and not be detectable by CT. Adenopathy in the splenic hilum and elsewhere in the abdomen is frequent.

Hematoma

Intrasplenic hematomas usually occur as a result of trauma, but may evolve spontaneously in a diseased spleen. Subcapsular hematomas appear as crescen-

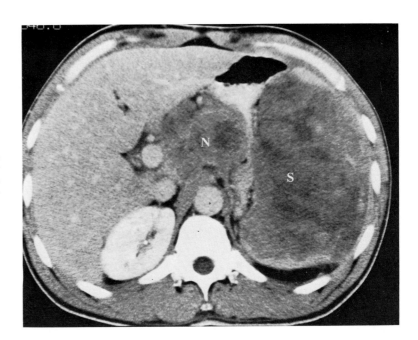

FIGURE 11–3. Lymphoma. Non-Hodgkin's lymphoma produces splenomegaly with a mottled low density area throughout the spleen (S) and massive adenopathy (N) in the upper abdomen.

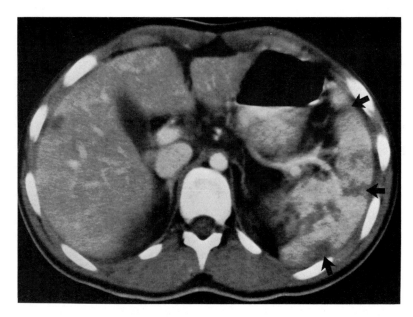

FIGURE 11–4. Shattered spleen. Multiple lacerations produce low density bands (arrows) extending through the spleen of this patient injured in a motor vehicle accident.

tic areas of hypodensity along the margin of the spleen, flattening or indenting the splenic parenchyma. Splenic lacerations are seen as low density bands or clefts traversing the splenic parenchyma (Fig. 11–4). Lacerations extend through the splenic capsule and are associated with perisplenic fluid collections and hemoperitoneum. Intrasplenic hematomas and splenic contusions appear as low density intrasplenic masses. CT can be effectively used to judge the severity of splenic injury in acute trauma. Splenic hematomas resolve gradually over months, with some leaving behind fibrous scars or calcifications.

Abscess

Abscesses occur uncommonly but result in a high mortality when untreated. Signs and symptoms may be vague. Diseased spleens are particularly susceptible to abscess formation when organisms are delivered hematogenously from distant foci of infection. Abscesses may also result from spread of infection from adjacent organs or from suppuration in a traumatic hematoma. They appear as single or multiple low density masses with ill-defined thick walls. They may contain gas or demonstrate fluid levels. Diagnosis is confirmed by aspiration. Treatment is by splenectomy or catheter drainage.

Metastases

Malignant melanoma, lung, breast, and ovarian carcinoma are the most common sources of splenic metastases. Most appear as ill-defined low density nodules (Fig. 11–5), but some form well-defined cystic masses.

Cysts

Cystic masses in the spleen may be caused by a wide range of conditions. Post-traumatic cysts (Fig. 11–6) are the final stage of intrasplenic hematomas

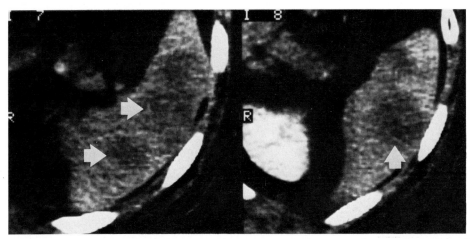

FIGURE 11–5. Spleen metastases. Metastases from malignant melanoma produce poorly marginated low density masses (arrows) in the spleen.

and make up the majority of splenic cysts. Internal debris and fluid levels are common. Calcification is found in the wall in 10%. Congenital epidermoid cysts are well-defined, spherical, and have irregular thick walls with peripheral trabeculations. Internal blood and debris are common. Echinococcal cysts may be indistinguishable from traumatic and epidermoid cysts, but are rare in the United States. Multiseptate appearance and calcification in the wall are common. Pancreatic fluid collections may gain access to the splenic parenchyma from the pancreatic tail by dissection through the splenic hilum.

Primary Tumors

Primary splenic tumors are rare. Benign hemangiomas are the most common. They vary from homogeneous solid to multicystic in appearance.

FIGURE 11–6. Post-traumatic splenic cyst. Liquefaction of an old hematoma resulted in formation of this cystic mass (arrow) in the splenic hilum. Note the calcification in the wall.

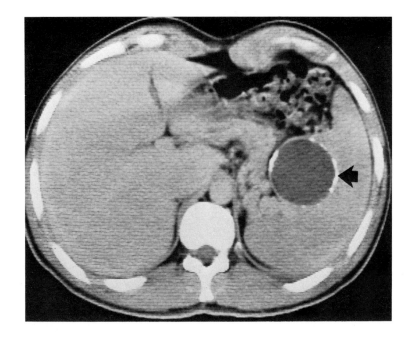

Calcification may be mottled and central or peripheral and curvilinear. Hemangiosarcomas are heterogeneous masses with mixed solid and cystic components.

SUGGESTED READING

Balcar I, Seltzer SE, Davis S, et al.: CT patterns of splenic infarction: A clinical and experimental study. Radiology, 151:723–729, 1984.

Balthazar EJ, Hilton S, Naidich D, et al.: CT of splenic and perisplenic abnormalities in septic patients. Am J Roentgenol, 144:53–56, 1985.

Beahrs JR, Stehens DH: Enlarged accessory spleens: CT appearance in postsplenectomy patients. Am J Roentgenol, 135:483–486, 1980.

Dachman AH, Ros PR, Murari PJ, et al.: Nonparasitic splenic cysts: A report of 52 cases with radiologic-pathologic correlation. Am J Roentgenol, 147:537–542, 1986.

Glazer GM, Axel L, Goldberg HI, et al.: Dynamic CT of the normal spleen. Am J Roentgenol, 137:343–346, 1981.

Meyer JE, Harris NL, Elman A, et al.: Large-cell lymphoma of the spleen: CT appearance. Radiology 148:199–201, 1983.

Mirvis SE, Whitley NO, Gens DR: Blunt splenic trauma in adults: CT-based classification and correlation with prognosis and treatment. Radiology, 171:33–39, 1989.

Piekarski J, Federle MP, Moss AA, et al.: Computed tomography of the spleen. Radiology, 135:683–689, 1980.

Ros PR, Moser RP Jr, Dachman AH, et al.: Hemangioma of the spleen: Radiologic-pathologic correlation in ten cases. Radiology, 162:73–77, 1987.

Scatamacchia SA., Raptopoulos V, Fink MP, et al.: Splenic trauma in adults: Impact of CT grading on management. Radiology, 171–725–729, 1989.

12

Kidneys

ANATOMY OF THE RETROPERITONEAL SPACE

Detailed understanding of the retroperitoneal fascial planes and compartments is a prerequisite for accurate interpretation of abdominal CT. The retroperitoneal space between the diaphragm and the pelvic brim is divided into anterior pararenal, perirenal, and posterior pararenal compartments by the anterior and posterior renal fascia (Fig. 12–1).

The anterior pararenal space extends between the posterior parietal peritoneum and the anterior renal fascia. It is bounded laterally by the lateroconal fascia, which is the continuation of the posterior lamina of the posterior renal fascia. The pancreas, duodenal loop, and ascending and descending portions of the colon are within the anterior pararenal space.

The anterior and posterior renal fascia encompass the kidney, adrenal gland, and perirenal fat within the perirenal space. The anterior renal fascia is thin and consists of one layer of connective tissue. The posterior renal fascia is thicker and consists of two layers of connective tissue. The anterior layer of the posterior renal fascia is continuous with the anterior renal fascia. The posterior layer of the posterior renal fascia is continuous with the lateroconal fascia forming the lateral boundary of the anterior pararenal space. The anterior and posterior layers of the posterior renal fascia may be separated by inflammatory processes extending from the anterior pararenal space (Fig. 14–2). The perirenal space is discontinuous across the midline due to fusion of the renal fascial layers with connective tissues surrounding the aorta and vena cava. The perirenal compartment narrows as it extends inferiorly to form an inverted cone shape. The ureter passes through the apex of the cone.

The posterior pararenal space is a potential space, usually filled only with fat, extending from the posterior renal fascia to the transversalis fascia. The posterior pararenal fat continues into the flank as the properitoneal fat stripe seen on plain films of the abdomen. The compartment is limited medially by the lateral edge of the psoas and quadratus lumborum muscles.

The kidneys are covered by a tight fibrous capsule which produces a sharp margin defined by perirenal fat on CT. Subcapsular collections of fluid or blood will compress and distort the renal parenchyma without affecting the perirenal fat. The perirenal fat extends into the renal sinus, outlining blood vessels and the renal collecting system. Connective tissue septae extend between the kidney and the renal fascia. These septae may be seen as prominent stranding

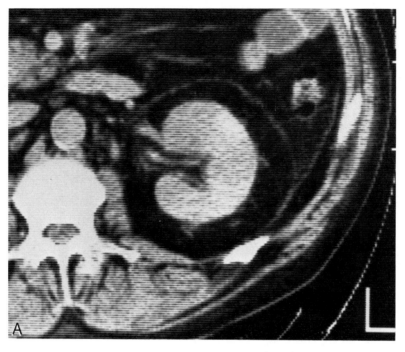

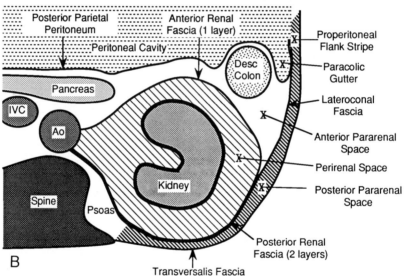

FIGURE 12–1. Retroperitoneal fascia. CT image of the left kidney (*A*) and diagrammatic representation (*B*) demonstrate the fascial planes and compartments of the retroperitoneal space.

densities in the perirenal fat when they are thickened by inflammation, hemorrhage, or ischemia. The renal arteries and veins can generally be identified from the great vessels to the kidneys. The right renal artery courses behind the vena cava. The left renal vein crosses between the aorta and the superior mesenteric artery.

Anatomic variants such as *horseshoe kidney* can be easily recognized on CT. With horseshoe kidney the lower poles are joined by an isthmus of fibrous tissue or functioning parenchyma. The kidneys are low in position and of abnormal axis.

TECHNIQUE

Because the kidneys actively concentrate contrast within the parenchyma, virtually all renal abnormalities are best seen on CT following contrast administration. The only indication to perform an unenhanced CT is to demonstrate calcifications and calculi which may be obscured by contrast. The kidneys are scanned with contiguous 10-mm-thick slices. We use 150 ml of contrast administered intravenously by power injector at 2.5 ml per second for 20 seconds followed by 1 ml per second for 100 seconds. Scanning is begun 30 seconds following initiation of contrast injection.

RENAL TUMORS

Renal Cell Carcinoma

Most solid renal masses in adults are renal cell carcinomas. Surgical excision is the only effective therapy, so preoperative CT staging of the extent of disease is important. Significant CT findings include the following:

Primary Tumor. Most are predominantly solid, but low density regions due to necrosis and hemorrhage are common (Fig. 12–2). Even strongly enhancing tumors are lower in density than enhanced renal parenchyma. Cystic and complex multilocular cystic forms are also seen. Stippled central or "eggshell" peripheral calcifications are seen in 10%. Visualization of tortuous vessels in the perirenal fat is evidence of the hypervascularity common in renal cell carcinoma.

Venous Invasion. Tumor growth into the renal vein occurs in 30% and extends into the vena cava in 5 to 10%. While venous invasion does not preclude curative surgical resection, its identification is crucial to surgical planning. Involved renal veins are enlarged, enhance poorly, and are filled with visible tumor

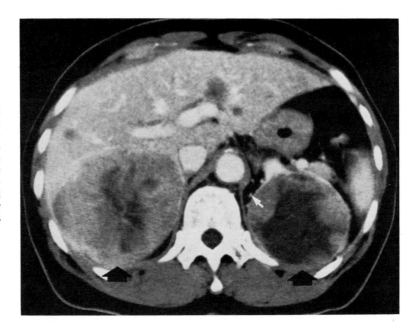

FIGURE 12–2. Bilateral renal cell carcinoma. An image through the upper abdomen demonstrates renal cell carcinomas (black arrows) arising from the upper poles of both kidneys. The low density regions within the tumors are areas of necrosis and hemorrhage. The white arrow shows enhancing tumor vessels in the perirenal fat.

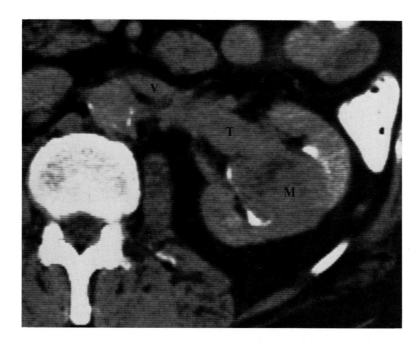

FIGURE 12–3. Renal carcinom **invading renal vein.** A renal ce carcinoma (M) arising within th renal sinus of the left kidney ex tends into the left renal vein (T The renal vein (V) is of normal siz anterior to the aorta, but is en larged and nodular in the portio of the vein containing tumor (T This tumor did not extend into the perirenal fat.

thrombus seen as nodular low density within the vein (Fig. 12–3). This nodular low density may extend into the vena cava all the way to the right atrium.

Tumor Spread.

1. Local extension is seen as strands or nodules of low density extending into the perirenal fat and to adjacent organs.

2. Lymphatic spread is evidenced by enlargement of renal hilar, pericaval, and periaortic nodes to 15 mm or more.

3. Hematogenous spread favors lung, bone, liver, adrenals, and the opposite kidney. CT of the chest and radionuclide bone scans are routine components of preoperative evaluation.

Interestingly, distant metastases will occasionally melt away with removal of the primary tumor. Late appearance of metastases as long as 20 years following "cure" is also seen.

Transitional Cell Carcinoma

Tumors arising from the epithelium of the renal collecting system account for 5 to 10% of renal tumors. Most (85%) are transitional cell carcinoma. The remainder are squamous cell carcinoma. Because hematuria is common, these tumors usually present earlier than renal cell carcinoma and thus are frequently smaller. CT findings include (Fig. 12–4)

Primary Tumor. Most appear as soft tissue density filling defects within the renal pelvis or within the renal sinus, distorting and compressing collecting structures. Enhancement is poor and calcifications are rare. Unenhanced CT numbers (15 to 30 H) are greater than unopacified urine but much less than even radiolucent calculi (150 to 200 H). CT is an excellent method to differentiate small tumors from calculi.

Tumor Spread.

1. Local spread is seen as low density tumor extension into or through the renal parenchyma and from the sinus into the perirenal fat.

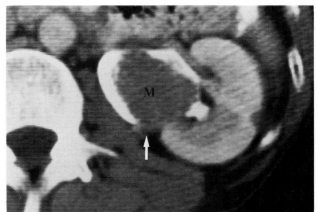

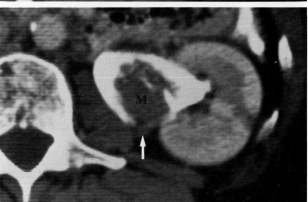

FIGURE 12–4. Transitional cell carcinoma. Two sequential images of the left kidney demonstrate a transitional cell carcinoma (M) occupying the renal pelvis. The tumor extends through the renal pelvis into the perirenal fat (arrows).

2. Lymphatic spread is seen as enlargement of regional nodes.

3. Synchronous tumors in the ipsilateral ureter and bladder should be searched for carefully.

Angiomyolipoma

CT reflects the composition of this benign tumor made up of varying amounts of blood vessel, smooth muscle, and fat. In 20% of cases, the angiomyolipomas are multiple, bilateral, and occur in patients with tuberous sclerosis. In 80%, the tumor is solitary, unilateral, and the patient is usually a middle-aged woman. Hemorrhage is the most frequent complication of the tumor. Because renal cell carcinomas do not contain fat detectable by CT, demonstration of fat content allows a specific diagnosis of angiomyolipoma (Fig. 12–5):

1. Fatty areas of tumor have attenuation values of -80 to -120 H.

2. Smooth muscle and vascular components of the tumor appear as nodules, whorls, and strands of soft tissue density within the fatty mass.

3. Hypervascular areas of the tumor may show striking contrast enhancement.

4. Tumors are commonly as small as 1 cm but may reach 20 cm and extend into perirenal tissues and lymph nodes.

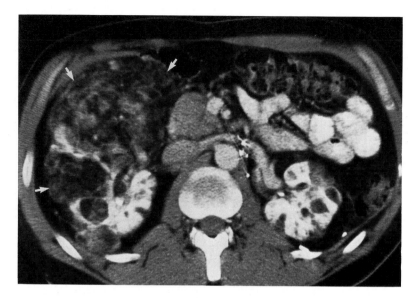

FIGURE 12–5. Bilateral angiomyolipomas. Both kidneys in this patient with tuberous sclerosis are extensively replaced by angiomyolipomas. The tumor (arrows) arising from the right kidney extends all the way to the anterior abdominal wall. Low density areas within the tumor are identical in density to subcutaneous and intra-abdominal fat, confirming the diagnosis of angiomyolipoma. Soft tissue density nodules and strands correspond to smooth muscle components of the tumor. Functioning renal parenchyma enhances brightly with contrast.

Renal Lymphoma

Lymphoma may present in the kidney as multiple parenchymal nodules (most common), invasion from perirenal disease, solitary solid mass, or diffuse infiltration causing renal enlargement. Signs that suggest lymphoma include bilaterality, extensive adenopathy, and splenomegaly.

RENAL CYSTIC DISEASE

Cystic Renal Masses

Cystic renal masses are an extremely common finding on abdominal CT. The challenge is to separate the ubiquitous simple cyst from a host of other cystic lesions.

Simple Cyst. Simple renal cysts are benign non-neoplastic fluid-filled masses that affect half the population over age 55. Small cysts are asymptomatic incidental findings. Large cysts (> 4 cm) occasionally cause hypertension, hematuria, pain, or ureteral obstruction. Multiple and bilateral cysts are common. Strict criteria which allow confident diagnosis of a renal mass as a simple cyst are

1. Sharp margination with the renal parenchyma
2. No perceptible wall
3. Homogeneous attenuation near water density (-10 to $+20$ H)
4. No evidence of enhancement following intravenous contrast administration.

Cysts smaller than 1 cm cause a problem in diagnosis because of volume averaging. Most of these can be confirmed as simple cysts by rescanning using thinner slices, by ultrasound, or by followup CT demonstrating no change. Thick walls may be simulated by imaging a beak of normal renal parenchyma abutting the cyst, or by the increased enhancement observed in compressed renal parenchyma adjacent to a cyst.

When a renal mass appears cystic but does not meet the criteria for simple cyst the following lesions should be considered:

Complicated Simple Cyst. Simple cysts may be complicated by hemorrhage, infection (Fig. 12–6), or calcification within the wall. Some may have internal septations. Multiple simple cysts adjacent to each other may appear as a complex mass. Observation over time or percutaneous aspiration biopsy may be required.

Renal Abscess. Pyelonephritis complicated by suppuration and liquefaction may result in formation of an abscess requiring drainage. On CT, abscesses appear as thick walled, low density fluid collections within the renal parenchyma. Gas is sometimes seen within the pus collection. The wall commonly enhances with contrast administration. Extension of infection into the perirenal space is not uncommon.

Renal Cell Carcinoma. Some renal carcinomas are comprised of multiple fluid-filled noncommunicating cystic spaces. Malignant tumor cells line the loculations. Rarely, renal carcinoma may arise within or adjacent to a simple renal cyst.

Multilocular Cystic Nephroma. This uncommon benign renal neoplasm is composed of cysts of varying size separated by connective tissue septa. They are seen in infants, young children, and middle-aged women. Surgical removal is usually necessary to differentiate it from renal carcinoma.

Multiple Renal Cysts

When multiple renal cysts are encountered the following conditions should be considered:

Multiple Simple Cysts. Simple cysts increase in frequency with age and are commonly multiple and bilateral. Patients over age 50 with no cysts in other organs, and who have no family history of renal cystic disease, are most likely to have multiple simple cysts.

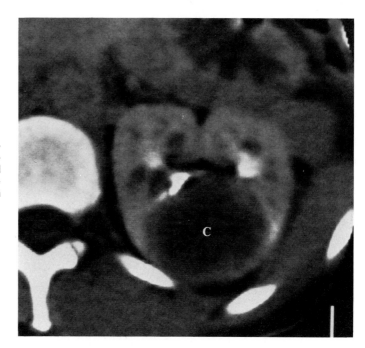

FIGURE 12–6. Infected renal cyst. This cystic renal mass (C) has poorly defined margination with the renal parenchyma and thickened, poorly defined walls. Percutaneous aspiration confirmed infection within a simple renal cyst.

Adult Polycystic Disease. The cortex and medulla of both kidneys are progressively replaced by multiple noncommunicating cysts of varying size in this common hereditary disorder transmitted as an autosomal dominant trait. While it may be detected in childhood, most cases present clinically with hypertension and renal failure between ages 30 and 50. CT findings become more pronounced as the disease progresses. Diagnostic findings include (Fig. 12–7)

1. Progressive replacement of renal parenchyma with cysts of varying size
2. Progressive bilateral increase in renal volume
3. Multiple cysts in the liver in 30 to 50%
4. Multiple cysts in the pancreas in 10%.

The renal cysts are commonly complicated by bleeding or infection, which causes thickening of the cyst walls and an increase in density of cyst fluid. Berry aneurysms are present in the circle of Willis in 10 to 15%. Adult polycystic disease is differentiated from other conditions by the presence of cysts in other organs, positive family history, presence of renal failure, and hypertension.

Multicystic Dysplastic Kidney. This is a nonhereditary renal dysplasia in which the kidney consists of multiple thin walled cysts held together by connective tissue. The involved kidney is functionless. At birth the involved kidney is greatly enlarged. With age the kidney progressively shrinks and often becomes calcified. Rarely, only a portion of one kidney may be involved. Bilateral multicystic dysplastic kidneys occur but are fatal at birth. The opposite kidney is affected by ureteropelvic junction obstruction or other anomaly in 30% of cases.

von Hippel – Lindau Syndrome. This is a genetically transmitted disorder characterized by retinal angiomas and cerebellar hemangioblastomas associated with abdominal cysts and tumors. Central nervous system abnormalities usually predominate. Abdominal findings (Fig. 12–8) include multiple renal and pancreatic cysts, small renal adenomas, and frequent multiple and bilateral renal adenocarcinomas. The hereditary pattern is autosomal dominant with variable expressivity often not manifest until between ages 20 and 50.

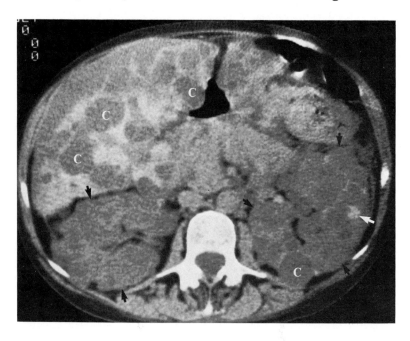

FIGURE 12–7. Adult polycystic disease. An unenhanced CT image of the upper abdomen demonstrates innumerable cysts (C) existing in the liver and replacing and enlarging both kidneys (black arrowheads). Residual renal parenchyma is seen as islands of higher density (white arrow) surrounded by cysts. Because renal failure is progressive, these patients are usually studied without intravenous contrast to avoid its nephrotoxic effects.

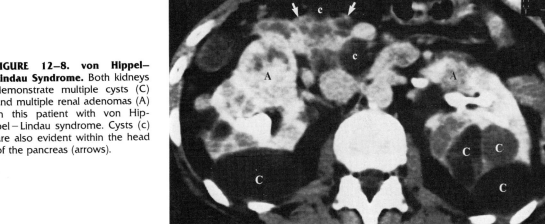

FIGURE 12–8. von Hippel–Lindau Syndrome. Both kidneys demonstrate multiple cysts (C) and multiple renal adenomas (A) in this patient with von Hippel–Lindau syndrome. Cysts (c) are also evident within the head of the pancreas (arrows).

Tuberous Sclerosis. This autosomal dominant syndrome combines multiple renal cysts and multiple and bilateral renal angiomyolipomas (Fig. 12–5) with cutaneous, retinal, and cerebral hamartomas. The renal lesions are commonly detected in infancy and childhood.

Renal Dialysis. Patients on maintenance hemodialysis commonly develop multiple cysts in their native kidneys. Multicentric renal adenomas and carcinomas develop in as many as 9% of patients.

STONES AND OBSTRUCTION

Stones

The major use of CT in renal stone disease is to differentiate radiolucent calculi from other causes of filling defects in the renal collecting system, such as tumor or hematoma. Even uric acid, xanthine, or cystine stones, which are radiolucent on plain film, appear high density on CT photographed for soft tissues. Most calculi have attenuation values in the range of 193 to 540 H (Fig. 12–9). Uroepithelial tumors have attenuation values of 20 to 46 H unenhanced and 64 to 84 H enhanced. Blood clots have attenuation values of 58 to 60 H similar to tumor, but can be observed to move with changes in patient position, or to disappear with time.

CT is a poorer detector of small calcified renal stones than is plain film. CT spatial resolution is greatly limited by volume averaging. When contrast is administered, stones in the renal collecting system are often obscured by contrast concentration in the urine. CT for renal calculi should be performed without contrast, and thin slices (5 mm or less) should be used.

Obstruction

The dilated collecting structures occurring with obstruction are readily demonstrated by CT, either without or with contrast. Dependent layering of

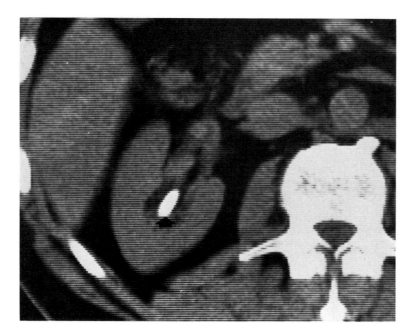

FIGURE 12–9. Uric acid stone. A CT image of the right kidney obtained without contrast administration demonstrates a pure uric acid stone (arrow) as a high density oval object in the renal sinus. CT attenuation measured 240 H. The stone appeared as an entirely radiolucent filling defect on an excretory urogram.

unopacified urine over heavier contrast material is commonly observed within dilated collecting structures. The affected kidney may show delayed contrast excretion. CT is effective in determining both the level and cause of obstruction by demonstrating calculi, tumor, or extrinsic mass. CT shows the parenchymal thinning that occurs with chronic obstruction.

RENAL TRAUMA

CT effectively demonstrates the exact nature and extent of renal injury and associated hematoma in trauma. Dynamic contrast-enhanced studies demonstrate the abnormalities best. The types of renal injury are:

Renovascular Injury. Failure of the kidney to enhance following intravenous contrast administration is evidence of vascular injury. If the entire kidney fails to enhance, occlusion of the renal artery due to intimal flap is suspected. Immediate surgical repair is generally needed. Angiography may be indicated since CT cannot demonstrate the specific anatomic lesion.

Renal Contusion. A patchy or "moth-eaten" pattern of enhancement which may be diffuse, lobar, or focal is evidence of renal contusion. This injury can be treated conservatively.

Subcapsular Hematoma. This is the most frequent type of renal injury due to blunt trauma. Blood collects beneath the renal capsule and flattens adjacent renal parenchyma. The perirenal space remains normal. This minor injury is managed conservatively.

Renal Laceration/Fracture. Blood in the perirenal space is evidence of renal laceration or fracture disrupting the renal capsule (Fig. 12–10). A lucent defect may be seen extending through the parenchyma. The kidney may be separated into two or more portions. Multiple clefts and fragments indicate a *shattered kidney*. Lack of enhancement of the renal fragments implies loss of blood supply to those fragments. If the collecting system is disrupted, contrast and urine spill into the perirenal space. The resulting fluid collection is often

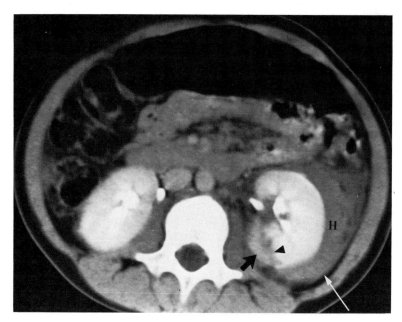

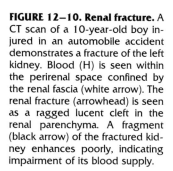

FIGURE 12–10. Renal fracture. A CT scan of a 10-year-old boy injured in an automobile accident demonstrates a fracture of the left kidney. Blood (H) is seen within the perirenal space confined by the renal fascia (white arrow). The renal fracture (arrowhead) is seen as a ragged lucent cleft in the renal parenchyma. A fragment (black arrow) of the fractured kidney enhances poorly, indicating impairment of its blood supply.

confined between the anterior and posterior leaves of renal fascia. Treatment depends upon the extent of injury and the condition of the patient.

SUGGESTED READING

Hartman DS, Davis CJ, Sanders RC, et al.: The multiloculated renal mass: Considerations and differential features. Radiographics, 7:29–52, 1987.

Love L, Meyers MA, Churchill RJ, et al.: Computed tomography of the extraperitoneal spaces. Am J Roentgenol, 136:781–789, 1981.

Newhouse JH, Prien EL, Amis ES Jr: Computed tomographic analysis of urinary calculi. Am J Roentgenol, 142:545–548, 1984.

Raptopoulos V, Kleinman PK, Marks S Jr, et al.: Renal fascial pathway: Posterior extension of pancreatic effusions within the anterior pararenal space. Radiology, 158:367–374, 1986.

Siegelman SS, Gatewood OMB, Goldman SM (eds): Computed Tomography of the Kidneys and Adrenals. Contemporary Issues in Computed Tomography, vol 3. New York, Churchill Livingstone, 1984.

Zeman RK, Cronan JJ, Rosenfield AT, et al.: Computed tomography of renal masses: Pitfalls and anatomic variants. Radiographics, 6:351–372, 1986.

13

Adrenal Glands

ANATOMY

The adrenal glands lie within the cone of renal fascia surrounded by the fat of the perirenal space. The right adrenal gland projects posteriorly from the inferior vena cava at the level where the vena cava enters the liver (Fig. 13–1). The right adrenal is medial to the right lobe of the liver and lateral to the right crus of the diaphragm just above the upper pole of the right kidney. The left adrenal (Fig. 13–2) lies medial and anterior to the upper pole of the left kidney, just lateral to the left crus of the diaphragm and posterior to the pancreas and splenic vessels.

On CT the adrenal glands have the shape of an inverted V or Y. Each limb is smooth in outline and uniform in thickness with straight or concave margins. Each limb is less than 10 mm in thickness and up to 3 cm in length. The entire gland is of uniform soft tissue density.

A major problem of adrenal CT is identifying normal and abnormal structures which simulate adrenal masses (Fig. 13–3). Masses arising from the upper pole of the kidney, tortuous splenic vessels, periadrenal portosystemic collaterals, pancreatic masses, and prominent splenic lobulations must all be differentiated from adrenal tumors. Strict attention to CT technique is the key to avoiding errors. Thin cuts (5 mm), and optimal administration of oral and intravenous contrast usually permit distinction of these various conditions.

TECHNIQUE

Screening examination of the adrenals can usually be performed using contiguous 10-mm-thick slices; however, fine detail and small tumors require 5-mm-thick slices at 5-mm or 3-mm intervals. Oral and intravenous contrast are always needed to produce an optimal study. We give 150 ml of 60% contrast by mechanical injector set at 2.5 ml per second for 20 seconds followed by 1 ml per second for 100 seconds. Scanning of the adrenals is begun 40 seconds after initiation of injection.

ADRENAL HYPERPLASIA

Hyperplasia typically enlarges both adrenal glands symmetrically without altering their shape (Fig. 13–4). The thickness of each limb exceeds 10 mm, and

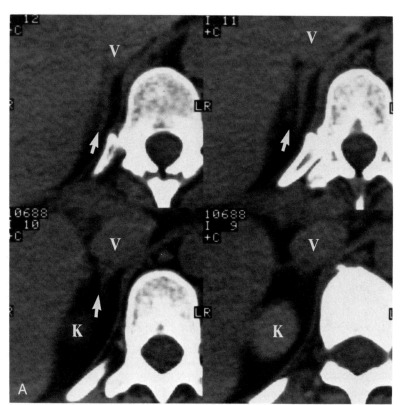

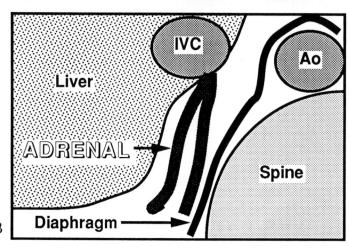

FIGURE 13–1. Normal right adrenal gland. The right adrenal (arrows) extends posteriorly from the inferior vena cava (V) between the right lobe of the liver and the right crus of the diaphragm, above the level of the upper pole of the right kidney (K). (*A*) Sequential 5-mm-thick CT slices of a normal right adrenal gland. (*B*) Diagrammatic representation of CT landmarks for the right adrenal gland. IVC = inferior vena cava; Ao = aorta.

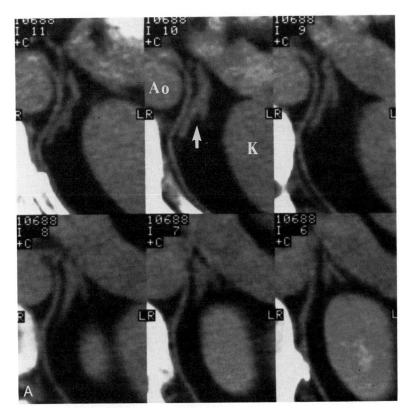

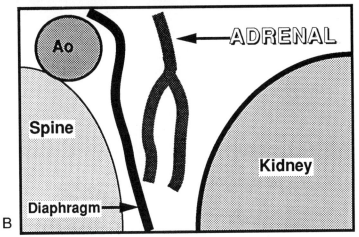

FIGURE 13–2. Normal left adrenal gland. The left adrenal (arrow) is imaged between the upper pole of the left kidney (K) and the aorta (Ao). (*A*) Sequential 5-mm-thick CT slices of a normal left adrenal gland. (*B*) Diagrammatic representation of CT landmarks for the left adrenal gland.

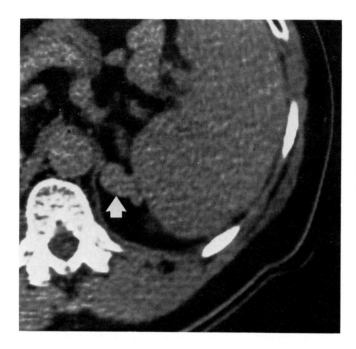

FIGURE 13–3. Perisplenic vessels. Enlarged portosystemic collateral vessels (arrow) in this patient with cirrhosis and hypertension simulate a left adrenal mass. Differentiation is made by optimizing intravenous contrast administration and carefully examining sequential images.

FIGURE 13–4. Adrenal hyperplasia. Both adrenal glands (arrows) demonstrate marked thickening of their limbs without focal masses.

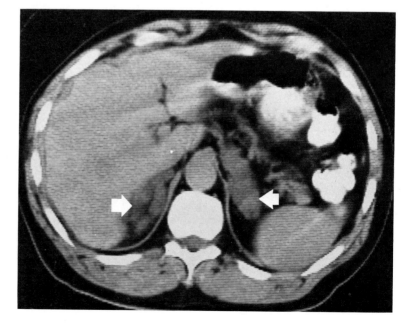

the glands appear unusually prominent. However, it is important to realize that the adrenals may be hyperfunctional in hormone secretion and even hyperplastic histologically without appearing enlarged or abnormal on CT.

Besides adrenal hyperplasia, enlarged adrenal glands may be caused by metastatic disease, granulomatous disease (tuberculosis or histoplasmosis), or bilateral adenomas in multiple endocrine neoplasia syndromes.

ADRENAL ADENOMA

Adrenal cortical adenomas may secrete hormones and be responsible for one of the syndromes listed below, or be nonfunctional and present as an incidental adrenal mass. Function cannot be determined from the CT appearance, although high cholesterol content makes some appear relatively lucent (Fig. 13–5). CT features of benign adrenal adenoma (Fig. 13–6) are

1. Small size, less than 4-cm diameter
2. Smooth, round, well-defined contour
3. Uniform soft tissue density without evidence of hemorrhage or necrosis
4. Minimal contrast enhancement
5. Calcifications uncommon.

Nonfunctional adrenal adenomas increase in incidence with age, and are commonly detected on routine CT examinations. Adrenal tumors which are less than 4 cm in size and have the appearance listed above can be considered benign and incidental if there is no evidence of excess hormonal function and no history of malignant disease. Routine followup at 3- to 6-month intervals for growth or change in appearance is recommended. Metastatic disease must be ruled out by percutaneous fine needle biopsy in patients with known malignancy. Adrenal masses larger than 6 cm in size should be considered for surgical removal because of risk of carcinoma.

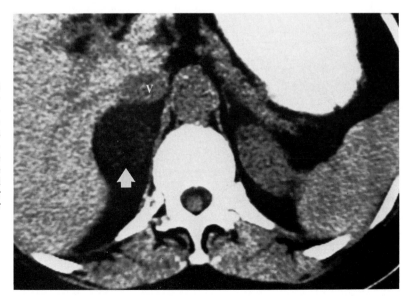

FIGURE 13–5. Benign adrenal adenoma—Conn's tumor. An aldosterone-producing benign adenoma (arrow) of the right adrenal is seen as a low density mass extending posteriorly from the inferior vena cava (V) between the liver and the right crus of the diaphragm. The high cholesterol content of this functioning tumor is believed to be responsible for its relatively low CT density.

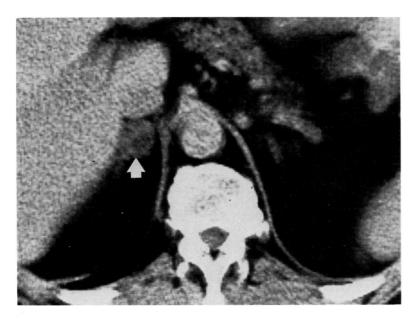

FIGURE 13–6. Benign adrenal adenoma. This benign adrenal adenoma (arrow) was found during CT staging of a squamous carcinoma of the lung. Its benign nature was confirmed by percutaneous CT-directed fine-needle biopsy. Benign adrenal adenomas are common findings even in patients with known malignancy.

ADRENAL CARCINOMA

Adrenal carcinomas are rare but highly malignant tumors with extremely poor prognosis. Five-year survival is almost zero. One-third to one-half are functional, most commonly producing Cushing's syndrome. The CT appearance of adrenal carcinoma (Fig. 13–7) is

1. Large size, averaging 12 cm median diameter, rarely smaller than 6 cm
2. Irregular, poorly defined contour
3. Large areas of internal hemorrhage, necrosis, and calcification
4. Rapid growth with invasion of adjacent organs and veins, including the inferior vena cava.

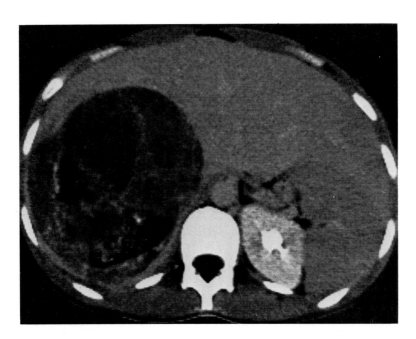

FIGURE 13–7. Adrenal carcinoma. This huge necrotic tumor replacing the right adrenal gland was discovered during evaluation for Cushing's syndrome in a 27-year-old woman.

ENDOCRINE SYNDROMES

Cushing's Syndrome

Cushing's syndrome results from excessive production of glucocorticoids. Approximately 70% of cases are due to adrenal hyperplasia resulting from pituitary adenoma or ectopic ACTH secretion. About 20% are due to adrenal adenoma, and 10% are due to adrenal carcinoma (Fig. 13–7). Most adenomas causing Cushing's syndrome are 2 to 3 cm or larger and are easily demonstrated on CT. Additional findings common with Cushing's syndrome are increased fat deposition in the subcutaneous tissues, abdomen, and liver.

Conn's Syndrome

Primary hyperaldosteronism is diagnosed clinically by the presence of hypertension, persistent hypokalemia, increased aldosterone, and decreased renin in the plasma. The role of CT is to identify the lesion. Eighty percent of cases are due to a solitary adrenal adenoma (Fig. 13–5), while 20% are due to adrenal hyperplasia. Surgical resection of adenoma is curative, while adrenal hyperplasia cases are treated medically. The difficulty is that the adenomas causing Conn's syndrome tend to be small with an average size of 1.8 cm. Optimal CT technique is required to demonstrate these small tumors.

Pheochromocytoma

Pheochromocytomas arise from the adrenal medulla and secrete catecholamines responsible for the clinical syndrome of hypertension, headaches, palpitations, and excessive sweating. Like primary hyperaldosteronism, the diagnosis is made by clinical evaluation, and the lesion is identified radiographically. Ninety percent of tumors arise from the adrenal. The tumor follows the "rule of 10's"; 10% are extra-adrenal, 10% are bilateral, and 10% are malignant. Most adrenal lesions can be demonstrated by CT:

1. Well-defined tumor usually larger than 2 cm
2. Contrast enhancement that may be uniform or nonuniform
3. Cystic degeneration, hemorrhage, necrosis, calcification common.

Multiple and bilateral tumors are generally seen in association with multiple endocrine neoplasia syndromes. Although extra-adrenal lesions have been found everywhere along the sympathetic chain from skull base to pelvis, most are in the abdomen along the course of the aorta or in the pelvis (Fig. 13–8).

Since pheochromocytoma is often sought but seldom present, the most appropriate CT strategy is to scan the adrenal alone as a screening exam. If no lesion is apparent then additional scanning is performed only when clinical diagnosis is secure.

ADRENAL METASTASES

The adrenals are a common site of metastatic deposits from common malignancies. Bilateral adrenal masses are usually metastases. The tumors may be any size, round or lobulated, homogeneous or inhomogeneous, calcified, or

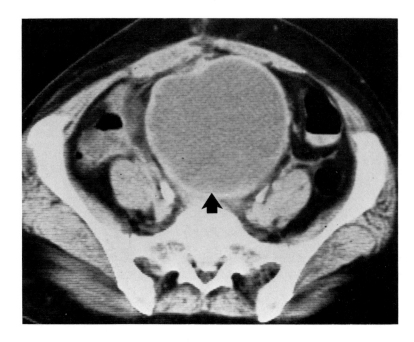

FIGURE 13–8. Pheochromocytoma. This pheochromocytoma (arrow) arose at the aortic bifurcation from the organ of Zuckerkandl. The tumor was benign, had a thick fibrous wall, and was filled with hemorrhagic fluid.

necrotic (Fig. 13–9). Despite the frequency and varied appearance of adrenal metastases, it should be noted that even in patients with known malignancy up to 50% of adrenal masses may be benign adenomas (Fig. 13–6). Percutaneous biopsy is needed for tissue diagnosis.

ADRENAL CYST

Adrenal cysts are uncommon lesions but can generally be diagnosed by CT, avoiding confusion with more significant lesions. Both true cysts with epithelial

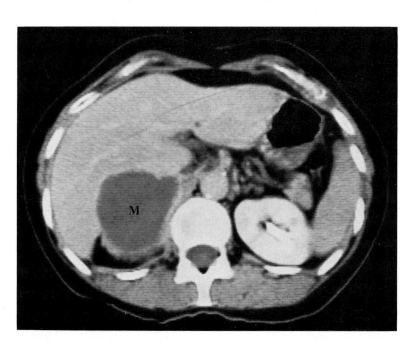

FIGURE 13–9. Necrotic adrenal metastasis. A large cell carcinoma of the lung metastasized to the right adrenal gland and produced this large cystic appearing mass (M). Note the lobulated contour, ragged margins, and thick walls. (Compare to Figure 13–10.)

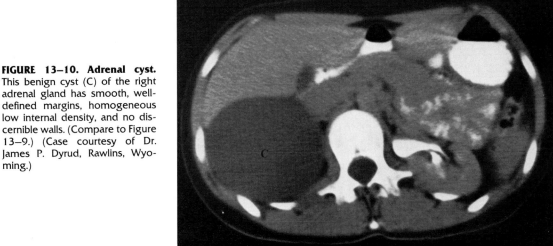

FIGURE 13–10. Adrenal cyst. This benign cyst (C) of the right adrenal gland has smooth, well-defined margins, homogeneous low internal density, and no discernible walls. (Compare to Figure 13–9.) (Case courtesy of Dr. James P. Dyrud, Rawlins, Wyoming.)

lining and pseudocysts resulting from adrenal hemorrhage occur. Both are seen as oval or round well-defined masses of uniform water density (Fig. 13–10). A calcified rim may be seen with pseudocysts. Ragged outline or thick walls suggests necrotic tumor (Fig. 13–9) rather than benign cyst.

ADRENAL MYELOLIPOMA

Myelolipomas are rare but radiographically interesting because we can usually make a specific diagnosis. They are nonfunctional tumors consisting of fat and bone marrow elements with no malignant potential. Characteristic CT findings are (Fig. 13–11) as follows

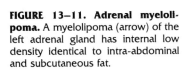
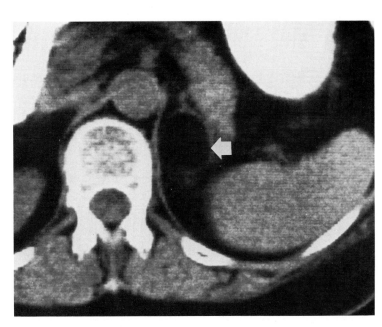

FIGURE 13–11. Adrenal myelolipoma. A myelolipoma (arrow) of the left adrenal gland has internal low density identical to intra-abdominal and subcutaneous fat.

1. Well-defined adrenal mass of any size up to 30 cm
2. Inhomogeneous central fat density (-30 to -100 H)
3. Relatively avascular, showing no contrast enhancement.

Fat density, not just low density, must be demonstrated to make a firm diagnosis. Necrotic tumors may have low density but not fat density.

SUGGESTED READING

Johnson CM, Sheedy PF II, Welch TJ, et al.: CT of the adrenal cortex. Semin Ultrasound CT MR, 6:241–260, 1985.
Johnson CM, Welch TJ, Hattery RR, et al.: CT of the adrenal medulla. Semin Ultrasound CT MR, 6:219–240, 1985.
Schultz CL: CT and MR of the adrenal glands. Semin Ultrasound CT MR, 7:219–233, 1986.

14

Pancreas

ANATOMY

The pancreas is situated within the anterior pararenal compartment of the retroperitoneal space, behind the left lobe of the liver and the stomach, and in front of the spine and great vessels (Fig. 14–1). The peritoneum lined lesser sac forms a potential space between stomach and pancreas. The pancreas somewhat resembles a question mark (?) turned on its left side with the hook portion formed by the pancreatic head and uncinate process as they lie cradled in the duodenal loop. The portal vein fills the center of the hook. The body and tail taper as they extend toward the splenic hilum. The pancreas is usually directed upward and to the left, although it may form an inverted U shape with the tail directed downward. Sequential CT slices must be mentally summated to assess the shape and size of the pancreas. The entire gland is 12 to 15 cm in length. Maximum dimensions for width are 3.0 cm for the head, 2.5 cm for the body, and 2.0 cm for the tail. The gland is larger in young patients and progressively decreases in size with age. The CT attenuation is uniform and approximately

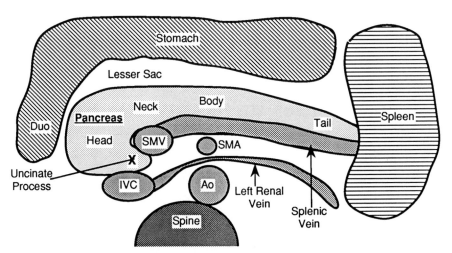

FIGURE 14–1. Pancreas anatomy. This diagram shows the CT landmarks for identification of the pancreas. The portal vein is formed behind the neck of the pancreas by the confluence of the splenic and superior mesenteric veins. The uncinate process of the pancreas extends between the superior mesenteric vein and the inferior vena cava. (SMV = superior mesenteric vein; SMA = superior mesenteric artery; IVC = inferior vena cava; Ao = aorta; Duo = descending duodenum.)

equal to muscle. Progressive infiltration of fat between the lobules of the pancreas gives it a feathery appearance with age. The pancreatic duct is best visualized with thin slices (5 mm). It measures 3 to 4 mm in width in the head and tapers smoothly to the tail.

The complex vascular anatomy about the pancreas must be understood to correctly interpret pancreatic CT. The splenic vein runs a straight course in the dorsum of the pancreas from the splenic hilum to its junction with the superior mesenteric vein just posterior to the neck of the pancreas. The plane of fat between the splenic vein and pancreas is commonly mistaken for the pancreatic duct. The splenic artery runs a markedly undulating course through the pancreas from the celiac axis to the spleen. Atherosclerotic calcifications are common in the splenic artery and are easily mistaken for pancreatic calcifications. The superior mesenteric artery (SMA) arises from the aorta dorsal to the pancreas and courses caudally, surrounded by a collar of fat. The superior mesenteric vein (SMV) courses cranially just to the right of the SMA until it joins the splenic vein to form the portal vein. The pancreatic head entirely surrounds this junction, with the uncinate process extending beneath the SMV and the inferior vena cava. The portal vein courses upward and rightward with the hepatic artery and common bile duct to the porta hepatis.

TECHNIQUE

Complete filling of the stomach and duodenal loop are essential for high quality pancreatic CT. Eight to 16 ounces of oral contrast are given immediately before scanning. Glucagon 0.1 mg by intravenous injection may be given to stop peristalsis in the duodenum and aid with bowel opacification. Intravenous contrast (150 ml) given rapidly by mechanical injector is routine. Scanning is done with contiguous 10-mm-thick slices for routine pancreatic survey. Detection of functioning islet cell tumors requires dynamic scanning with contiguous 5-mm-thick slices obtained during rapid contrast infusion.

ACUTE PANCREATITIS

Inflammation of the pancreas damages acinar tissue and leads to focal disruption of small ducts, resulting in leakage of pancreatic juice. The absence of a capsule around the pancreas allows easy access of pancreatic secretions to surrounding tissues. Pancreatic enzymes digest through fascial layers to spread to multiple anatomic compartments.

The diagnosis of pancreatitis is made clinically. CT may be normal in mild cases. The role of CT is to document the presence and severity of complications. CT findings are as follows:

Pancreatic changes:

1. Focal or diffuse enlargement of the pancreas
2. Decrease in density due to edema
3. Blurring of the margins of the gland due to inflammation

Peripancreatic changes:

1. Stranding densities in fat and blurring of fat planes
2. Thickening of retroperitoneal fascial planes

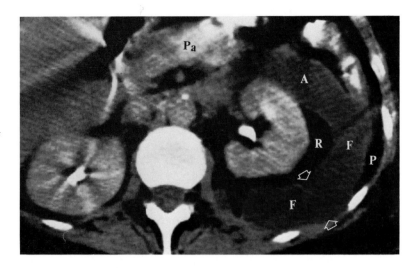

FIGURE 14–2. Acute pancreatitis—renal halo. Pancreatic fluid (F) and inflammation extend from the pancreas (Pa) in the anterior pararenal space (A) to a retrorenal position between the leaves of the posterior renal fascia (open arrows). Note that the perirenal space (R) and the posterior pararenal space (P) are spared. (Compare this to Figure 12–1.)

Complications:

1. Fluid collections: pancreatic, peripancreatic, within retroperitoneal compartments, and often widespread throughout the abdomen (Fig. 14–2)

2. Necrosis: liquefaction of portions of the gland (Fig. 14–3)

3. Phlegmon: mass-like enlargement of the pancreas due to edema and inflammation

4. Abscess: bacterial growth within necrotic tissues (Fig. 14–4)

5. Hemorrhage: due to erosion of blood vessels or bowel

6. Pancreatic ascites: leakage of pancreatic juice into the peritoneal cavity

7. Pseudocyst: persisting, walled-off collection of pancreatic fluid and debris (Fig. 14–5).

CHRONIC PANCREATITIS

Recurrent and prolonged bouts of inflammation cause progressive parenchymal atrophy and proliferation of fibrous tissue. Both exocrine and endocrine

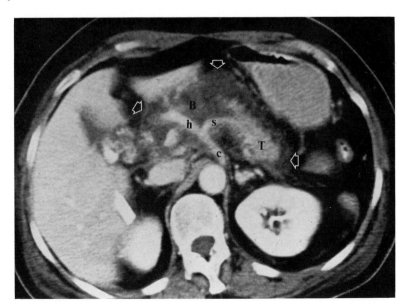

FIGURE 14–3. Pancreatic necrosis. The tail (T) of the pancreas enhances normally but the head and body (B) of the pancreas have undergone liquefactive necrosis and are replaced by fluid density. Edema and inflammation (open arrows) cause fluid density in the pancreatic bed and in the fat surrounding peripancreatic blood vessels. (c = celiac axis; s = splenic artery; h = common hepatic artery.)

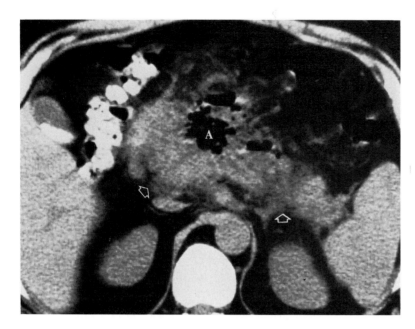

FIGURE 14–4. Pancreatic abscess. Pancreatic abscess in a 63-year-old man with a penetrating duodenal ulcer. An extensive gas collection (A) occupies the pancreatic bed. The margins of the pancreas are blurred by the inflammatory process (open arrows).

function are progressively impaired. CT evidence of chronic pancreatitis includes the following (Fig. 14–6)

1. Dilatation of the pancreatic duct often in a beaded pattern
2. Decrease in visible pancreatic tissue due to parenchymal atrophy
3. Calcifications varying from tiny stippled to coarse
4. Fluid collections, both intra- and extrapancreatic
5. Focal enlargement of the pancreas due to benign inflammation and fibrosis (Fig. 14–7)
6. Dilatation of the biliary duct due to fibrosis or mass in the pancreatic head
7. Fascial thickening and stranding in the peripancreatic fat.

Differentiating an inflammatory mass from pancreatic carcinoma is frequently difficult and usually requires biopsy (Fig. 14–7). Calcifications occur most frequently in chronic alcoholic pancreatitis.

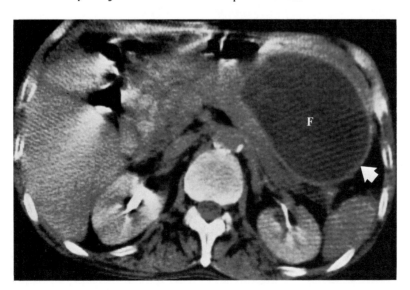

FIGURE 14–5. Pancreatic pseudocyst in the lesser sac. A huge fluid collection (F) persists in the lesser sac 6 weeks following an episode of alcohol-induced pancreatitis. Note the well-defined wall (arrow).

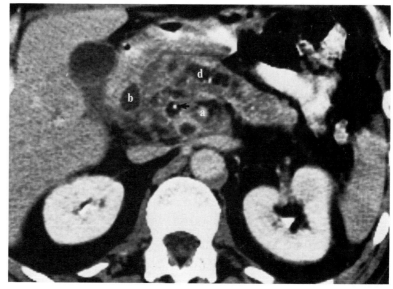

FIGURE 14–6. Chronic pancreatitis. Chronic pancreatitis is seen in a 55-year-old alcoholic male. The pancreatic duct (d) is enlarged, tortuous, and beaded in contour. The common bile duct (b) is also dilated. Speckled calcifications (arrow) are seen within the pancreas. Inflammatory changes cause increased density in the fat surrounding the superior mesenteric artery (a).

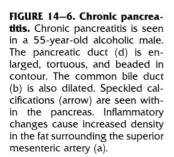

PANCREATIC CARCINOMA

Pancreatic adenocarcinoma is a highly lethal tumor with surgical resection offering only the slightest hope of long-term cure. CT plays a pivotal role in preoperative staging, separating those patients who have obviously unresectable tumors from the 10 to 15% who have potentially resectable tumors. Unfortunately, most of those who undergo aggressive resection still eventually die of their disease. Criteria for CT staging include

Signs of potential resectability (Fig. 14–8):

1. Isolated pancreatic mass with or without dilatation of the bile and pancreatic ducts

2. Combined bile-pancreatic duct dilatation without an identifiable pancreatic mass (pancreatic duct > 5 mm in head or > 3 mm in tail; common bile duct > 9 mm)

Signs of unresectability (Fig. 14–9):

1. Extension of tumor beyond the margins of the pancreas
2. Tumor involvement of contiguous organs

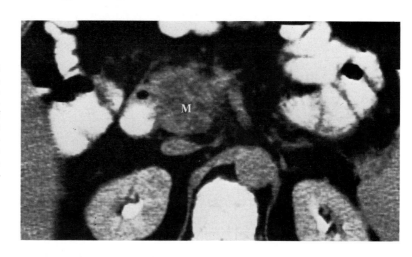

FIGURE 14–7. Benign pancreatic mass due to pancreatitis. Chronic pancreatitis is the biopsy-proven cause of this inhomogeneous mass (M) in the head of the pancreas. The margins of the mass are indistinct. The appearance of this mass is indistinguishable from that in pancreatic carcinoma. (Compare to Figures 14–8 and 14–9.)

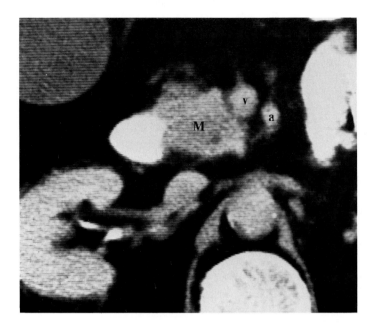

FIGURE 14—8. Resectable pancreatic carcinoma. This small tumor (M) caused obstruction of both the pancreatic and common bile ducts in a 72-year-old male presenting with painless jaundice. The collar of fat surrounding the superior mesenteric artery (a) is uninvolved. The superior mesenteric vein (v) enhances normally, indicating patency.

3. Enlarged regional lymph nodes (> 1.5 cm)
4. Encasement or obstruction of peripancreatic arteries or veins
5. Metastases to the liver
6. Ascites, which is usually evidence of peritoneal carcinomatosis.

ISLET CELL TUMORS

Most islet cell tumors produce identifiable hormones and present with specific endocrine syndromes. Hormones secreted by islet cells include insulin,

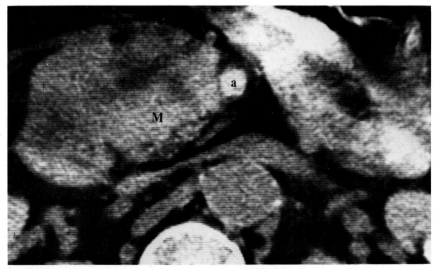

FIGURE 14—9. Unresectable pancreatic carcinoma. This CT image of a mass (M) in the head of the pancreas demonstrates several signs that indicate the tumor is unresectable. The collar of fat around the superior mesenteric artery (a) is infiltrated by adjacent tumor. The superior mesenteric vein, normally seen just to the right of the artery, is not identifiable. At autopsy the vein was invaded and occluded by tumor.

gastrin, glucagon, somatostatin, and vasoactive intestinal polypeptide. The tumors are generally small (0.4 to 4.0 cm) and require meticulous attention to CT technique to be detected. Most small islet cell tumors cannot be identified on precontrast scans. The characteristic feature of small tumors is transient circumscribed contrast enhancement that follows bolus contrast administration (Fig. 14–10). Rapid scan acquisition is needed to maximize contrast effect. This technique takes advantage of the hypervascularity demonstrated by most tumors. Functioning islet cell tumors may be either benign or malignant.

Nonfunctioning islet cell tumors are larger (6 to 20 cm) and present clinically with mass effect. About 25% are malignant. Features which help differentiate islet cell malignancy from pancreatic adenocarcinoma are unusually large tumor size, the presence of calcifications, and contrast enhancement of the tumor.

CYSTIC LESIONS

Pseudocyst. By far the most common cystic lesion in and around the pancreas, pseudocysts are collections of pancreatic fluid that have become encapsulated within fibrous walls. On CT they appear as low density fluid masses with well-defined walls of variable thickness and occasional calcifications.

Abscess. Any fluid collection in or around the pancreas is a potential abscess in a patient with fever. Its CT appearance may be indistinguishable from sterile pseudocyst. Air within the fluid collection is strong evidence of the presence of infection. Diagnosis is confirmed by aspiration.

True Pancreatic Cyst. True cysts are well-defined, fluid-filled, epithelial-lined masses with walls of variable thickness. Multiple congenital true cysts are seen in the pancreas in patients with adult polycystic disease and von Hippel–Lindau syndrome (see Fig. 12–8). Acquired retention cysts are due to focal obstruction of the pancreatic duct system.

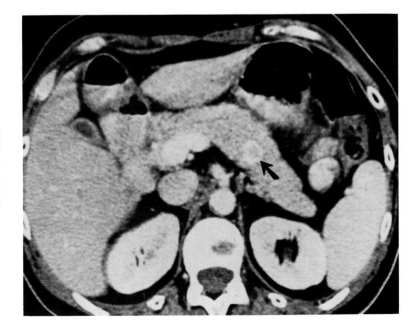

FIGURE 14–10. Insulinoma. A 1.8-cm insulin-producing islet cell tumor (arrow) is seen a circular area of intense enhancement in the distal body of the pancreas. The patient is a 62-year-old woman with hypoglycemia and increased serum insulin.

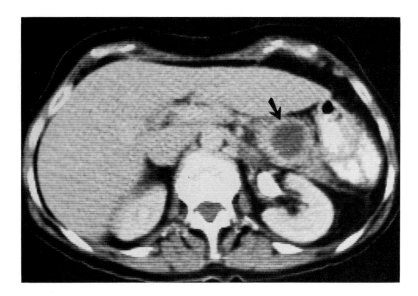

FIGURE 14–11. Cystic adenocarcinoma. CT scan through the tail of the pancreas demonstrates a cystic mass (arrow) with irregular thick walls. Although no septations are identifiable by CT, several were evident on the pathologic specimen.

Cystic Tumors. Cystic pancreatic tumors are classified as serous microcystic adenoma, which is benign, and mucinous (macrocystic) cystadenoma/cystadenocarcinoma, which is potentially or frankly malignant. Malignant tumors have a significantly better prognosis than pancreatic adenocarcinoma. On CT, both types appear as multicystic masses with a variable amount of solid component. Septations and cyst walls may be up to 1 cm thick. Benign microcystic lesions typically have six or more cysts of 2 cm or smaller size. Potentially malignant macrocystic tumors typically have fewer cysts (< 6) which are larger in size (> 2 cm) (Fig. 14–11).

TRAUMA

Traumatic injury to the pancreas is uncommon but has a high morbidity and is commonly clinically occult. Blunt abdominal trauma, often due to child abuse, is the most common cause of pancreatitis in children. The body of the pancreas may be compressed against the spine and is prone to contusion, laceration, transection, pancreatitis, and focal hemorrhagic necrosis. CT signs of pancreatic injury include pancreatic enlargement, fluid collections, and lucent defects representing lacerations. Since tissue displacement may be minimal, lacerations are difficult to identify. Unexplained thickening of the anterior renal fascia is a CT clue to possible pancreatic injury.

SUGGESTED READING

Freeny PC, Marks WM, Ryan JA, et al.: Pancreatic ductal adenocarcinoma: Diagnosis and staging with dynamic CT. Radiology, 166:125–133, 1988.

Günther RW: Ultrasound and CT in the assessment of suspected islet cell tumors of the pancreas. Semin Ultrasound CT MR, 6:261–275, 1985.

Jeffrey RB Jr, Federle MP, Crass RA: Computed tomography of pancreatic trauma. Radiology, 147:491–494, 1983.

Johnson CD, Stephens DH, Charboneau JW, et al.: Cystic pancreatic tumors: CT and sonographic appearance. Am J Roentgenol, 151:1133–1138, 1988.

Luetmer PH, Stephens DH, Ward EM: Chronic pancreatitis: Reassessment with current CT. Radiology, 171:353–357, 1989.

Siegelman SS (ed): Computed Tomography of the Pancreas. Contemporary Issues in Computed Tomography, vol 1. New York, Churchill Livingstone, 1983.

15

Gastrointestinal Tract

ESOPHAGUS

Anatomy

The esophagus is a muscular tube that extends from the cricopharyngeus muscle at the level of the cricoid cartilage to the stomach. The major portion of its length is within the middle mediastinum. A cervical portion extends from C-6 vertebral body to the thoracic inlet. A short abdominal segment extends below the diaphragm to the gastroesophageal junction. The esophagus is lined by squamous epithelium but lacks a serosal covering. The lack of serosal covering allows early invasion of esophageal tumors into periesophageal tissues.

On CT the esophagus appears as an oval of soft tissue density often containing air or contrast material within its lumen. When distended the wall of the esophagus should not exceed 3 mm in thickness (Fig. 15–1). In the neck and upper thorax, the esophagus courses between the trachea and the spine. In the lower thorax, the esophagus courses to the right of the descending aorta between the left atrium and the spine. The esophagus enters the abdomen through the esophageal hiatus and courses to the left to join the stomach. The edges of the diaphragmatic crura forming the esophageal hiatus are seen as often prominent, teardrop-shaped structures (Fig. 15–2) partially surrounding the esophagus.

CT complements endoscopic and barium studies of the esophagus by demonstrating the esophageal wall and adjacent structures. However, CT does not evaluate the mucosa, and the findings produced by both neoplastic and inflammatory conditions may appear identical. CT is excellent for determining the extent of disease, but is not specific for its nature.

Technique

The esophagus is studied using contiguous 10-mm-thick slices from the level of the larynx to the stomach. When esophageal tumors are evaluated, scanning is continued through the liver to look for metastases. Oral contrast is given to distend the stomach and the gastroesophageal junction. Intravenous contrast is useful to evaluate mediastinal vessels and varices. Attempts to fully distend the esophagus during CT scanning are not consistently successful.

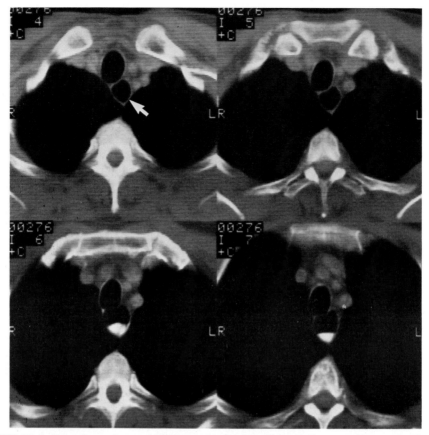

FIGURE 15–1. Normal esophagus. Multiple sequential slices through the normal upper esophagus in a patient with a distal obstructing tumor demonstrate the normally thin wall (arrow).

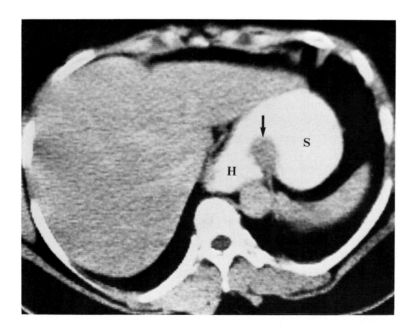

FIGURE 15–2. Hiatus hernia. A portion of the stomach (S) extends through the esophageal hiatus to form a hiatal hernia (H). Note the prominent teardrop-shaped soft tissue mass (arrow) formed by the margin of the diaphragm at the esophageal hiatus.

Hiatus Hernia

Hiatus hernia is a protrusion of any portion of the stomach into the thorax. On CT hiatus hernia appears as a contrast- or air-filled mass continuous with the stomach, lying within and above the esophageal hiatus (Fig. 15–2). The edges of the esophageal hiatus are often widely separated, exceeding 15 mm in width. The major reason to recognize a hiatus hernia is to avoid mistaking it for a tumor.

Esophageal Carcinoma

Because of the lack of serosal covering, carcinoma spreads beyond the esophagus early in its course, resulting in a poor prognosis. Ninety percent of tumors are squamous cell carcinoma with the remaining 10% being adenocarcinoma arising in Barrett's esophagus in the distal esophagus. It must be recognized that the CT findings in esophageal carcinoma may be duplicated by benign disease. Diagnosis depends upon biopsy. CT is done to assess the extent of disease and identify those patients whose lesions are unresectable.

The CT findings in esophageal carcinoma include (Fig. 15–3)

1. Irregular thickening of the wall of the esophagus >3 mm
2. Eccentric narrowing of the lumen
3. Dilatation of the esophagus above the area of narrowing
4. Invasion of periesophageal tissues: fat, aorta, trachea
5. Metastases to mediastinal lymph nodes and liver.

Esophageal Leiomyoma

Leiomyomas are the most common benign tumors of the esophagus. They are asymptomatic until they are very large. As submucosal tumors they are easily differentiated from carcinoma by endoscopy but are difficult to differentiate by CT. On CT they appear as smooth, well-defined masses of uniform soft tissue

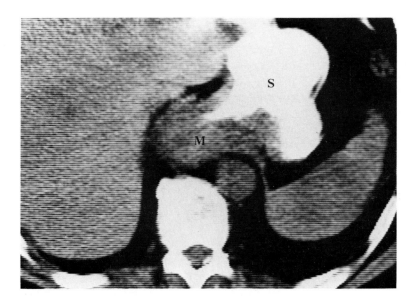

FIGURE 15–3. Esophageal carcinoma. A squamous cell carcinoma (M) of the distal esophagus extends into the proximal stomach (S). (Compare to Figure 15–4.)

density. The esophageal wall is eccentrically thickened and the lumen is deformed. Large, well-defined masses are much more likely to be leiomyoma than carcinoma.

Esophageal Varices

Varices cause thickening of the esophageal wall that may be indistinguishable from tumor or inflammation without contrast. The key to CT diagnosis is vascular enhancement, best demonstrated by giving bolus contrast injection combined with rapid CT scanning. Signs of cirrhosis, portal hypertension, and other portosystemic collaterals may also be present.

Esophagitis

Esophagitis results in circumferential thickening of the esophageal wall, usually without disruption of the periesophageal tissues. Strictures are seen as areas of luminal narrowing with dilatation of the esophagus above the lesion. Severe esophagitis may lead to perforation, mediastinitis, and abscess.

Esophageal Perforation

Esophageal perforation may be traumatic, iatrogenic postinstrumentation, or may result from neoplasm or inflammation. Since it may be lethal, prompt recognition is essential. CT signs include fluid collections and air within the mediastinum, widening of the mediastinum, hydro- and pneumothorax.

STOMACH

Anatomy

The posteriorly located gastric fundus is seen on the highest CT sections through the dome of the diaphragm. The esophagus joins the stomach a short distance below the fundus. A prominent pseudotumor caused by thickening of the gastric wall due to incomplete distention is often present near the gastroesophageal junction (Fig. 15–4). Additional distension with more air or contrast will eliminate this pseudotumor. The body of the stomach sweeps toward the right. The antrum crosses the midline of the abdomen between the left lobe of the liver and the pancreas to join the duodenal bulb in the region of the gallbladder.

The normal gastric wall should not exceed 5 mm in thickness when the stomach is well distended. Rugal folds are commonly visualized even with good distension. Like the esophagus, both benign and malignant conditions produce similar CT findings. CT is performed to document the extent of extraluminal disease.

Technique

The stomach must be filled with positive contrast or distended with air for optimal assessment by CT. Six to 8 ounces (200 to 300 ml) of oral contrast

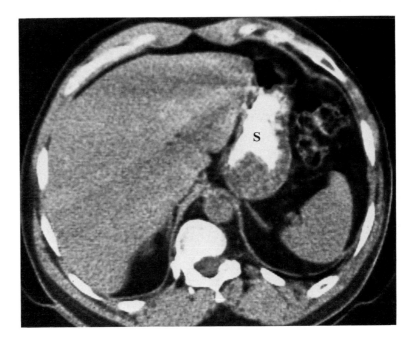

FIGURE 15–4. Pseudotumor at gastroesophageal junction. The wall of the stomach (S) is thickened and nodular due to poor distension. Subsequent images obtained after administration of additional oral contrast material demonstrated normal gastric wall thickness. (Compare to Figure 15–3.)

are routinely given to fill the stomach just before the patient lies down on the CT couch. Distension of the stomach with air may be obtained by giving a dose of gas-producing crystals, such as are used for air contrast barium studies, with 10 to 15 ml of water instead of the opaque contrast. The patient can be repositioned to optimize distension of the various portions of the stomach with air. Scanning is performed using contiguous 10-mm-thick slices.

Thickened Gastric Wall

Thickening of the gastric wall (Fig. 15–5), either focal or diffuse, is an important but nonspecific sign of gastric disease. With good technique, which

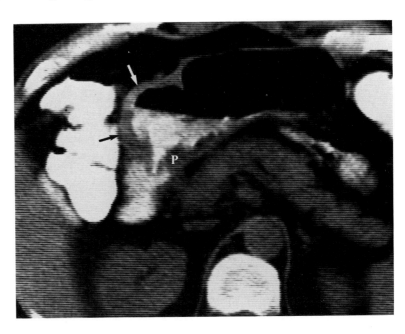

FIGURE 15–5. Gastric lymphoma. Lymphoma thickens the gastric wall in the region of the antrum (arrows). This finding is nonspecific and may be due to both inflammatory and neoplastic conditions. (P = pylorus.)

includes aggressive distension of the stomach with air or contrast, wall thickening greater than 5 mm can be considered abnormal. Causes include carcinoma, lymphoma, gastric inflammation (peptic or Crohn's disease), perigastric inflammation (pancreatitis), and radiation.

Gastric Carcinoma

CT is used to stage disease and identify tumors that are not surgically resectable. CT findings are (Fig. 15–6)

1. Soft tissue density intraluminal mass lesion, calcifications rare
2. Focal or diffuse, nodular or irregular thickening of the gastric wall
3. Extension of tumor into the perigastric fat
4. Adenopathy in the celiac region and gastrohepatic ligament
5. Metastases in the liver.

Gastric Lymphoma

The stomach is the most common site of involvement for primary gastrointestinal lymphoma (Fig. 15–5). CT findings are similar to adenocarcinoma. However, lymphoma tends to cause more dramatic thickening of the stomach wall (exceeding 3 cm) and often involves more than one region of the gastrointestinal tract. The perigastric fat is rarely invaded. Adenopathy is generally much more widespread with lymphoma.

Gastric Leiomyoma/Leiomyosarcoma

Leiomyoma, leiomyoblastoma, and leiomyosarcoma arise from the smooth muscle of the gastric wall and grow as submucosal, subserosal, or exophytic tumors. They grow silently and may reach large size before presenting

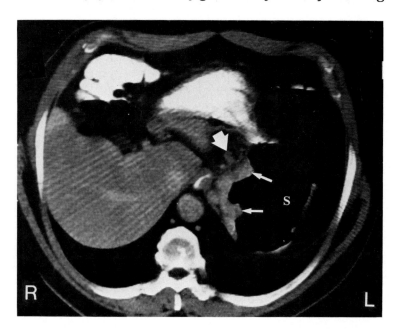

FIGURE 15–6. Gastric carcinoma. This patient was scanned prone to optimally distend the gastric fundus (S) following administration of gas-producing crystals. The image is inverted to maintain standard anatomic orientation. A gastric carcinoma caused nodular thickening of the gastric wall (small arrows). Tumor extension through the wall, suggested by the soft tissue densities (large arrow) in the perigastric fat, was confirmed at surgery.

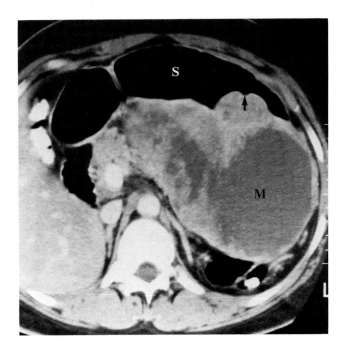

FIGURE 15–7. Gastric leiomyosarcoma. A leiomyosarcoma arising in the posterior wall of the stomach (S) is seen as a huge heterogeneous mass (M) with multiple low density areas within it. Note the ulcer crater (arrow) within the mass.

clinically with ulceration and GI bleeding. Histologic criteria for differentiating benign from malignant tumors are not foolproof. The diagnosis of malignancy is based upon size, gross appearance, and behavior of the tumor. Benign lesions are smaller (4 to 5 cm average size), homogeneous in density, and enhance diffusely and symmetrically. Malignant lesions (Fig. 15–7) are larger (12 cm average size) and markedly heterogeneous, with multiple low density regions and irregular enhancement patterns. Deep ulcerations may be evident.

Gastric Varices

Gastric varices occur as a result of portal hypertension. They appear as well-defined clusters of rounded and tubular densities in or adjacent to the wall of the stomach. Bright enhancement with intravenous contrast clinches the diagnosis. CT signs of liver disease and other portosystemic collaterals are often present.

SMALL BOWEL

Anatomy

The duodenum extends from the pylorus to the ligament of Treitz, forming the familiar C-loop. The duodenum becomes retroperitoneal at the right free edge of the hepatoduodenal ligament, closely related to the neck of the gallbladder. The descending duodenum passes to the right of the pancreatic head to just below the uncinate process where it turns to the left. The horizontal portion crosses anterior to the inferior vena cava and aorta, and posterior to the superior mesenteric vein and artery. The fourth portion ascends just left of the aorta to the ligament of Treitz, where it becomes the intraperitoneal jejunum.

The jejunum occupies the left upper abdomen, while the ileum lies in the right lower abdomen and pelvis. Jejunal loops are feathery with distinct folds. Ileal loops are featureless with thin walls. Opacification of the lumen with oral contrast is essential to adequately evaluate the bowel. Unopacified small bowel may mimic adenopathy and abdominal masses. The small bowel mesentery contains many vessels which are easily visualized when outlined by fat.

The normal luminal diameter of the small bowel does not exceed 3 cm. The normal wall thickness is less than 3 mm.

Technique

Opacification of the small bowel with oral contrast agent is mandatory for high quality abdominal CT. It is virtually impossible to administer too much oral contrast. A 1 to 3% concentration of oral contrast is optimal for CT. This concentration is obtained by adding 3 ml of 60% oral contrast solution to 100 ml of water. We give 400-ml doses of this mixture 12 hours, 2 hours, 30 minutes, and immediately before CT scanning. To study the small bowel we obtain sequential 10-mm-thick slices through the abdomen and pelvis. When the duodenum is the organ of primary interest, administration of 0.1 mg of glucagon intravenously is helpful in stopping peristalsis and distending the bowel. Intravenous contrast is optional.

Small Bowel Edema and Wall Thickening

Like the other portions of the GI tract, edema and wall thickening (Fig. 15–8) are nonspecific signs seen in a wide variety of disease states. Considerations include inflammatory disease, ischemia, trauma, hypoalbuminemia, lymphatic obstruction, and tumor. CT findings include dilatation of the bowel lumen, thickening of the mucosal folds, and haziness of the bowel wall.

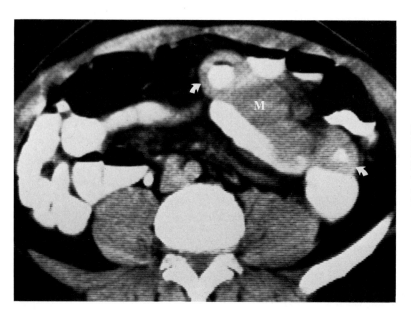

FIGURE 15–8. Small bowel lymphoma. CT image through the lower abdomen demonstrates loops of ileum with markedly thickened walls (arrows) and adenopathy producing a mass (M) in the small bowel mesentery.

Small Bowel Diverticuli

Small bowel diverticuli may cause unusual collections of fluid, air, contrast material, or soft tissue density in the fat and tissues adjacent to the bowel. These must not be mistaken for abscesses, pancreatic pseudocysts, or tumors. Rescanning the patient will often demonstrate a significant change in the appearance of diverticuli.

Small Bowel Tumors

Both benign and malignant small bowel neoplasms are uncommon. On CT they appear as nonspecific soft tissue mass or wall thickening. CT is useful in demonstrating extraluminal tumor growth, involvement of adjacent structures, adenopathy, and complications such as fisulae or necrosis. Histologic types include adenocarcinoma, lymphoma, carcinoid, and metastases.

Crohn's Disease

Crohn's disease is characterized by inflammation of the bowel mucosa, bowel wall, and mesentery with marked submucosal edema. These features are nicely reflected in the CT appearance (Fig. 15–9):

1. Circumferential thickening of the bowel wall up to 1 to 2 cm
2. Low density inner ring of submucosal edema
3. Diffuse haziness and increased density of the mesenteric fat
4. "Skip areas" of normal bowel intervened between diseased segments
5. Fistulae and sinus tracts between bowel loops, or to the bladder, adjacent muscle, or the skin surface
6. Mesenteric abscesses containing fluid, air, or contrast material.

CT is excellent in documenting the extraluminal extent of disease.

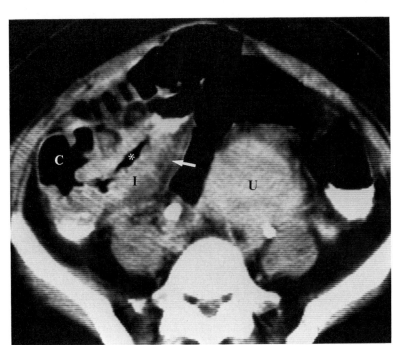

FIGURE 15–9. Crohn's disease. This image demonstrates the CT equivalent of the "string sign" characteristic of Crohn's disease. The wall of the terminal ileum (I) is markedly thickened, narrowing the lumen (*). The inflammatory changes extend into the surrounding fat (arrow). Histologic examination following resection confirmed transmural inflammation with multiple granulomas. (C = cecum; U = fundus of the uterus.)

Mesenteric Mass

Soft tissue masses in the small bowel mesentery are most commonly due to lymphoma (Fig. 15–8). Diffuse histiocytic lymphoma commonly involves the stomach and small bowel, which may demonstrate focal nodular or circumferential wall thickening. Mesenteric involvement may consist of enlarged individual mesenteric nodes or large confluent masses. Lymphomatous masses characteristically "sandwich" mesenteric vessels between thin layers of spared mesenteric fat.

Other causes of mesenteric masses include metastases, carcinoid tumor, and mesenteric fibromatosis. Metastases tend to be multiple and small. Carcinoid tumors characteristically incite a prominent fibrotic response. Mesenteric fibromatosis produces well-defined homogeneous solid masses.

APPENDIX

Anatomy

The normal appendix is rarely identified on routine CT of the abdomen. When seen it has the ring-like or tubular appearance of a bowel loop but is only about half the transverse diameter of small bowel. Recognizing its origin from the cecum confirms its identification. The origin of the appendix is between the ileocecal valve and the cecal apex, always on the same side of the cecum as the valve. Air and contrast material in the appendix are normal findings.

Appendicitis

CT is particularly useful in identifying complications like phlegmon and periappendiceal abscess. Uncomplicated appendicitis cannot be ruled out by CT. CT findings in appendicitis are

1. Appendicolith appearing as a ring-like or homogeneous calcification in the right lower quadrant within the appendiceal lumen or adjacent to a perforated appendix (diagnostic of appendicitis)
2. Periappendiceal phlegmon seen as an indurated soft tissue mass greater than 20 H
3. Periappendiceal abscess seen as a liquefied mass less than 20 H
4. Thickened wall of distended appendix (rarely seen).

CT is highly accurate in differentiating phlegmon from abscess. Phlegmons and abscesses less than 3 cm generally resolve on antibiotic treatment, while abscesses larger than 3 cm require surgical or catheter drainage.

Mucocele of the Appendix

Mucocele refers to a distended appendix filled with mucus. Most cases are due to benign proximal obstruction, although some are due to mucus-secreting adenocarcinoma. On CT they appear as cystic masses with thin walls which may be calcified. Size is variable, up to 15 cm. Pseudomyxoma peritonei is an interesting complication that manifests as mucinous ascites and gelatinous implants throughout the abdomen cavity fixating bowel loops and causing mass effect.

COLON AND RECTUM

Anatomy

The colon is easily identified by its haustral markings when it is distended by air or contrast. Mottled fecal material also serves as a marker of the colon and rectum. The scout view of the abdominal CT should be inspected to determine the general outline and location of the colon. The cecum generally occupies the iliac fossa, although because of its long mesentery it may be found almost anywhere in the abdomen. Its identity is confirmed by recognizing the ileocecal valve or appendix. The ascending colon occupies a posterior and lateral position in the right flank. The hepatic flexure makes one or more sharp bends near the undersurface of the liver and gallbladder. The transverse colon sweeps across the abdomen on a long and mobile mesentery. Because of its anterior position the transverse colon is usually filled with air when patients are supine on the CT couch. The splenic flexure makes one or more tight bends below the spleen. The descending colon extends caudally down the left flank. Remember that the ascending and descending portions of the colon are retroperitoneal. The peritoneum sweeps over their anterior surfaces and extends laterally to form the gutters which distend with fluid when ascites is present. The sigmoid colon begins in the left iliac fossa and extends a variable distance cranially before it dives toward the rectum. The sigmoid becomes the rectum at the level of the third sacral segment. The rectum distends to form the rectal ampulla and then abruptly narrows to form the anal canal.

The peritoneum covering the anterior surface of the rectum extends to the level of the vagina, forming the rectovaginal pouch of Douglas. In males the peritoneum extends to 2.5 cm above the prostate to form the rectovesical pouch. Three anatomic compartments are important to recognize when staging rectal carcinoma (see Fig. 16–1): (1) the peritoneal cavity above the peritoneal reflections, (2) the subperitoneal compartment between the peritoneum and the levator ani muscle forming the pelvic diaphragm, and (3) the triangular ischiorectal fossa inferior and lateral to the levator ani. The lower two-thirds of the rectum are extraperitoneal.

On CT the thickness of the wall of the normal colon does not exceed 5 mm.

Technique

For routine scanning, the rectum and colon can usually be adequately opacified by giving contrast agents orally. However, when detailed examination of the colon is needed, air contrast techniques are preferred. Preliminary bowel preparation is carried out identical to preparation for a barium enema. Just prior to CT scanning, an enema tube is placed in the rectum after digital rectal examination. The colon is insufflated with approximately 20 puffs of air or to the limit of patient comfort. Scanning is then carried out through the entire abdomen and pelvis. Intravenous contrast is optional. When diverticulitis is suspected, colon opacification is obtained entirely by oral contrast administration beginning 12 hours prior to scanning.

Colorectal Carcinoma

Seventy percent of colon cancers occur in the rectosigmoid region. The remainder are scattered fairly evenly throughout the rest of the colon. Colon cancer spreads by (1) direct extension due to penetration of the colon wall, (2) lymphatic drainage to regional nodes, (3) hematogenous routes through portal veins to the liver, and (4) intraperitoneal seeding. About half of colon cancer recurrences occur at the site of the original tumor (Fig. 15–10), while the remainder recur at distant sites. CT scans should survey the entire abdomen and pelvis to stage and followup colon carcinomas. While barium enemas and colonoscopy are the primary modalities for initial detection of colorectal cancer, CT is the screening procedure of choice for detection of recurrences. CT signs of colon carcinoma include (Fig. 15–11)

1. Focal lobulated soft tissue mass in colon
2. Localized thickening of the bowel wall (> 5 mm)
3. Irregular lumen surface
4. Extension of linear soft tissue densities or discrete mass into pericolic fat or adjacent organs
5. Regional adenopathy
6. Liver metastases.

The tumor is desmoplastic and commonly causes narrowing of the lumen and bowel obstruction. Calcifications in the primary tumor and metastases occur with mucinous adenocarcinoma. Soft tissue masses within the peritoneal cavity may represent colon cancer spread or recurrence. Following abdominoperineal resection for rectal cancer, presacral soft tissue densities (Fig. 15–12) may be recurrent tumor and commonly require percutaneous biopsy for confirmation.

Colon Lymphoma

Colon lymphoma is less common than gastric or small bowel lymphoma but has a striking and fairly characteristic CT appearance:

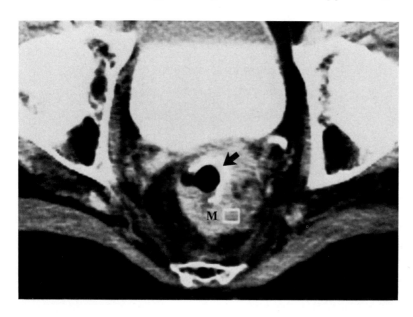

FIGURE 15–10. Recurrence of rectal carcinoma. A CT slice through the rectum at the level of anastomosis marked by metallic staples (arrow) demonstrates an eccentric soft tissue mass (M). Surgery confirmed recurrence of rectal carcinoma.

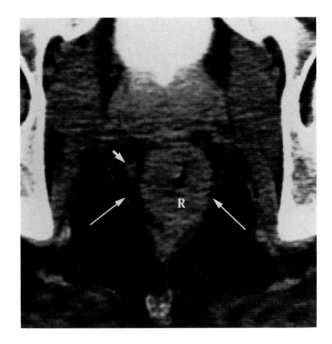

FIGURE 15–11. Rectal carcinoma. A circumferential rectal carcinoma (R) markedly thickens the rectal wall and narrows the lumen. A soft tissue nodule (short arrow) indicates spread of tumor into the perirectal fat. The levator ani muscle (long arrows) separates the rectum and perirectal fat from the ischiorectal fossae.

1. Marked thickening of the bowel wall often exceeding 5 cm
2. Homogeneous soft tissue mass without calcification or necrosis
3. Minimal to no enhancement of the mass with intravenous contrast
4. Regional and diffuse adenopathy, often massive.

Lymphoma characteristically causes much larger soft tissue masses than does carcinoma. The absence of desmoplastic reaction is typical and the colon lumen is commonly dilated rather than constricted at the site of tumor involvement. Bowel obstruction is uncommon.

Colon Lipoma

CT can be used to make a specific and noninvasive diagnosis of colon lipoma by demonstrating homogeneous fat density within a sharply defined

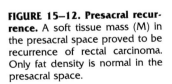

FIGURE 15–12. Presacral recurrence. A soft tissue mass (M) in the presacral space proved to be recurrence of rectal carcinoma. Only fat density is normal in the presacral space.

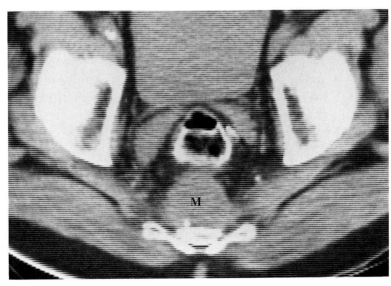

colonic tumor. Most lipomas are 2 to 3 cm in size, round or ovoid, and are clinically silent. Some may bleed or be a cause of intussusception.

Diverticulitis

Since most diverticula occur along the mesenteric surface of the colon, perforation due to diverticulitis is confined initially to between the leaves of the mesocolon. The inflammatory mass that forms is both extraluminal and extra-peritoneal. CT is better suited to documentation of this extraluminal disease than is barium enema. Colon opacification with contrast can be achieved by oral administration without the potential trauma of an enema. Diverticula are easily visualized on CT as small rounded collections of air, feces, or contrast material outside of the lumen. Thickening of the muscular wall of the colon is commonly present. Diverticulitis causes the following signs (Fig. 15–13):

1. Focal symmetric, usually circumferential, thickening of the bowel wall (> 5 mm)
2. Pericolic inflammatory soft tissue mass often containing fluid, air, contrast, or fecal material
3. Linear stranding densities in pericolic fat representing inflammatory changes
4. Sinus tracts and fistulas to adjacent organs or skin represented by linear fluid or air collections.

Abscess formation may be extensive. Obstruction of the colon or urinary tract may result from the inflammatory process.

Thickening of the Colon Wall

Just as in the other portions of the GI tract, thickening of the bowel wall is nonspecific and may result from a variety of insults. The colon wall is abnormally thickened (Fig. 15–14) when it exceeds 3 mm with the lumen distended or 5

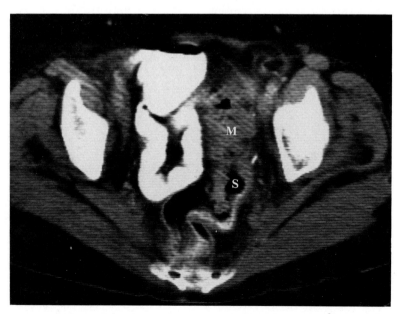

FIGURE 15–13. Diverticulitis. Diverticulitis of the sigmoid colon (S) produces a soft tissue mass (M) that narrows the lumen and extends into adjacent tissues. CT is excellent for demonstrating the nature and extent of an extraluminal mass.

FIGURE 15–14. Ischemic colitis. The wall of the ascending colon (large arrow) is circumferentially thickened owing to bowel ischemia. Compare the normal thickness of the wall of unaffected portions of the transverse colon (small arrow).

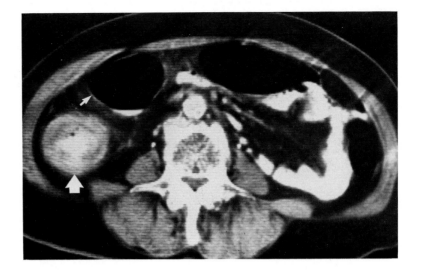

mm when the lumen is collapsed. Differential considerations include inflammatory colitis, necrotizing colitis, ischemia, radiation, and tumor including carcinoma and lymphoma. Correlation with clinical history and other findings is needed to differentiate these conditions.

SUGGESTED READING

Balthazar EJ, Gordon RB: CT of appendicitis. Semin Ultrasound CT MR, 10:326–340, 1989.

Fishman EK, Jones B (eds): Computed Tomography of the Gastrointestinal Tract. Contemporary Issues in Computed Tomography, vol 9. New York, Churchill Livingstone, 1988.

Jeffrey RB Jr, Federle MP, Tolentino CS: Periappendiceal inflammatory masses: CT-directed management and clinical outcome in 70 patients. Radiology, 167:13–16, 1988.

Marx MV, Balfe DM: Computed tomography of the esophagus. Semin Ultrasound CT MR, 8:316–348, 1987.

Megibow AJ, Balthazar EJ: Computed Tomography of the Gastrointestinal Tract. St. Louis, CV Mosby, 1986.

Silverman PM, Baker ME, Cooper C, et al.: Computed tomography of mesenteric disease. Radiographics, 7:309–320, 1987.

Stone EE, Brant WE, Smith G: Computed tomography of duodenal diverticula. J Comput Assist Tomogr, 13:61–64, 1989.

16

Pelvis

ANATOMY

The true (lesser) pelvis is divided from the false (greater) pelvis by an oblique plane extending along the pelvic brim from the sacral promontory to the symphysis pubis. The true pelvis contains the bladder, pelvic ureters, and prostate and seminal vesicles in the male, or vagina, uterus, and ovaries in the female. The false pelvis is open anteriorly and is bounded laterally by the iliac fossae. It contains small bowel loops, and the ascending, descending, and sigmoid portions of the colon.

Muscle groups form prominent anatomic landmarks on CT. The psoas muscle extends from the lumbar vertebra through the greater pelvis to join with the iliacus arising from the iliac fossa. The iliopsoas exits the pelvis anteriorly to insert on the lesser trochanter of the femur. The obturator internus lines the interior surface of the lateral walls of the true pelvis (Fig. 16–1). Involvement of this muscle by pelvic tumors precludes surgical resection of the tumor. The piriformis muscle arises from the anterior sacrum and exits the pelvis through the greater sciatic foramen to insert on the greater trochanter of the femur. The piriformis forms a portion of the lateral wall of the true pelvis. The pelvic diaphragm, composed of the levator ani anteriorly and the coccygeus posteriorly, stretches across the pelvis to separate the pelvic cavity from the perineum (Fig. 16–1). The pelvic diaphragm is penetrated by the rectum, urethra, and vagina.

The pelvis is divided into three major anatomic compartments (Figs. 16–1, 16–2). The *peritoneal cavity* extends to the level of the vagina, forming the pouch of Douglas in females, or to the third sacral level, forming the rectovesical pouch in males. The *extraperitoneal space* of the pelvis is continuous with the retroperitoneal space of the abdomen. Pathologic processes from the pelvis may spread preferentially into the retroperitoneal compartments of the abdomen. The retropubic space (of Retzius) is continuous with the posterior pararenal space and the extraperitoneal fat of the abdominal wall (Fig. 16–6). Fascial planes also allow communication with the scrotum and labia. The *perineum* lies below the pelvic diaphragm. On CT the most obvious portion of the perineum is the ischiorectal fossa. This fossa is seen as a triangular area of fat density extending between the obturator internus laterally, the gluteus maximus posteriorly, and the anus and urogenital region medially.

The arteries and veins define the location of the major lymphatic node chains in the pelvis. The aorta and vena cava divide to form the common iliac vessels at the level of the top of the iliac crest. The common iliac vessels divide

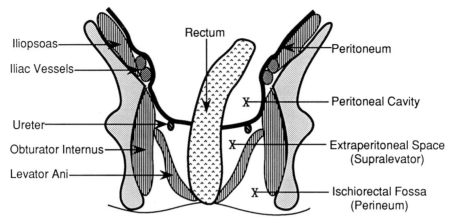

FIGURE 16–1. Compartments of the pelvis. Diagram of a posterior coronal section at the level of the rectum demonstrates the major anatomic compartments of the pelvis.

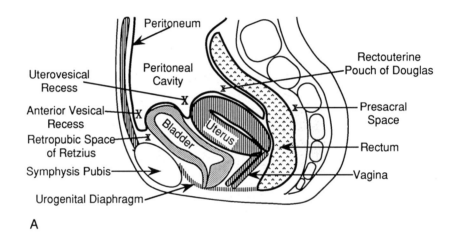

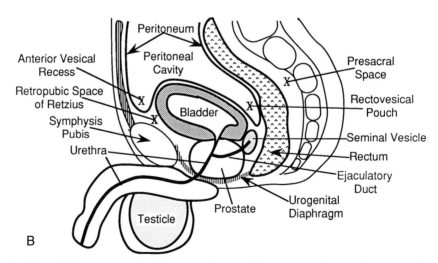

FIGURE 16–2. Pelvic organs and pelvic compartments. Diagrams of midline sagittal planes through a female *(A)* and a male *(B)* pelvis demonstrate the pelvic compartments and peritoneal recesses and their relationships to pelvic organs.

at the pelvic brim, marked on CT by the transition between the convex sacral promontory and the concave sacral cavity. The internal iliac vessels course posteriorly across the sciatic foramen, dividing rapidly into many small branches. The external iliac vessels course anteriorly adjacent to the iliopsoas to exit the pelvis at the inguinal ligament. Pelvic lymph nodes are classified with their accompanying vessels, and are correspondingly named the common iliac, internal iliac, and external iliac nodal chains (Fig. 16–3). The obturator nodes are satellites of the external iliac chain and course along the midportion of the obturator internus. Pelvic lymph nodes are considered pathologically enlarged when they exceed *15 mm* in any dimension.

The bladder is best appreciated on CT when filled with urine or contrast. The normal bladder wall does not exceed 5 mm thickness when the bladder is distended. The dome of the bladder is covered by peritoneum, while its base and anterior surface are extraperitoneal (Fig. 16–2). The ureters course anterior to the psoas, cross over the common iliac vessels at the pelvic brim, and insert into the bladder trigone on either side of the cervix or prostate.

The vagina is seen in cross section as a flattened ellipse of soft tissue density between the bladder and rectum. An inserted tampon will outline the cavity of the vagina with air density and is useful in marking the vagina for pelvic CT. The level of the cervix is recognized by the transition from the elliptic shape of the vagina to the round shape of the cervix. Contrast-containing ureters are frequently identified in close proximity to the cervix. The uterus is seen as a homogeneous, smooth-outlined oval of soft tissue density. The myometrium is highly vascular, causing the uterus to enhance more than most pelvic organs. Estimation of size of the uterus is very difficult on CT because of variations in position and flexion of the uterus, and the amount of bladder filling. The broad ligament is a sheet-like fold of peritoneum that drapes over the uterus and can be seen as it extends to the pelvic side walls. Between the leaves of the broad ligament are the fallopian tubes, uterine and ovarian vessels, and pelvic ureter. The *parametrium* is the connective tissue between the leaves of the broad ligament contiguous with the lateral aspect of the uterine body and cervix. Determination of tumor extension into the parametrium is an important part of tumor staging. Normal ovaries may be difficult to identify on CT. Because they are very mobile, they may be anywhere in the pelvis. They appear as oval soft tissue densities, approximately $2 \times 3 \times 4$ cm in size. The presence of cystic follicles allows positive identification as ovaries.

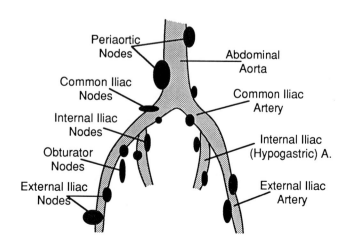

FIGURE 16–3. Pelvic lymph nodes. Diagram of the aortic bifurcation and the iliac arteries illustrates the classification and naming of pelvic lymph nodes.

The normal prostate gland is seen at the base of the bladder as a rounded soft tissue body up to 4 cm in maximal diameter. A well-defined plane of fat separates the prostate from the obturator internus. This fat plane may be invaded by carcinoma. Denonvilliers' fascia provides a particularly tough barrier between the prostate and rectum, preventing spread of disease from one organ to the other. The paired seminal vesicles produce a characteristic bowtie-shaped soft tissue mass in the groove between the bladder base and the prostate (Figs. 16–2B, 16–5). Normal testicles are easily identified in the scrotum as homogeneous oval structures 3 to 4 cm in diameter. The spermatic cord can be recognized in the inguinal canal as a thin walled oval structure of fat density containing small dots representing the vas deferens or spermatic vessels.

TECHNIQUE

Ideal technique for CT imaging of the pelvis requires optimal bowel opacification. We give 500 ml of dilute contrast orally the evening preceding the examination, and repeat the dose 45 to 60 minutes before the examination. We routinely distend colon and rectum by placing a tube in the rectum and insufflating with 20 puffs of air, or to the limit of patient comfort. Women are asked to place a tampon in the vagina. All patients are asked to avoid urination for 30 to 40 minutes before the examination to allow bladder filling. Intravenous contrast is routinely given by mechanical injector at 2.5 ml per second for 20 seconds followed by 1.0 ml per second for 100 seconds for a total dose of 150 ml of 60% contrast. Scanning through the pelvis is performed with contiguous 10-mm-thick slices. We routinely screen the abdomen as well, using 10-mm-thick slices at 15- to 20-mm intervals in patients with known or suspected pelvic malignancy. To optimize contrast enhancement we scan the pelvis first, then the abdomen.

BLADDER

Bladder Carcinoma

Bladder cancer may be superficial and confined to the mucosa. However, with invasion of the bladder wall musculature, risk of spread to regional and distant nodes increases. As the number and size of nodal metastases increase, so does the risk of hematogenous spread to bone and lung. Most malignant bladder tumors are transitional cell carcinomas, which carry a risk of multiple synchronous tumors in the ipsilateral ureter and renal collecting system. CT findings are as follows (Figs. 16–4, 16–5):

1. The primary tumor appears as a focal thickening of the bladder wall, or as a soft tissue mass projecting into the bladder lumen. CT is poor at differentiating superficial tumors from those that have invaded the bladder wall.

2. Perivesical spread is seen as soft tissue density in the perivesical fat. Extension to the pelvic side wall precludes complete surgical resection.

3. Pelvic lymph nodes larger than 15-mm size are considered positive for metastatic disease. Smaller nodes are unlikely to be involved.

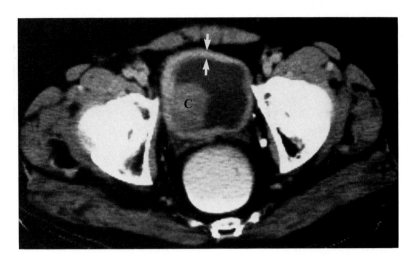

FIGURE 16–4. Bladder transitional cell carcinoma. A papillary transitional cell carcinoma (C) arose from the right lateral wall of the bladder in a 62-year-old man. The tumor infiltrated the bladder wall, but did not extend into the perivesical fat. Note the distinct fat plane separating the bladder from the pelvic side wall. The bladder wall (arrows) is thickened owing to benign prostate hypertrophy.

Bladder Trauma

Rupture of the bladder occurs in 10% of patients with pelvic fractures. In most cases the bladder is lacerated by a spicule of fractured bone, and urine (and contrast) leak into the extraperitoneal space. Intraperitoneal rupture of the bladder occurs as a result of blows to the lower abdomen when the bladder is distended. Either type of rupture is effectively demonstrated by CT following contrast administration either intravenously or by bladder catheter. However, the bladder must be well distended to demonstrate small ruptures. With intraperitoneal rupture, contrast is seen within the peritoneal cavity surrounding bowel loops and extending into the pericolic gutters. Most extraperitoneal ruptures (Fig. 16–6) leak into the retropubic space and may extend along fascial planes to the abdominal wall, retroperitoneal compartments of the abdomen, and, most commonly, into the scrotum and thigh.

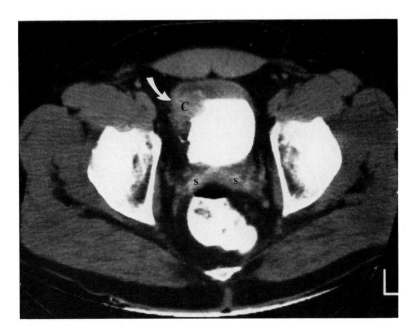

FIGURE 16–5. Bladder transitional cell carcinoma. CT image of a 45-year-old man with gross hematuria demonstrates a transitional cell carcinoma (C) that extends (arrow) through the bladder wall into the perivesical fat. (s = seminal vesicles.)

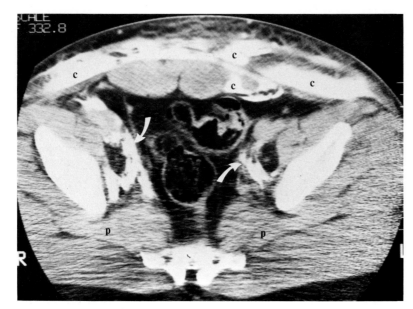

FIGURE 16–6. Extraperitoneal bladder rupture. CT slice at the level of the sciatic foramina in a patient with multiple pelvic fractures demonstrates the extraperitoneal dissection of contrast from a ruptured bladder. Contrast collections are seen along the iliac vessels (arrows) and in the fascial planes of the anterior abdominal wall (c). (p = piriformis muscle coursing through the sciatic foramen.)

UTERUS

Leiomyoma

Leiomyomas are found in up to 40% of women over age 30. As frequent incidental findings, their CT features should be recognized. On CT they appear as soft tissue masses that may be hypodense, isodense, or hyperdense relative to enhanced myometrium (Fig. 16–7). Coarse calcifications within the mass are both common and characteristic. Diffuse enlargement of the uterus and lobulation of its contour are common. Pedunculated leiomyomas may appear as adnexal rather than uterine masses. Leiomyomas cannot be accurately differentiated from much less frequent leiomyosarcomas by CT appearance alone.

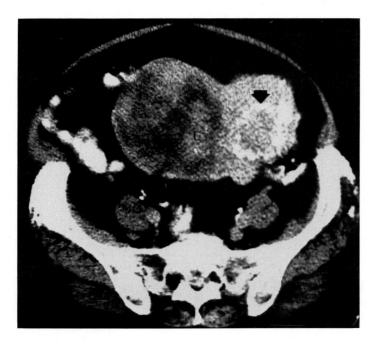

FIGURE 16–7. Uterine leiomyoma. Numerous leiomyomas infiltrate and enlarge the uterus (U). The tumors demonstrate hypodense areas of necrosis and characteristic dense calcification (arrow).

Carcinoma of the Cervix

CT is used to stage cervical carcinoma, document response to therapy, and detect recurrence. Most cervical malignancies are squamous cell carcinomas that spread primarily by direct extension to adjacent organs and tissues. Lymphatic spread to regional nodes is common. Hematogenous spread to lung, bone, and brain is uncommon and occurs late in the course of disease. CT findings are as follows (Figs. 16–8, 16–9)

1. The primary tumor may enlarge the cervix (> 3 cm diameter) or be seen as a hypodense mass within the normally homogeneous cervix. Fluid collections in the endometrial cavity are common due to tumor obstruction of the cervix.

2. Direct extension is seen as thick, irregular tissue strands or masses fanning out from the cervix into the parametrium, the ureters, the vagina, or to the pelvic side walls (obturator internus).

3. Enlarged lymph nodes (> 15 mm) are strong evidence of metastatic involvement, but cervical carcinoma will commonly involve nodes without enlarging them. These involved nodes cannot be differentiated from benign nodes by CT.

4. Recurrences appear as soft tissue masses anywhere in the pelvis but most commonly at the top of the vaginal vault in patients who have undergone hysterectomy. Enlarged nodes are also suspicious for recurrence. Percutaneous biopsy is frequently needed to confirm the diagnosis.

Endometrial Carcinoma

Adenocarcinoma of the endometrium is the most common invasive gynecologic malignancy. CT evaluation is useful as an adjunct to clinical staging, especially in patients with advanced disease or who are difficult to examine. The tumor spreads first by invasion of the myometrium, then by lymphatic channels to regional nodes, or by direct extension through the uterine wall to parametrial tissues. When the uterine serosa is penetrated, diffuse peritoneal spread may

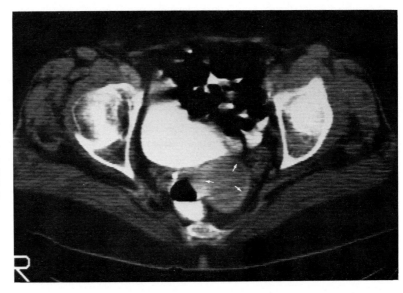

FIGURE 16–8. Cervical carcinoma. A cervical carcinoma, confined to the cervix, is seen as a round hypodense mass within the cervix. The margins of the tumor (arrows) are smooth and well-defined and do not extend into the paracervical tissue. Contrast enhancement is usually needed to visualize the tumor within the cervix.

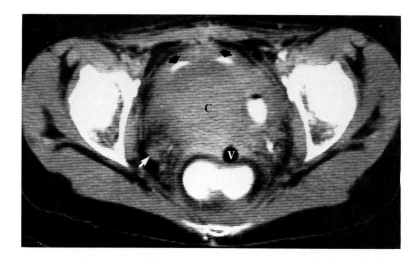

FIGURE 16–9. Cervical carcinoma. CT image at the level of the cervix demonstrates a large cervical carcinoma (C) that has spread into the parametrium and upper vagina. The vagina is marked by a tampon (V). Enlarged internal iliac nodes containing metastatic tumor are also evident (white arrow). The bladder (black arrows) is compressed and distorted by tumor.

occur. Hematogenous spread to lung, bone, liver, and brain is much more common with endometrial than cervical cancer. Since the tumor is isodense with uterine tissue on unenhanced CT, all studies should be performed with intravenous contrast. CT features include the following

1. The primary tumor appears as a hypodense mass in the endometrial cavity or myometrium. The uterine cavity is frequently fluid-filled due to tumor obstruction. The uterus may be greatly enlarged.

2. Parametrial invasion and sidewall extension has the same appearance as cervical carcinoma.

3. Enlarged pelvic lymph nodes indicate tumor involvement. However, as with other pelvic tumors, CT will miss microscopic nodal metastases that do not enlarge the nodes.

4. Tumor recurrences appear as pelvic soft tissue masses or nodal enlargement. Most recurrences occur within 2 years.

OVARY

Ovarian Cancer

Ovarian malignancy encompasses a wide range of histologic tumor types, but most share a common pattern of spread and similar range of CT appearances. Two-thirds of ovarian cancers are cystic, 25% are bilateral, and 85% are endocrinologically nonfunctional. The primary route of tumor spread is diffusion through the peritoneal cavity. Direct extension to pelvic organs, lymphatic spread to nodes, and hematogenous spread to lung, liver, and bone also occur. CT staging of the original tumor tends to be less useful than in other gynecologic malignancy because most patients will go to surgical exploration regardless of the CT findings, and CT will commonly miss even extensive peritoneal seeding. Important CT findings include the following (Fig. 16–10)

1. The primary tumor is usually cystic with thick irregular walls, internal septations, and prominent soft tissue components. Uniformly solid tumors and mixed cystic/solid tumors also occur.

2. Peritoneal implants are seen as soft tissue nodules on peritoneal surfaces or as "omental cake" separating bowel from the anterior abdominal wall (Fig. 17–2).

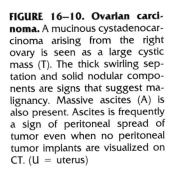
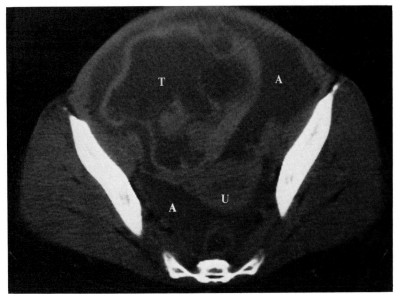

FIGURE 16–10. Ovarian carcinoma. A mucinous cystadenocarcinoma arising from the right ovary is seen as a large cystic mass (T). The thick swirling septation and solid nodular components are signs that suggest malignancy. Massive ascites (A) is also present. Ascites is frequently a sign of peritoneal spread of tumor even when no peritoneal tumor implants are visualized on CT. (U = uterus)

3. The presence of ascites usually indicates peritoneal spread even if peritoneal tumor nodules are not visualized.

4. Lymphatic metastases usually follow gonadal lymphatics, skipping pelvic nodes, to involve nodes at the renal hilum.

Benign Adnexal Masses

While ultrasound is the primary imaging modality for female pelvic masses, adnexal masses may be discovered incidentally on CT. CT may also be used to further characterize difficult examinations. A few conditions to consider are

1. **Functional Ovarian Cyst:** Benign ovarian cysts are common incidental findings. On CT they are well-defined, thin-walled, and have homogeneous internal density near that of water. Atypical cysts can be followed with ultrasound to determine if they resolve after one or two menstrual cycles.

2. **Benign Cystic Teratoma:** The presence of fat, teeth, bone, hair, or fat-fluid levels allows definitive CT diagnosis in most cases.

3. **Ovarian Cystadenoma:** Benign ovarian tumors tend to have regular thin walls, fine septations, no solid components, and no associated ascites. Definitive differentiation of benign from malignant cystic ovarian tumors is not possible with CT.

4. **Endometriosis/Tubo-ovarian Abscess:** These two conditions have an identical CT appearance. Both cause complex cystic pelvic masses, frequently with high density fluid components. Inflammation and fibrosis are prominent. Multiple pelvic organs may be incorporated into the mass. Differentiation from malignancy is usually not possible by imaging methods.

PROSTATE
Prostate Cancer

Prostate cancer is the second most common malignancy in males. Prostate carcinoma spreads by direct extension to periprostatic tissues and the seminal vesicles. Lymphatic spread is similar to bladder cancer, with early involvement of regional pelvic nodes and later involvement of para-aortic and inguinal nodes. Hematogenous spread to the axial skeleton via vertebral veins is particularly characteristic. CT does not demonstrate intraprostatic architecture and is poor at demonstrating intraprostatic tumor. CT findings are (Fig. 16–11)

    1. Enlargement of the prostate due to benign prostatic hypertrophy cannot be differentiated from enlargement due to carcinoma by CT scan. Nodules or stranding densities in the periprostatic fat are signs of tumor extension.

    2. Asymmetry of the seminal vesicles suggests tumor invasion. Bladder involvement is very difficult to detect accurately. Rectal invasion is rare.

    3. Nodes larger than 15 mm are usually involved with metastatic tumor.

TESTICLES

Testicular Cancer

    For the radiologist, the long list of pathologic types of testicular tumors can be easily separated into seminomas and nonseminomas. Seminomas are

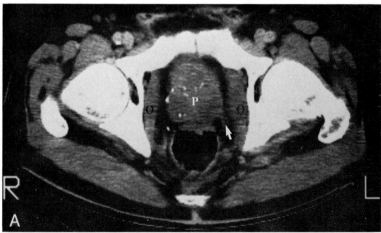

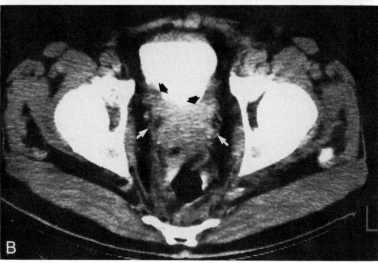

FIGURE 16–11. Prostate carcinoma. CT images through the prostate gland *(A)* and through the bladder base *(B)* demonstrate signs of direct extension of prostate carcinoma into adjacent tissues. The prostate gland (P) is enlarged and nodular and has ill-defined margins. The tumor has invaded both the seminal vesicles and the bladder base (black arrows). Periprostatic stranding densities (white arrows) indicate invasion of adjacent fat. However, the tumor does not extend into the obturator internus muscle (O). Calcifications in the prostate are associated with coexisting benign prostate hypertrophy.

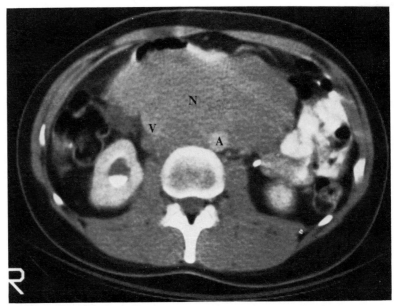

FIGURE 16–12. Metastatic testicular carcinoma. Teratocarcinoma of the testicle, metastatic to para-aortic nodes, causes massive adenopathy (N). The inferior vena cava (V) is anteriorly and laterally displaced by the adenopathy. The aorta (A) is nicely demonstrated by contrast enhancement. The right kidney demonstrates mild dilatation of the collecting system with a contrast-urine level.

treated with orchiectomy and radiation and generally do not require retroperitoneal node dissection. Nonseminomas are treated with orchiectomy or chemotherapy, and generally do require retroperitoneal node dissection. Lymphatic spread of tumor is most common with nodal involvement following an orderly ascending pattern. Initial spread is along gonadal lymphatics following testicular veins to renal hilar nodes (Fig. 16–12). Alternatively, lymphatic metastases may follow the external iliac chain to the para-aortic nodes. Internal iliac and inguinal nodes are rarely involved. Lymphatic spread to mediastinum and hematogenous spread to the lungs rarely occur without para-aortic disease, except for choriocarcinoma, which spreads hematogenously early. CT is excellent for initial tumor staging and for detection of recurrences.

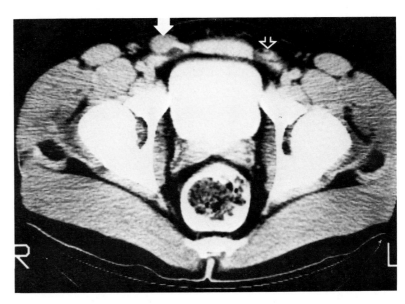

FIGURE 16–13. Undescended testicle. An undescended testicle (closed arrow) is seen in the right inguinal canal near the internal inguinal ring. A normal spermatic cord (open arrow) in the inguinal canal is seen on the left.

Undescended Testicles

Undescended testicles may be located anywhere along the course of testicular descent from the lower pole of the kidney to the superficial inguinal ring. The undescended testis appears as an oval soft tissue density up to 4 cm in size (Fig. 16–13). Undescended testes are usually atrophic. CT detection of intra-abdominal testes requires optimal bowel opacification and intravenous contrast to opacify normal structures. Testes in the inguinal canal can be easily identified on CT as long as you know where to look. The inguinal canal runs an oblique, medially directed course through the flat muscles of the abdominal wall between the deep and superficial inguinal rings. The deep inguinal ring is located midway between the anterior superior iliac spine and the symphysis pubis. The superficial inguinal ring is located just above the pubic crest.

SUGGESTED READING

Pozniak M, Petasnick JP, Matalon TAS, et al.: Computed tomography in the differential diagnosis of pelvic and extrapelvic disease. Radiographics, 5:587–610, 1985.
Sawyer RW, Walsh JW: CT in gynecologic pelvic diseases. Semin Ultrasound CT MR, 9:122–142, 1988.
Walsh JW (ed): Computed Tomography of the Pelvis. Contemporary Issues in Computed Tomography, vol 6. New York, Churchill Livingstone, 1985.

17

Peritoneal Cavity, Vessels, and Nodes

PERITONEAL CAVITY

Anatomy

The various recesses and spaces of the peritoneal cavity are best recognized on CT when ascites is present (Fig. 17–1). Identifying the precise compartment that an abnormality occupies goes a long way toward identifying the nature of the abnormality. While all the spaces of the peritoneal cavity potentially communicate with one another, diseases such as abscess tend to loculate within one or more specific locations. The right subphrenic space communicates around the liver with the anterior subhepatic and posterior subhepatic (Morison's) space. The left subphrenic space communicates freely with the left subhepatic space. The right and left subphrenic spaces are separated by the falciform ligament and do not communicate directly. The lesser sac is the isolated peritoneal compartment between the stomach and the pancreas (see Fig. 14–1). It communicates with the rest of the peritoneal cavity (greater sac) via the foramen of Winslow.

The right subphrenic and subhepatic spaces communicate freely with the pelvic peritoneal cavity via the right paracolic gutter. The phrenicocolic ligament prevents free communication between the left subphrenic and subhepatic spaces and the left paracolic gutter. Free fluid, blood, infection, and peritoneal tumors commonly settle in the pelvis because the pelvis is the most dependent portion of the peritoneal cavity and it communicates with both sides of the abdomen.

The small bowel mesentery suspends the jejunum and ileum, and contains branches of the superior mesenteric artery and vein, as well as mesenteric lymph nodes. The mesentery extends like a fan obliquely across the abdomen from the ligament of Trietz in the left upper quadrant to the region of the right sacroiliac joint. Disease originating from above the ligament is directed toward the right lower quadrant. Disease originating from below the ligament has open access to the pelvis.

The greater omentum is a double layer of peritoneum which hangs from the greater curvature of the stomach and descends in front of the abdominal viscera. The greater omentum encloses fat and a few blood vessels. It serves as fertile ground for implantation of peritoneal metastases.

225

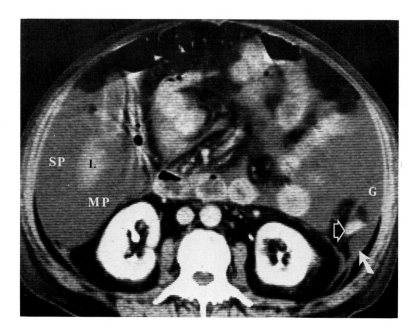

FIGURE 17–1. Ascites. CT image through the midabdomen at the level of the tip of the liver (L) demonstrates low density ascites filling the peritoneal cavity and outlining the peritoneal recesses. The right subphrenic space (SP) is seen to communicate freely with Morison's pouch (MP), the right subhepatic space. The right subphrenic/subhepatic space continues caudad to the pelvis as the right paracolic gutter. The left paracolic gutter (G) is seen to extend three-quarters of the way around the descending colon (open arrow), forming a deep recess (closed arrow).

Fluid in the Peritoneal Cavity

Fluid in the peritoneal cavity varies greatly in composition and may originate from many different sources. Ascites refers to accumulation of serous fluid within the peritoneal cavity and may result from cirrhosis, hypoproteinemia, congestive heart failure, or venous obstruction. Exudative ascites is associated with inflammatory processes such as pancreatitis, peritonitis, and bowel perforation. Hemoperitoneum is an important sign of abdominal injury in blunt trauma. Neoplastic ascites is caused by intraperitoneal tumor. Chylous ascites may be due to obstruction or traumatic injury to the thoracic duct or cisterna chyli. Urine and bile may spread through the peritoneal cavity due to obstruction or injury to the urinary or biliary tracts.

When the anatomy of the peritoneal cavity is known, recognition of fluid density within its recesses on CT is easy. With free peritoneal fluid, bowel loops tend to float to the central abdomen.

Paracentesis is required for precise differentiation of the exact type of fluid present in the peritoneal cavity. However, CT can offer some clues. Serous ascites has an attenuation value near water (-10 to $+15$ H), and tends to accumulate in the greater peritoneal space, sparing the lesser sac. On the other hand, exudative ascites due to pancreatitis tends to preferentially accumulate within the lesser sac. Acute bleeding into the peritoneal cavity has a higher attenuation value, averaging 45 H, and usually above 30 H. Blood tends to accumulate in greatest amount about the site of hemorrhage. Exudative and neoplastic ascites have intermediate attenuation values which overlap both serous ascites and blood.

Loculations of peritoneal fluid due to benign or malignant adhesions may simulate cystic abdominal masses. Tense loculated ascites may accumulate in confined spaces like the lesser sac and compress and displace bowel loops. Loculated ascites, however, tends to conform to the general shape of the space it occupies. Cystic masses make their own space, cause greater displacement of adjacent structures, and have more varied internal consistency. *Pseudomyxoma peritonei* is an unusual complication of mucocele of the appendix or of mucinous cystadenocarcinoma manifested by filling of the peritoneal cavity with gelatinous mucin. The mucinous fluid is typically loculated and causes scalloping and mass effect on the liver and adjacent bowel. Septations, mottled densities, and calcification within the fluid may be seen on CT.

Free Peritoneal Air

Free air within the peritoneal cavity is an important sign of a perforated viscus but may be surprisingly difficult to recognize on CT. The diagnosis is based upon recognizing that the air is outside of the bowel lumen. Images photographed at "lung windows" (window level −400 to −600 H, window width 500 to 1000 H) should be routinely examined for free intraperitoneal air. Unsuspected pneumothorax may also be detected using this technique on abdominal CT scans obtained because of abdominal trauma.

Peritoneal Tumor Implants

Diffuse metastatic seeding of the peritoneal cavity occurs commonly with abdominopelvic tumors. The most common tumors to spread by this method are ovarian carcinoma in females, and stomach, pancreas, and colon carcinoma in males. The preferential sites for tumor implantation are the pouch of Douglas, the right paracolic gutter, and the greater omentum. CT findings with peritoneal tumor seeding are (Fig. 17–2)

1. Ascites, frequently loculated
2. Tumor nodules on the parietal peritoneal surface
3. "Omental cake"—thickened nodular greater omentum displacing bowel away from the anterior abdominal wall
4. Tumor nodules in the mesentery
5. Thickening and nodularity of the bowel wall due to serosal tumor implant.

Minute implants, which may be painfully obvious and diffuse at surgery, are commonly missed by CT due to their small size. The presence of ascites in patients with known abdominopelvic tumor, especially ovarian carcinoma, should be regarded as suspicious for peritoneal seeding. Calcification of tumor implants may aid in their CT identification.

Peritoneal Mesothelioma

Approximately 20% of mesotheliomas arise within the abdomen. On CT, mesothelioma causes diffuse irregular thickening of the peritoneal surfaces. Nodules and globular thickening are commonly evident. Multilocular cystic forms of the tumor also occur. Ascites is present in most cases.

Abscess

CT is commonly requested to search and destroy abdominal abscesses. Once found, percutaneous aspiration confirms the diagnosis and provides

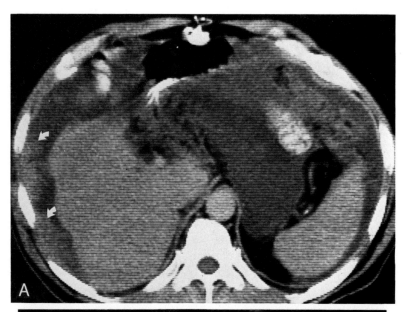

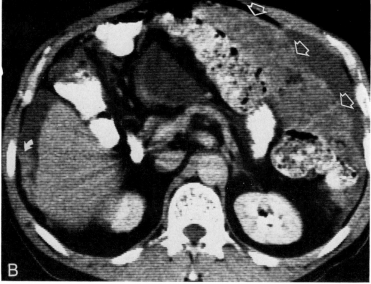

FIGURE 17–2. Peritoneal implants and omental cake. CT images through the upper *(A)* and lower *(B)* portions of the liver demonstrate peritoneal metastases due to colon carcinoma. Tumor metastases (closed arrows) on the parietal peritoneum are seen as soft tissue density masses projecting into peritoneal fluid. Tumor implants on the greater omentum (open arrows) produce a soft tissue density pancake, "omental cake," separating bowel from the anterior abdominal wall.

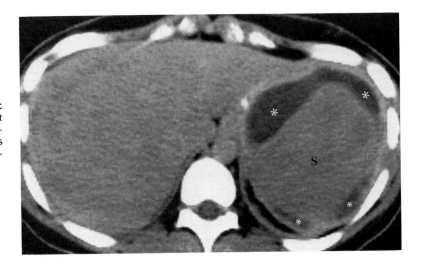

FIGURE 17–3. Left subphrenic abscess. An abscess in the left subphrenic recess of the peritoneal cavity is seen as loculations of the fluid density (*) surrounding the spleen (S).

material for culture. Image-directed catheter placement is commonly used for drainage ("pus-busting"). Most abscesses occur as complications of abdominal trauma, surgery, or bowel perforation. Intraperitoneal abscesses are commonly located in the pelvic cavity and the subphrenic and subhepatic spaces. CT features of abscess are (Figs. 17–3, 17–4)

1. Loculated fluid collection, often with internal debris and fluid-fluid levels

2. Commonly, definable walls, often irregularly thickened.

3. Presence of gas within the fluid collection, which is strongly indicative of abscess

4. Thickening of fascia and obliteration of fat planes due to inflammation

5. Ascites, pleural effusions, and lower lobe pulmonary infiltrates, commonly accompanying abdominal abscesses.

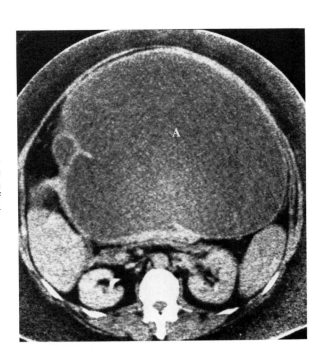

FIGURE 17–4. Huge abdominal abscess. Image obtained through the midabdomen in a very obese patient demonstrates a huge cystic mass (A) with well-defined thick walls. This mass contained 14 L of purulent green fluid that grew *Streptococcus agalactiae.*

Any fluid collection within the abdomen is suspect in patients who are clinically suspicious for abscess. Fine needle aspiration is a safe and definitive way to exclude or confirm the diagnosis.

Large Abdominal Cystic Masses

Large cystic masses in the abdomen commonly present challenges in diagnosis (Fig. 17–4). Differential considerations include

1. Abscess
2. Loculated ascites
3. Pancreatic pseudocyst
4. Ovarian cyst/cystic tumor
5. *Lymphoceles* are cystic masses containing lymphatic fluid that occur as complications of surgery or trauma that disrupts lymphatic channels. They may appear days to years after surgery. They may be of any size.
6. *Cystic lymphangiomas* are congenital counterparts of lymphoceles. They are believed to arise due to congenital obstruction of lymphatic channels. *Mesenteric cysts* are cystic lymphangiomas of the mesentery. *Omental cysts* are less common lymphangiomas of the greater omentum.

VESSELS

Anatomy

The abdominal aorta descends anterior to the left side of the spine to its bifurcation at the level of the iliac crest. The normal aorta does not exceed 3 cm in diameter and tapers progressively as it proceeds distally. The inferior vena cava (IVC) lies to the right of the aorta. Its shape varies from round to oval to slit-like depending upon breath-holding technique and intravenous fluid balance. The celiac axis originates from the anterior aspect of the aorta at the level of the aortic hiatus in the diaphragm (see Fig. 14–3). The superior mesenteric artery (SMA) originates anteriorly from the aorta 1 cm below the celiac axis. The renal arteries arise from the lateral aspect of the aorta within 1 cm of the SMA.

A number of vascular anomalies must be recognized to avoid misinterpretation as abnormalities. Duplication of the IVC may be identified, extending between the left common iliac vein and the left renal vein on the left side of the aorta. Left renal veins may course posterior instead of anterior to the aorta, or duplicated left renal veins may course both anterior and posterior to the aorta. The intrahepatic segment of the IVC may be absent with drainage continuing to the superior vena cava via the azygos system.

Technique

Scanning of the aorta and vena cava is routinely performed using contiguous 10-mm-thick slices following both oral and intravenous contrast. In cases of suspected aneurysm rupture or inflammatory aneurysm, both pre- and postinfusion scans should be obtained. Acute higher density hemorrhage is more obvious on preinfusion scans. Demonstration of enhancement of the periaortic tissue confirms the diagnosis of inflammatory aneurysm.

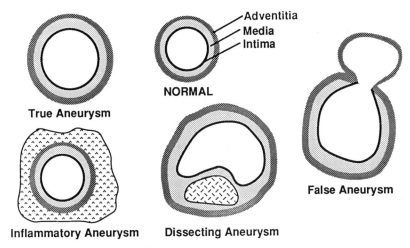

True Aneurysm

NORMAL

Adventitia
Media
Intima

False Aneurysm

Inflammatory Aneurysm   Dissecting Aneurysm

FIGURE 17–5. Types of aneurysms. Diagram illustrating the major types of aneurysms.

Aneurysm

Aneurysms are defined as circumscribed dilatations of an artery. An aneurysm of the abdominal aorta is present when the diameter of the aorta exceeds 3 cm or when the aorta fails to taper as it proceeds distally. CT provides more comprehensive evaluation of aneurysms than does ultrasound. Several types of aneurysms are defined (Fig. 17–5):

1. A *true aneurysm* (Fig. 17–6) involves all 3 layers of the aortic wall (intima, media, and adventitia). The risk of rupture increases dramatically when the diameter exceeds 5 cm (Fig. 17–7).

2. A *pseudoaneurysm* or *false aneurysm* is a perforation of the aorta, usually due to trauma or surgery, with the hematoma confined within the adventitia or surrounding fibrous tissue.

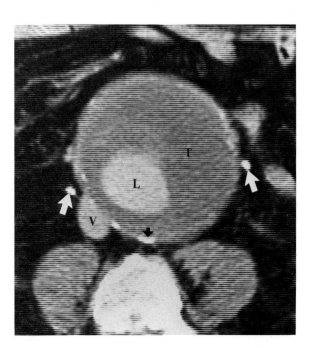

FIGURE 17–6. Abdominal aortic aneurysm. CT shows a 10-cm aneurysm of the abdominal aorta, which is lined with thrombus (T). The patent lumen (L) enhances with contrast. The intima can be identified by the presence of calcification (black arrow). The ureters (white arrows) are seen in close proximity to the aneurysm. Clinically silent ureteral obstruction is one of the complications of abdominal aortic aneurysm. (V = inferior vena cava.)

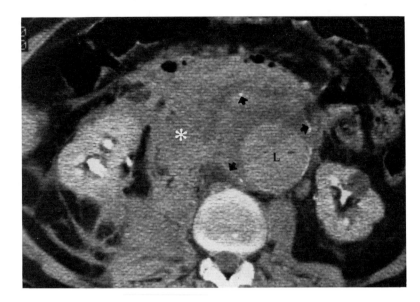

FIGURE 17–7. Rupture of an abdominal aortic aneurysm. Blood (*) from rupture of an aortic aneurysm dissects through the retroperitoneal space and displaces the right kidney. The wall of the aneurysm is identified by calcification (arrows). The lumen (L) shows contrast enhancement.

3. An *inflammatory aneurysm* (Fig. 17–8) is characterized by perianeurysmal fibrosis and increased difficulty of surgical repair.

Aneurysms of the iliac artery (Fig. 17–9) are usually clinically silent, but rupture is common and has a high mortality. Most occur in association with aortic aneurysms.

Venous Thrombosis

Venous thrombi may be bland, septic, or associated with tumor invasion. CT signs of thrombosis include increased venous diameter, low density intralu-

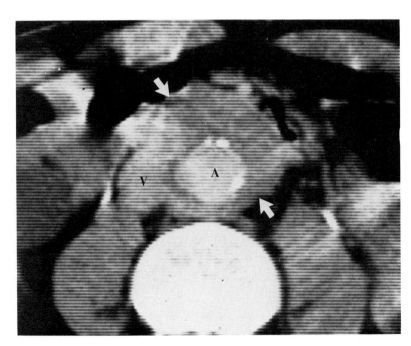

FIGURE 17–8. Inflammatory aneurysm. The abdominal aorta (A) is surrounded by a collar of inflammatory tissue (arrows). The aorta is only minimally dilated to 3.2 cm, but it has a thick wall that is calcified. (V = inferior vena cava.)

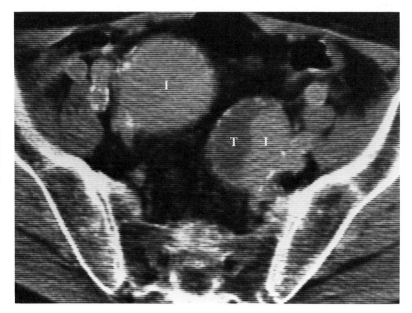

FIGURE 17–9. Bilateral iliac artery aneurysms. CT slice through the pelvis demonstrates bilateral aneurysms of the common iliac arteries (I). The left iliac artery aneurysm contains a larger thrombus (T).

minal filling defects, and surrounding rim of high density contrast. Flow artifacts and layering of contrast may mimic thrombosis. Extrinsic displacement and compression may also be difficult to differentiate from thrombosis. Tumors most likely to extend into the inferior vena cava are renal, hepatic, and adrenal carcinomas.

NODES

Anatomy

Normal lymph nodes are oblong in shape and homogeneous in CT attenuation. Most are oriented parallel to their accompanying vessels. Abdominoaortic nodal groups surround the aorta and IVC and are commonly involved in abdominal and pelvic malignancy. Visceral nodes drain adjacent organs and include mesenteric, hepatic, splenic, and pancreaticoduodenal nodal groups.

Technique

Both intravenous and oral contrast are essential for accurate identification of nodal disease. We routinely scan the abdomen and pelvis with 10-mm-thick slices at 15-mm intervals when searching for adenopathy.

Nodal Metastases

We consider nodes to be pathologically enlarged when they exceed 15 mm in largest dimension in the abdomen and pelvis or 6 mm in largest dimension in the retrocrural region. Multiple 10-mm nodes in the abdomen or pelvis are considered suspicious. Interpretation must always be made in clinical context. Even minimally enlarged nodes should be viewed with suspicion when present in an area where a known malignancy is highly likely to metastasize.

Unfortunately, involvement of nodes with metastatic tumor does not usually change the CT attenuation of the node, and in some cases will not enlarge the node sufficiently to be interpreted as pathologic by size criteria. Nodes can be enlarged due to benign disease (false positive interpretation), or can be of normal size and yet be involved (false negative interpretation). Low attenuation within enlarged nodes is seen uncommonly and usually represents central necrosis. Calcification of nodes may occur with some calcifying tumors or with tumor necrosis following treatment.

Lymphoma

Lymphomas are divided into Hodgkin's and non-Hodgkin's types. Hodgkin's lymphoma (HL) accounts for about 40 percent of the total, and tends to spread in an orderly contiguous manner. Non-Hodgkin's lymphoma (NHL) is a mixed group of diseases with a confusing array of constantly changing names and classifications. Noncontiguous spread and involvement of the gastrointestinal tract are characteristic of NHL. CT features of lymphoma in the abdomen and pelvis include:

1. Multiple enlarged individual nodes
2. Coalescence of enlarged nodes to form rounded multilobular masses which may encase vessels, displace organs, and obstruct ureters (Fig. 17–10).

Conglomerate nodal masses are typical of lymphoma and are rarely seen with other conditions.

AIDS

Full-blown acquired immunodeficiency syndrome (AIDS) is characterized on abdominal CT by signs of intra-abdominal opportunistic infections, non-Hodgkin's lymphoma, and Kaposi's sarcoma:

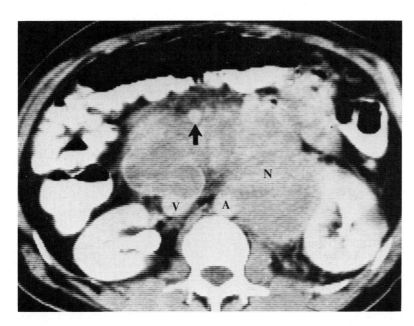

FIGURE 17–10. Confluent retroperitoneal adenopathy. CT scan at the level of the renal hila in a patient with lymphoma presenting with a recent-onset left varicocele. Conglomerate adenopathy (N) extends from the periaortic region, displacing the left kidney laterally. The left testicular and renal veins were enveloped and occluded by the mass, resulting in the left varicocele. The superior mesenteric artery (arrow) is anteriorly displaced. (A = aorta; V = inferior vena cava.)

1. Adenopathy involving the retroperitoneal, pelvic, and mesenteric nodes is due to lymphoma, Kaposi's sarcoma, or infection, especially *Mycobacterium avium-intracellulare.*

2. Focal thickening of bowel wall is due to opportunistic infections of the gastrointestinal tract or focal masses of Kaposi's sarcoma.

3. Hypodense lesions in the liver and spleen are usually due to lymphoma.

AIDS-related complex (ARC) presents on abdominal CT as a triad of mild adenopathy, splenomegaly, and perirectal inflammation. Nodes in the abdomen and pelvis are enlarged to 5- to 10-mm in size as part of the benign lymphadenopathy syndrome. Adenopathy larger than 15 mm suggests development of lymphoma or Kaposi's sarcoma and is considered an indication for percutaneous biopsy. Perirectal inflammation is seen as soft tissue stranding densities in the perirectal fat due to chronic proctitis.

SUGGESTED READING

Dodds WJ, Foley WD, Lawson TL, et al.: Anatomy and imaging of the lesser peritoneal sac. Am J Roentgenol, 144:567–575, 1985.

Jeffrey RB, Nyberg DA, Bottles K, et al.: Abdominal CT in acquired immunodeficiency syndrome. Am J Roentgenol, 146:7–13, 1986.

Kellman GM, Alpern MB, Sandler MA, et al.: Computed tomography of vena caval anomalies with embryologic correlation. Radiographics, 8:533–556, 1988.

LaRoy LL, Cormier PJ, Matalon TAS, et al.: Imaging of abdominal aortic aneurysms. Am J Roentgenol, 152:785–792, 1989.

Meyers MA: Dynamic Radiology of the Abdomen. Normal and Pathologic Anatomy, 3rd ed. New York, Springer-Verlag, 1988.

Walkey MM, Friedman AC, Sohotra P, et al.: CT manifestations of peritoneal carcinomatosis. Am J Roentgenol, 150:1035–1041, 1988.

Yeh H-C, Shafir MK, Slater G, et al.: Ultrasonography and computed tomography in pseudomyxoma peritonei. Radiology, 153:507–510, 1984.

THE MUSCULOSKELETAL 3
SYSTEM

18

Musculoskeletal System

The use of CT in the musculoskeletal system has been markedly affected by the introduction of magnetic resonance imaging (MRI). Many applications of CT have diminished or even been eliminated as a result of MRI; nevertheless, CT continues to play an important role in musculoskeletal diagnostic imaging. This chapter will examine the use of CT in the musculoskeletal system with the exception of lumbar spine disc disease and stenosis.

TRAUMA

CT has proven to be extremely important in trauma, both in the axial (central) and the appendicular (peripheral) skeleton. CT should be used in almost any instance of trauma in which plain films do not clearly depict the full extent of the bony pathology. Because of its ability to demonstrate cross-sectional anatomy and then display any additional plane with reformations, CT has almost completely replaced conventional tomography in evaluating trauma to the skeleton.

Axial Skeleton (Spine)

All spinal trauma with neurologic deficits should be examined with CT to fully evaluate the amount of bony abnormality, regardless of what the plain films demonstrate. Obviously the patient's condition will not always allow this; however, it should be considered in every case. If no neurologic deficits are present, plain films are usually sufficient. However, if the plain films are nondiagnostic or raise questions that cannot be answered by the clinical exam, CT should be performed.

It is not necessary to do a myelographic enhanced CT if MRI is available; however, it is usually recommended if no MRI can be obtained and the status of the cord is in question. In the lumbar spine a myelo/CT is rarely necessary.

Slice thickness will vary depending on the anatomic location in the spine, the number of vertebral body levels to be examined, and the need for reformations. In general, thin slices (1.5 mm) will allow for more acceptable reformations, but cannot be recommended over large areas of the spine due to the enormous number of slices that would be taken. Contiguous 3-mm slices are usually employed throughout the spine with good results in most instances.

A typical example of a cervical spine fracture that is more completely evaluated with CT is a Jefferson fracture, i.e., a burst fracture of the C-1 ring (Fig. 18–1). Any vertebral body fractures with retropulsed fragments in the central canal should be examined with CT (Fig. 18–2).

It is not unusual to have an underlying bony abnormality that allows minor trauma to result in a fracture. An example of this is a pathologic fracture through a vertebral body with eosinophilic granuloma (Fig. 18–3). CT can demonstrate the extent of bony involvement as well as show the soft tissue mass. MRI would demonstrate these findings; however, if life-support equipment or external stabilization is required, MRI might not be possible.

In the lumbar spine a common post-traumatic entity that is clearly shown with CT is spondylolysis. Although many claim it is necessary to use reformations to identify the pars defects, they can be easily seen by examining the midvertebral body axial slice. This can be found by using the lateral "scout" view or by finding the basivertebral plexus, which is always in the posterior aspect of the midvertebral body. On this slice the lamina should be a continuous bony ring; any defect is a pars break (spondylolysis) (Fig. 18–4). Occasionally the pars defect

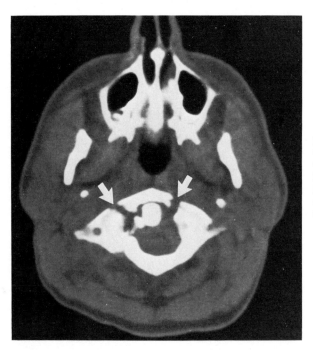

FIGURE 18–1. Jefferson fracture. An axial slice through the first cervical (C-1) vertebra in this patient with trauma shows several obvious fractures of the bony ring (arrows) that were not appreciated on the plain film. CT often reveals fractures not visible by conventional radiography and should be used in all spinal fracture cases.

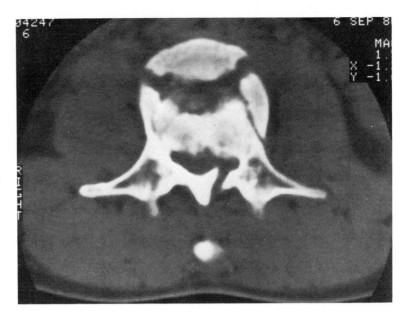

FIGURE 18–2. Vertebral body fracture. An axial cut through the L-2 vertebral body in this victim of an automobile accident shows a stellate fracture of the body, but, more importantly, it shows a displaced fracture of the lamina, with part of the lamina extending into the central canal.

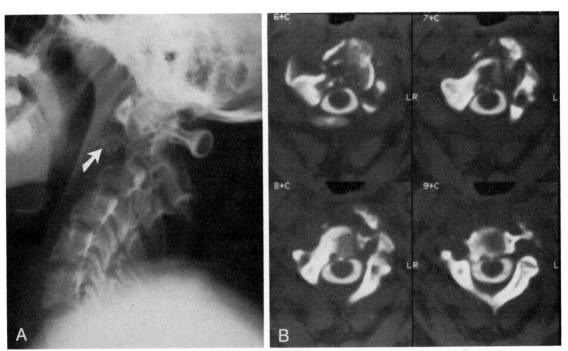

FIGURE 18–3. Eosinophilic granuloma with a fracture. (*A*) A lateral cervical spine film in this 12-year-old with neck pain shows the C-2 vertebral body to be disrupted with an apparent large fragment extending into the retropharyngeal space (arrow). (*B*) An axial metrizamide CT cut through the C-2 body shows a comminuted fracture of the body with some impression on the cord. This was secondary to eosinophilic granuloma.

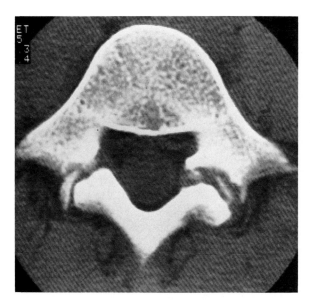

FIGURE 18–4. Spondylolysis. This axial CT cut through the center of L-5 reveals linear breaks in the lamina bilaterally, which can be mistaken for normal facets. On a midbody cut, such as this, the lamina should be an unbroken bony ring. The facets barely seen posterior to the pars break will be visible on adjacent cuts.

is very smooth and bilaterally symmetric so that it resembles normal facet joints and is overlooked. For this reason, any break in the bony ring that occurs on the slice that has the basivertebral plexus is a spondylolysis until proven otherwise.

A very uncommon but serious sequella of spondylolysis is a fibrocartilaginous buildup that can occur at the pars defect or fracture site to such a degree that it encroaches on the thecal sac or nerve roots (Fig. 18–5). If not recognized, a surgical fusion across that level would result in missing what could be the main cause of the patient's complaints. This fibrocartilaginous mass has been likened to excess callus across a fracture in a long bone that occurs if it is not immobilized. Whatever the etiology, it is rare but should be searched for in every instance of spondylolysis that is studied with CT.

A fracture that is often mistaken for metastatic disease is a stress fracture of the sacrum. This is found primarily in two types of patients—patients with osteoporosis and patients with prior irradiation. They present with low back or

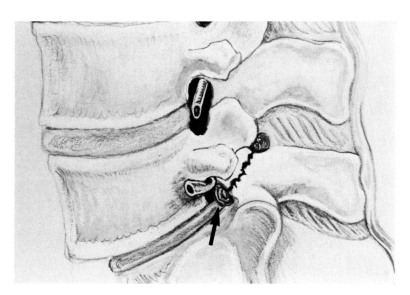

FIGURE 18–5. Fibrocartilaginous mass at pars break. This drawing shows how a fibrocartilaginous mass (arrow) at a pars break can impinge on a nerve root in the neuroforamen.

sacral pain and have patchy sclerosis of one or both sacral alae on plain films (Fig. 18–6A). A radionuclide bone scan is characteristic and should be pathognomonic because of its geographic appearance throughout half or all of the sacrum (Fig. 18–6B). A CT is often done to confirm the diagnosis of a stress fracture or to convince a disbelieving clinician. CT will demonstrate a fracture in most, but not all, cases (Fig. 18–6C).

Appendicular Skeleton

Any complex joint, such as the hip or shoulder, can hide multiple fractures or loose bodies on routine plain film examination and should be considered for CT imaging. The wrist and ankle are also imaged more completely with CT, as are the sacroiliac (S-I) joints.

CT of the hip is routinely done in most centers when loose bodies are considered, whether or not the plain films are positive (Fig. 18–7). In instances

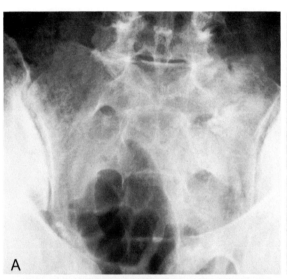

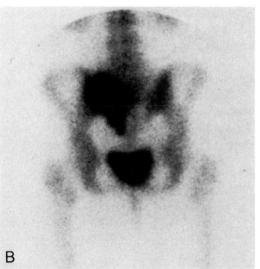

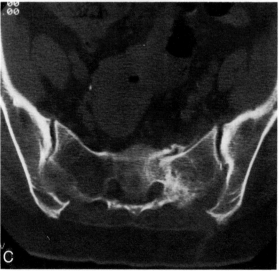

FIGURE 18–6. Sacral stress fracture. (*A*) An anteroposterior plain film of the sacrum in this elderly woman with pain shows faint patchy sclerosis throughout the left sacral ala. This could easily represent metastatic disease. (*B*) A posterior view of a radionuclide bone scan shows a geographic pattern of increased uptake, corresponding to the left sacral ala and body. This is a characteristic appearance for a sacral stress fracture. (*C*) A CT scan through the sacrum reveals a left-sided sacral fracture with reactive sclerosis in the ala.

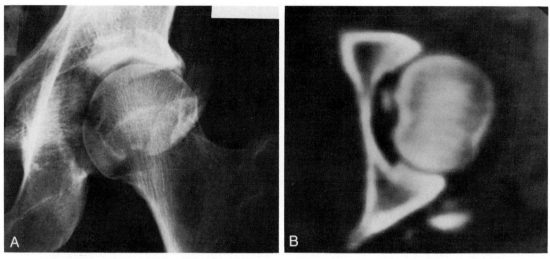

FIGURE 18–7. Hip fracture with loose body. (*A*) A plain film of the hip in this patient with trauma to the pelvis shows a large bony fragment just lateral to the acetabulum. This fracture fragment is most commonly seen with a posterior rim fracture. (*B*) A CT scan through the hip shows not only the posterior rim fracture, as expected from the plain film, but also a loose body in the joint medial to the femoral head. CT is excellent for showing free fragments in joints.

where metal might be present in the joint (bullets, shrapnel, or fixation pins or screws from surgery), CT can still be employed with useful information almost always obtained in spite of metallic streak artifacts (Figs. 18–8, 18–9). Reformations often will diminish the metallic streak artifact, making interpretation less difficult.

CT can be very useful in children with congenital dislocation of the hip (CDH). Plain films will usually suffice for making the initial diagnosis, but after the patient is placed in abduction in a spica cast it can be very difficult using plain films to confirm that the femoral head is relocated (Fig. 18–10). CT can show the femoral head position with minimal radiation dose to the patient. MRI can do the same thing, but it can be difficult to get the patient in a spica cast fixed in abduction into the small aperture of the MRI unit.

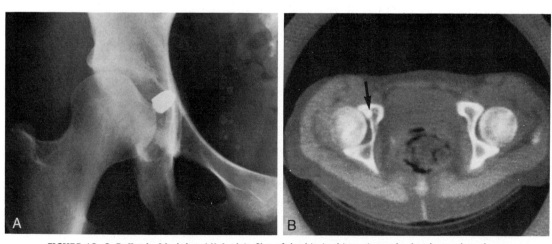

FIGURE 18–8. Bullet in hip joint. (*A*) A plain film of the hip in this patient who has been shot shows a bullet overlying the hip joint. Plain films did not reveal the intra- (versus extra-) articular position of the bullet. (*B*) A CT scan through the hips shows a faint track of the bullet in the femoral head, but the bullet itself is clearly outside of the joint, embedded in the anterior column (arrow).

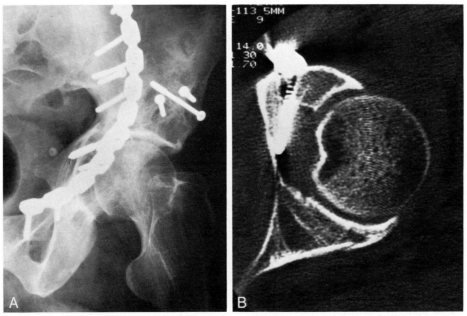

FIGURE 18–9. Metallic screw in hip joint. (*A*) Internal fixation of the pelvis was performed on this patient following multiple fractures suffered in an automobile accident. He now presents with hip pain that was thought to be secondary to inadvertent placement of one or more of the screws into the joint. Plain films did not resolve the issue. (*B*) A CT scan through the hip revealed that one of the screws had indeed been placed in the joint. In spite of the metallic nature of the screws and plate and the streak artifacts, a diagnostic CT study was obtained.

Fractures of the shoulder, with or without dislocation, are studied with CT only if the plain films do not clearly show all the abnormalities, or if it is felt that some aspect of the anatomy is not depicted (Figs. 18–11, 18–12).

In the wrist, CT has been shown to be very adept at demonstrating fractures that are not seen on plain films (Fig. 18–13). A radionuclide bone scan can be helpful in pinpointing the area of concern, which can then be imaged in fine detail with thin section CT slices, as opposed to performing thicker slices through the entire wrist (Fig. 18–14).

In the ankle, as in the wrist, a positive bone scan can often reduce the area scanned and allow thinner slices to be used. A frequent use of CT in the ankle is in tarsal coalition. The most common site for coalition is at the calcaneonavicular joint. The next most common locations are at the talonavicular joint and the middle facet of the talocalcaneal joint (Fig. 18–15). It is often difficult to diagnose a coalition if there is a fibrous rather than a bony fusion, but usually there will be enough associated bony abnormalities to allow a diagnosis to be made (Fig. 18–16).

CT can be very helpful in ankle fractures and in evaluating displacement of the peroneal tendons from their normal position behind the fibula. It has also been used to diagnose tendonitis or rupture of the posterior tibial tendon, usually seen in patients with rheumatoid arthritis. Most centers prefer MRI over CT for tendon evaluation. An ankle fracture that can be confusing on plain films is avulsion of the anterior inferior tibiofibular ligament, called a fracture of Tillaux. A bony fragment off the tibia is avulsed, but its location, whether it is anterior or posterior, can be difficult to ascertain on plain films (Fig. 18–17A–C). CT will demonstrate the fragment's position and can be performed quickly and inex-

Text continued on page 251

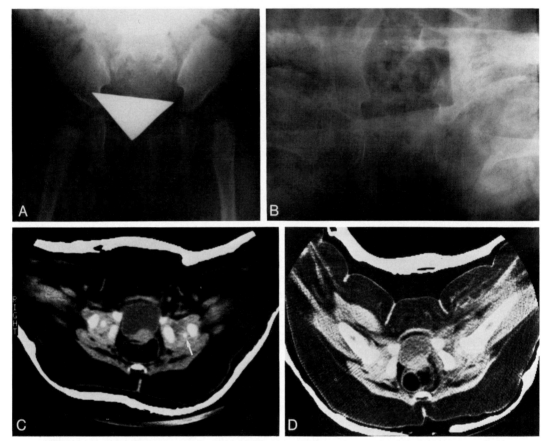

FIGURE 18–10. Congenital dislocation of the hip. (A) An anteroposterior plain film shows left-sided congenital dislocation of the hip in this infant. (B) A plain film obtained after the child was placed in an abduction spica cast fails to show whether the left hip is adequately reduced. (C) A CT scan through the hips shows the left femoral capital epiphysis to be posteriorly dislocated (arrow). This is a critical diagnosis, since the patient must be kept casted in this position for months. Obviously, if the hip remains dislocated, the casting is useless. (D) After removal of the first cast and manual reduction of the hip, a CT scan shows the hip to be reduced in the second spica cast.

FIGURE 18–11. Glenohumeral Joint fracture. (*A* and *B*) Two cuts through a fractured scapula reveal that the fracture extends into the articular portion of the glenoid and to the anterior portion of the scapula. The plain films failed to show the full extent of the fracture.

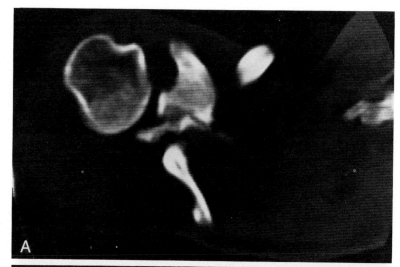

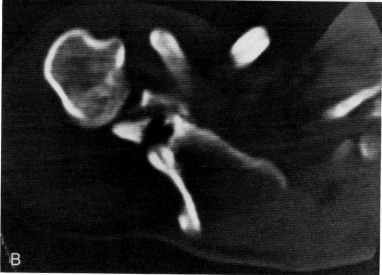

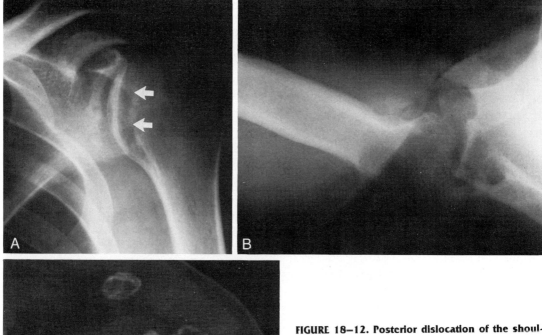

FIGURE 18–12. Posterior dislocation of the shoulder. (*A*) An anteroposterior plain film of the shoulder in this patient with chronic shoulder pain reveals a vertical lucency (arrows) that has been termed a "trough" sign, which is indicative of an impaction from a posterior dislocation. (*B*) An axillary view shows that the humeral head is posteriorly dislocated. (*C*) A CT scan through the shoulder gives a better look at the impacted humeral head and shows an avulsion from the scapula.

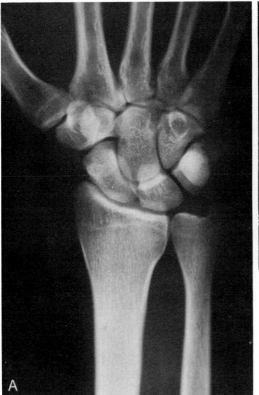

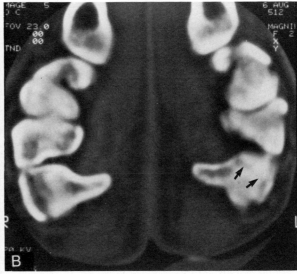

FIGURE 18–13. Fractured hamate bone. (*A*) A plain film of the wrist in this patient who fell on an outstretched hand failed to reveal an abnormality. Oblique views and a carpal tunnel view for the hook of the hamate were all negative. (*B*) A CT scan of the wrist shows a fracture of the body of the hamate bone (arrows) that extended through the entire hamate on several cuts.

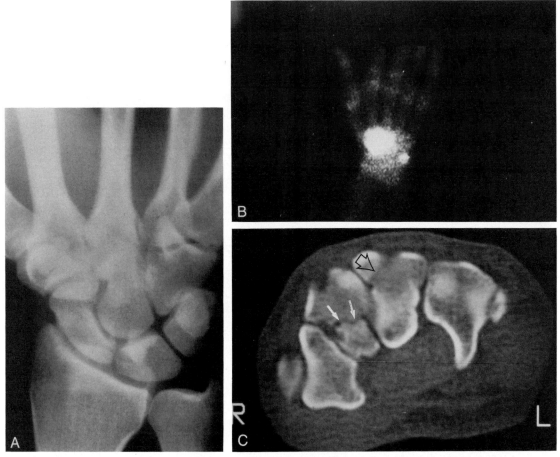

FIGURE 18–14. Fractured multangular with negative plain films and positive bone scan. (*A*) This karate devotee suffered continuous wrist pain following a workout. The anteroposterior plain film, obliques, and conventional tomograms were negative. (*B*) A radionuclide bone scan showed increased radionuclide uptake over the pisiform and at the base of the second and third metacarpals. (*C*) A CT scan of the wrist revealed a fracture of the lesser multangular bone (arrows). The lucency through the capitate (open arrow) is a joint space and illustrates how difficult it can be to separate normal anatomy from pathology in the small joints of the wrist and ankle. Both wrists or ankles should be imaged together so that one can compare the normal joint with the abnormal one.

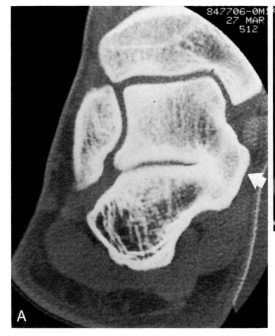

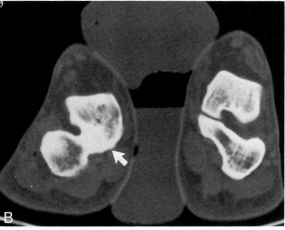

FIGURE 18–15. Tarsal coalition at the talocalcaneal joint. (*A*) An axial CT scan through the ankle in this patient with painful flat feet shows a bony bridge between the talus and the calcaneus (arrow). (*B*) The coalition (arrow) is more easily appreciated when the normal ankle is shown.

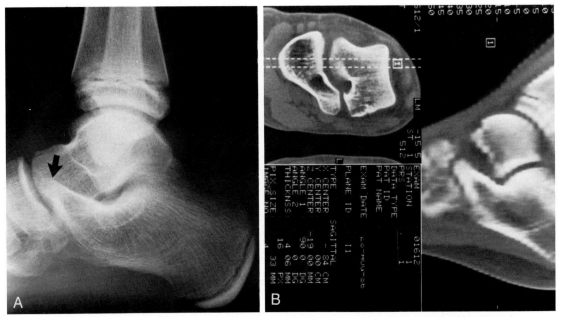

FIGURE 18–16. Fibrous tarsal coalition at the calcaneonavicular joint. (*A*) A lateral plain film of the ankle in this patient with painful flat feet shows a prominent anterior process of the calcaneus (arrow). (*B*) A CT scan through the ankle with a sagittal reformation shows the prominent anterior process to better advantage and shows that there is not a bony ankylosis. This is consistent with a fibrous coalition.

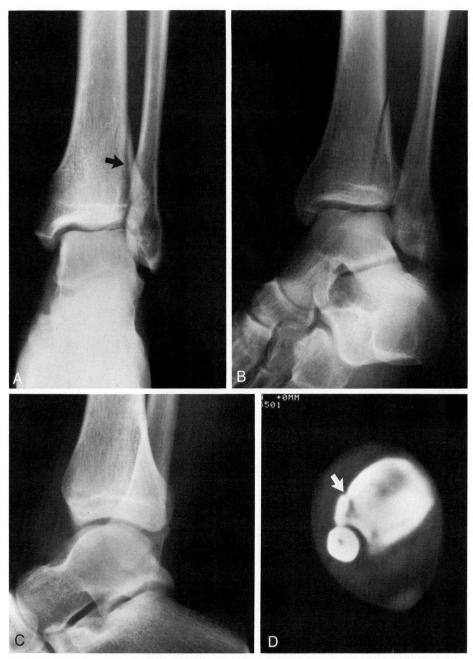

FIGURE 18–17. Fracture of Tillaux. (*A*) An anteroposterior film and (*B*) an oblique plain film of the ankle show a fracture of the lateral aspect of the distal tibia (arrow), but the lateral view (*C*) fails to show if it is anteriorly or posteriorly located. Because internal fixation was planned, it was considered essential to know the exact location of the fracture. (*D*) A CT scan through the distal tibia shows the fracture to be anteriorly located (arrow). This is consistent with an avulsion of the anterior inferior tibiofibular ligament and has been termed a fracture of Tillaux.

pensively (Fig. 18–17D). In children, the distal tibial physis fuses incrementally from medial to lateral with the lateral portion, which is attached to the anterior inferior tibiofibular ligament, susceptible to an avulsion injury called a juvenile Tillaux fracture. This is basically a Salter type 3 injury.

Facial trauma can be difficult to assess with plain films, and CT should be considered in almost all instances of facial trauma when fractures are suspected. Orbital blowout fractures, Le Fort's fractures, and countless other types of facial fractures are often seen with CT and not appreciated on plain films. Mandibular and temporomandibular joint fractures should also be studied with CT when plain films are inconclusive.

Tumors and Infection

MRI is without question superior to CT in evaluating tumors of the musculoskeletal system. Although it is true that CT is better than MRI at evaluating subtle cortical abnormalities, in reality it is seldom necessary to improve on the resolution that MRI affords. In addition to passable bony evaluation, MRI is unsurpassed at showing the extent of tumors in the medullary bone and in the soft tissues. What then is the role of CT in tumors? Not much!

CT can be helpful in diagnosing bony involvement of multiple myeloma prior to plain film findings. CT of the spine will show a "Swiss cheese" pattern of lytic myeloma (Fig. 18–18). In longstanding myeloma the pattern is considerably different. The few remaining normal trabeculae undergo compensatory hypertrophy and the resulting appearance is of thick, sclerotic bony struts with

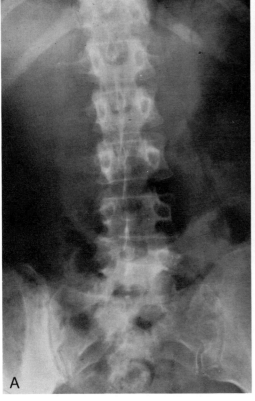

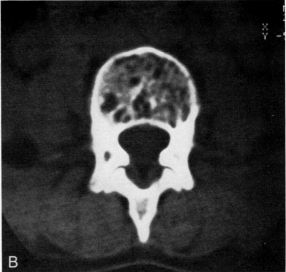

FIGURE 18–18. Multiple myeloma. (A) An anteroposterior film of the lumbar spine was taken in this patient with known myeloma to see if bony involvement was present. The plain films were all considered normal except for mild osteopenia. (B) A CT scan through a lumbar vertebral body shows diffuse lytic lesions consistent with multiple myeloma. This is a typical appearance for multiple myeloma in the spine and almost always precedes plain film findings.

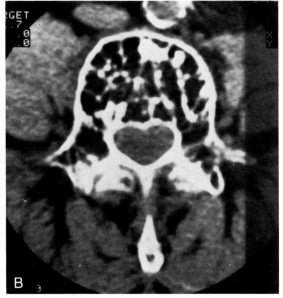

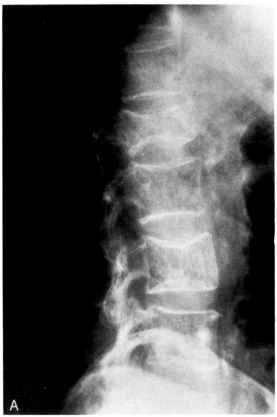

FIGURE 18–19. Chronic multiple myeloma. (*A*) A lateral plain film of the spine in this patient with myeloma shows marked osteopenia and a partial collapse of the L-2 vertebral body. (*B*) A CT scan through one of the noncollapsed lumbar bodies shows dense trabecular struts that are hypertrophied. They are separated by multiple cystic areas. This is a characteristic appearance for chronic myeloma with compensatory hypertrophy of the remaining trabeculae. It has an appearance similar to scans of Paget's disease and hemangioma.

lytic areas in between (Fig. 18–19). This pattern resembles spinal hemangioma (Fig. 18–20) except that the hypertrophied trabecular struts in hemangioma are much more ordered and symmetric.

CT plays a very valuable role in cases of suspected osteoid osteoma. (Is it a tumor? Is it an infection? Is it a virus? Is it a dessert topping? Nobody really knows, least of all me, but since it is most often confused with tumors and

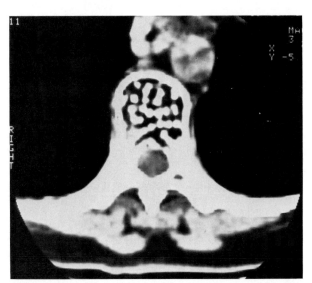

FIGURE 18–20. Hemangioma. A CT scan through a vertebral body hemangioma reveals strikingly dense, hypertrophied trabeculae that are arranged in a columnar fashion. Note the symmetry to this pattern, as compared to that of chronic myeloma.

osteomyelitis it will be discussed with them.) CT can show the location of the nidus, which will facilitate its removal by the surgeon. This is especially useful in complex joints such as the hip (Fig. 18–21) or in the spine (Fig. 18–22). It is important to remember that seeing a small lucency surrounded by sclerosis is not an absolute for the nidus of an osteoid osteoma. Osteomyelitis with a small abscess can have an identical appearance. The nidus of an osteoid osteoma often partially calcifies and can then resemble a sequestrum in osteomyelitis (Figs. 18–23, 18–24). CT, plain films, and even MRI can appear identical in both osteoid osteoma and osteomyelitis, with or without a sequestrum; therefore, a differential diagnosis of both entities should be given when a lesion with this appearance is found. Radionuclide bone scan can usually differentiate between osteoid osteoma and osteomyelitis by noting a "double density" sign at the nidus of the osteoid osteoma. This is caused by the increased affinity for the radionuclide by the hypervascular nidus. The surrounding reactive new bone takes up the radionuclide to a lesser degree than the nidus. In osteomyelitis a small abscess will be photopenic on radionuclide exam.

CT plays an important role in osteomyelitis by finding sequestrations (Fig. 18–25). The finding of a sequestration has both a diagnostic and a therapeutic significance. The diagnostic significance is that only three entities have been described in association with a sequestration. These are osteomyelitis, eosinophilic granuloma (Fig. 18–26), and fibrosarcoma (Fig. 18–27). As mentioned above, a partially calcified nidus of an osteoid osteoma can have the identical appearance as osteomyelitis with a sequestrum. All four entities should be considered when a sequestrum is encountered. The therapeutic significance is that the presence of a sequestrum usually requires surgical removal. Antibiotics alone will generally not suffice, as the sequestration does not have a blood supply and will not have the antibiotics delivered to it.

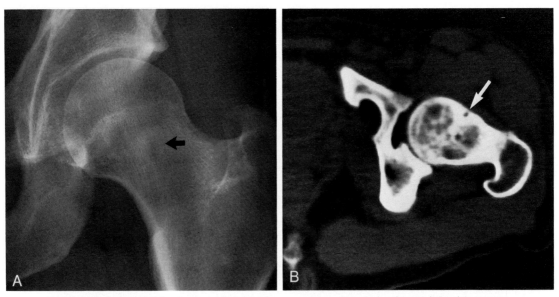

FIGURE 18–21. Osteoid osteoma. (*A*) A faint lucency with surrounding sclerosis (arrow) is present in the femoral neck of this 20-year-old with hip pain. A radionuclide bone scan showed marked increased uptake at this spot, which supported the diagnosis of an osteoid osteoma. (*B*) A CT scan through this area shows a sclerotic lesion with a lucency (arrow) consistent with the nidus of an osteoid osteoma. The CT scan shows the anterior position of the lesion which helps the surgeon plan an approach. This was removed and found to be an osteoid osteoma.

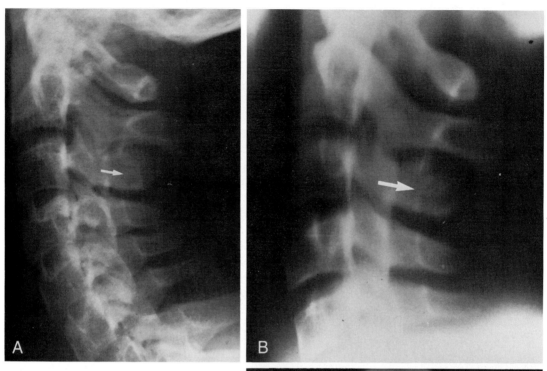

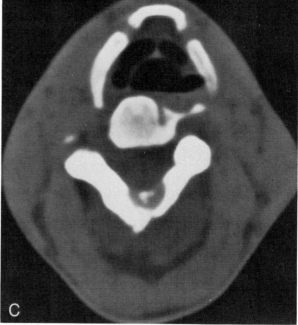

FIGURE 18–22. Osteoid osteoma. (*A*) A lateral cervical spine film in this young patient with neck pain shows an area of subtle sclerosis with absence of the normal spinolaminal line at C-3 (arrow). (*B*) A conventional tomogram of this area confirms the absent spinolaminal line (arrow), but is otherwise noncontributory. (*C*) An axial CT scan through the C-3 vertebra reveals a lucency with a small calcific center, which was found at surgery to be an osteoid osteoma. Osteomyelitis with a sequestrum could have an identical appearance.

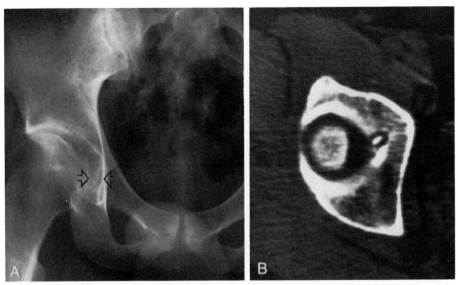

FIGURE 18–23. Osteoid osteoma with calcified nidus. (*A*) This young patient presented with hip pain and a widened teardrop measurement (arrows) on the right, as compared to the left. A hip aspiration ruled out an infectious process. (*B*) An axial CT scan of the hip showed an acetabular lucency with a central calcific density consistent with either osteomyelitis with a sequestrum or an osteoid osteoma with a partially calcified nidus. At surgery this was found to be an osteoid osteoma.

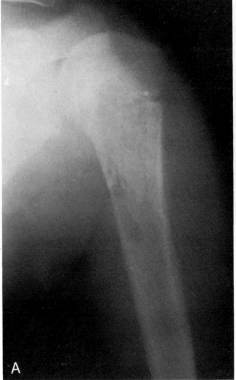

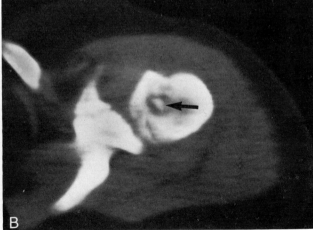

FIGURE 18–24. Osteomyelitis. (*A*) An anteroposterior plain film of the upper humerus in this child with pain and swelling shows a faint permeative pattern in the bone with periostitis. The differential diagnosis includes osteomyelitis, Ewing's sarcoma, and eosinophilic granuloma. (*B*) A CT scan of the humerus shows a lytic lesion with a bony sequestrum (arrow). This narrows the diagnosis to osteomyelitis and eosinophilic granuloma, since Ewing's sarcoma will not have a sequestrum. Biopsy showed this to be osteomyelitis. Because a sequestrum was known to be present, the surgeons chose to remove the sequestrum rather than just treat with antibiotics.

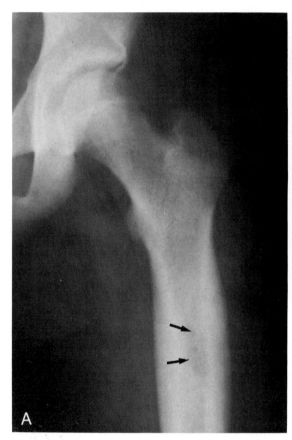

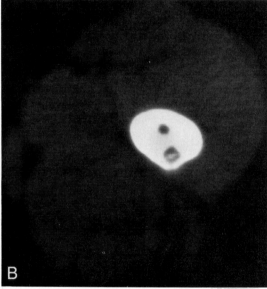

FIGURE 18–25. Sequestration in osteomyelitis. (*A*) An anteroposterior plain film of the proximal femur in this child with pain shows an area of diffuse sclerosis and cortical thickening with a faint lucency in the intramedullary portion (arrows). (*B*) A CT scan of the femur reveals a lucency with a calcific central portion. Some felt this was a partially calcified nidus in an osteoid osteoma, while others felt it was a sequestration in osteomyelitis. Either process could have this appearance. At biopsy this was found to be a sequestration in osteomyelitis.

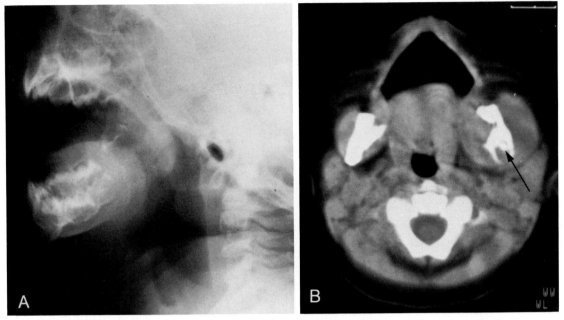

FIGURE 18–26. Sequestration in eosinophilic granuloma. (*A*) This 2-year-old presented with a painful, swollen jaw, and the plain film that was taken showed some destruction of the mandible near the angle of the jaw. Infection, Ewing's sarcoma, osteogenic sarcoma, neuroblastoma, and eosinophilic granuloma were diagnostic considerations. (*B*) A CT scan through the jaw revealed a destructive lesion that involved much of the mandible. A sequestration (arrow) was found, which limits the differential diagnosis to osteomyelitis and eosinophilic granuloma. At biopsy this was found to be eosinophilic granuloma.

A "tumorous" condition that can be mistaken for a malignancy both radiographically and histologically is myositis ossificans. It is imperative that a biopsy not be performed if myositis ossificans is a consideration because it can resemble a sarcoma to the pathologist and result in unnecessary radical surgery. The plain film finding that is virtually pathognomonic for myositis ossificans is peripheral calcification (Fig. 18–28). Often it is difficult to characterize the calcification as either central or peripheral on plain films; CT can help determine the location of the calcification and avert a biopsy in some instances (Fig. 18–29).

Miscellaneous Uses

There are several additional uses of CT in the musculoskeletal system that do not fall into any neat category other than "miscellaneous." These include examination of the sacroiliac joints, measurements, temporomandibular joint examination, CT arthrography of the shoulder, and bone densitometry. Bone densitometry will not be covered here, as there are several different techniques employed, and it is beyond the scope of this text.

Sacroiliac Joints

Plain film examination of the S-I joints can be extremely difficult to interpret due to the anatomic obliquity of the joints themselves and the thick overlying soft tissues. If the diagnosis or treatment of the patient rests on the appearance of the S-I joints (and it is not always so) then CT is a more reliable imaging

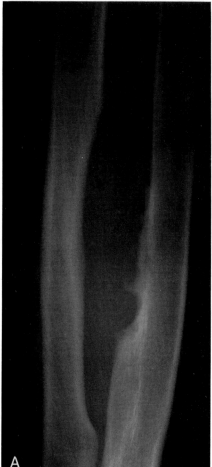

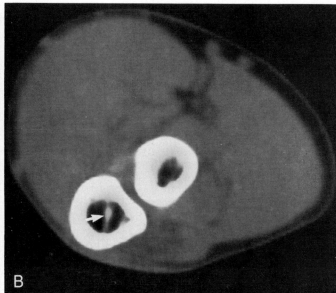

FIGURE 18–27. Sequestration in fibrosarcoma. (*A*) A plain film of the forearm shows a destructive lesion of the ulna with some aggressive periostitis. (*B*) A CT scan through the lesion revealed a sequestrum (arrow), which limited the differential diagnosis to eosinophilic granuloma, fibrosarcoma, and osteomyelitis. At surgery this was found to be a fibrosarcoma.

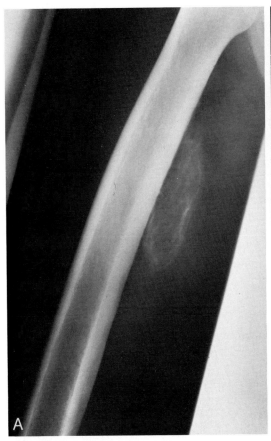

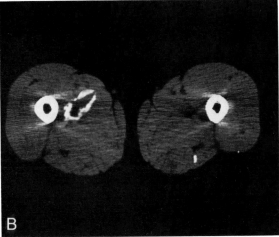

FIGURE 18–28. Myositis ossificans. (*A*) A plain film of the thigh in this young surgeon with pain and swelling shows a calcific mass that could be myositis ossificans or a parosteal osteosarcoma. The patient could not recall any recent trauma to this area. (*B*) A CT scan through the mass shows definite peripheral, circumferential calcification, which is characteristic for myositis ossificans. A planned biopsy was canceled, since myositis can mimic a sarcoma histologically.

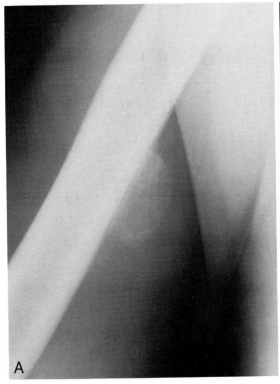

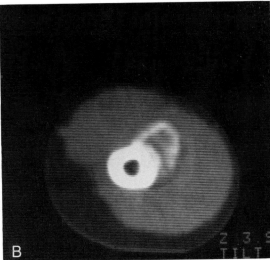

FIGURE 18–29. Myositis ossificans. (*A*) A plain film of the humerus in this patient with a painful mass shows a faintly calcified mass adjacent to the humerus with some periostitis present. Myositis ossificans and parosteal osteosarcoma were thought to be the main considerations. (*B*) A CT scan through the mass shows definite circumferential calcification, which indicates myositis ossificans. No biopsy was taken, since myositis can simulate a sarcoma histologically.

technique than plain films. It certainly is more reproducible, more sensitive, and more accurate than plain films and gives the patient less radiation. If the protocol is streamlined, it can be performed rapidly and at a relatively low cost, making it cost effective.

To steamline the protocol and diminish the number of cuts necessary to cover the S-I joints, reverse the gantry so that it is at a steep angle parallel to the S-I joints (Fig. 18–30). This is just opposite to the direction the gantry is angled when trying to scan parallel to the L-5/S-1 disc. Eight to ten 3-mm- or 5-mm-thick slices are obtained, which cover the S-I joints as seen on the lateral scout film.

S-I joint sclerosis and erosions can be identified with much more clarity than on plain films (Fig. 18–31). The iliac side of the joint invariably has more sclerosis than the sacral side; however, this should not be confused with osteitis condensans ilii. It must also be remembered that degenerative joint disease (DJD) can cause erosions in the S-I joints and mimic a spondyloarthropathy or an infection (Fig. 18–32). It has been shown that erosions and sclerosis in the S-I joints, as shown with CT, increase with aging to the point that patients over the age of 40 often have S-I joint abnormalities.

Measurements

Almost any measurement that is done with plain films, such as pelvimetry and scanograms for leg-length discrepancy, can be done more accurately and with considerably less radiation by using CT. There are few more thankless tasks in skeletal radiology than trying to read a poorly exposed scanogram of the legs with a barely discernible ruler between the patient's legs and trying to give accurate measurements of leg length. The measurements can be easily and accurately obtained with CT by taking an AP scout film of the extremities and

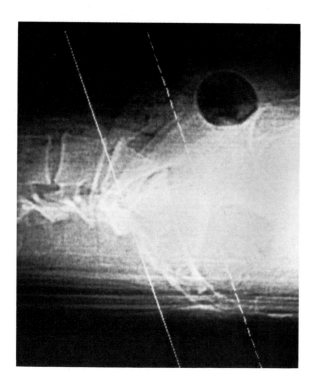

FIGURE 18–30. Scout film for sacroiliac joints. This lateral scout view of the sacrum shows how the cursors are angled parallel to the sacroiliac joints. Eight to ten 3- to 5-mm thick slices are then taken to cover the extent of the joints.

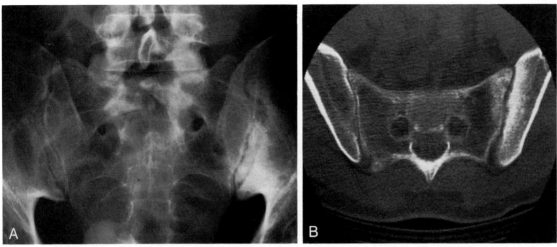

FIGURE 18–31. CT of the sacroiliac joints in psoriasis. (*A*) An anteroposterior plain film of the pelvis demonstrates left-sided sacroiliac joint sclerosis and erosions. It was not clear whether the right side was minimally involved. (*B*) A CT scan shows the left-sided changes nicely and shows that the right joint is definitely not involved.

placing cursor points on the bony landmarks for measurement (Fig. 18–33). The computer gives the distance measurements between the chosen points. This technique has been shown to have reproducibility and accuracy, but it suffers from not being able to have the patient weight-bearing. Most of the time a weight-bearing exam is not necessary; however, if a weight-bearing exam is a necessity then a CT scanogram cannot replace the conventional scanogram. The radiation dose from the CT scanogram has been estimated at 50 to 100 times less than a conventional scanogram. The cost of a CT scanogram is less than a conventional scanogram because of the low cost of the scout views, which comprise the imaging portion of the exam.

Pelvimetry is a frequent source of consternation for many radiologists because of the difficulty seeing the bony landmarks and ruler markings, as well as the reluctance to order repeat films to improve the quality because of the

FIGURE 18–32. CT of the sacroiliac joints in degenerative joint disease. A CT scan of the sacroiliac joints in this patient shows some minimal sclerosis and definite erosions in the right joint. A small erosion is also present in the left joint. These changes could be due to any inflammatory arthritis or a spondyloarthropathy, but these were due to DJD. This patient has extensive osteoarthritis in his spine and large joints. This is a typical appearance of DJD in the sacroiliac joints.

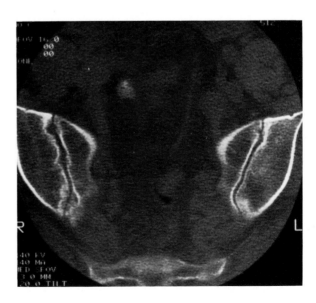

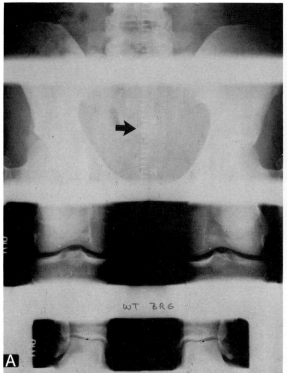

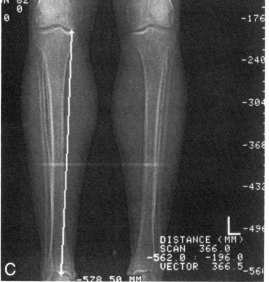

FIGURE 18–33. CT scanogram. (*A*) This conventional plain film scanogram shows how difficult it can be to visualize the ruler (arrow) on all the images. It could not be seen at all on the images of the knees and ankles. (*B*) A scout view of the femurs shows the cursor placement at the proximal and distal femur on the right with a distance measurement of 44.2 cm given between the two points. (*C*) A scout view of the tibias in the same patient with cursors placed on the medial tibial plateau and on the plafond. The measurement of the distance between the cursors is 36.6 cm. These measurements are repeated on the opposite leg and compared.

radiation dose to this sensitive population. CT eliminates all these concerns. An AP and a lateral scout view are obtained. From these the pelvic inlet can be measured (Fig. 18–34). A single axial CT slice is taken at the level of the fovea of the femoral heads, which will allow measurement across the ischial spines. This technique is accurate, reproducible, and has a radiation dose 30 times less than conventional pelvimetry. The entire exam takes 10 minutes or less to complete, therefore it should be cost-effective.

Temporomandibular Joint

For several years CT was used to replace temporomandibular joint (TMJ) arthrography in multiple institutions. CT compares favorably with arthrography in diagnosing an anteriorly displaced disc. However, MRI is far superior to CT in demonstrating displaced discs as well as other joint pathology and is considered

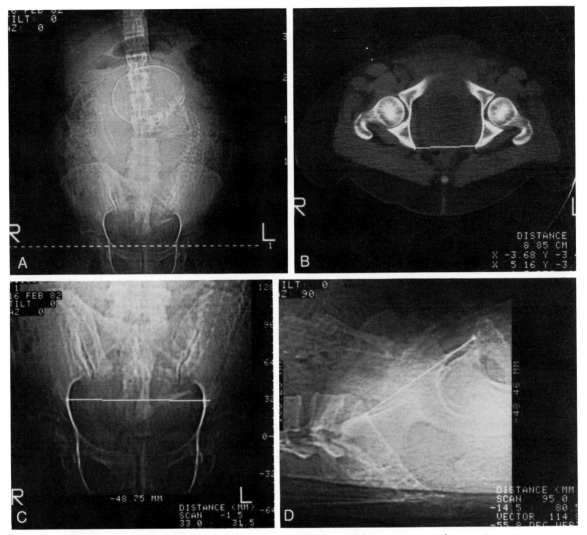

FIGURE 18–34. CT pelvimetry. For pelvimetry measurements it is necessary to take an anteroposterior and a lateral scout view of the pelvis, and a single axial CT slice. The anteroposterior scout view is used to find the femoral head fovea, throught which a cursor is placed (*A*) for a single axial slice. On the single axial slice thru the fovea of the femoral heads the measurement of the ischial spines is made (*B*). In this patient that measurement is 8.85 cm. The anteroposterior scout view is also used to measure the pelvic inlet (*C*). In this patient the inlet measured 48.75 mm. The lateral scout view is then used to measure the pelvic inlet from the sacrum to the symphysis pubis (*D*). This measured 48.46 mm in this patient.

by most to be the procedure of choice for imaging the disc. CT is still very useful for imaging bony abnormalities of the TMJ.

The temporomandibular joint is very difficult to image with conventional techniques because of its position in the dense, bony glenoid fossa. With CT, the TMJ is clearly depicted and many joint abnormalities that are not appreciated on plain films are easily diagnosed.

Commonplace abnormalities such as DJD and fractures are often not well visualized on plain films, yet are shown clearly with CT. A less common abnormality that often goes undiagnosed because plain films fail to demonstrate it is coronoid process hyperplasia (Fig. 18–35). This is a congenital hypertrophy

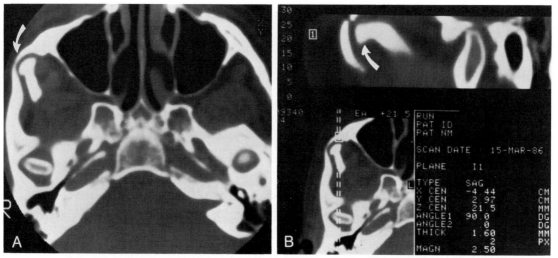

FIGURE 18–35. Coronoid process hyperplasia. (A) An axial CT scan of the temporomandibular joints in this patient with joint pain and inability to fully open her mouth shows a large bony protuberance eroding the right zygomatic arch (arrow). This bony protuberance is a hypertrophied coronoid process that is mechanically impinging on the zygoma, thereby limiting mouth opening. (B) A sagittal reformation through the right TMJ shows the hypertrophied coronoid process (arrow) to be larger than the condyle.

of one or both coronoid processes that can limit mouth opening by impinging against the zygomatic arch. Once recognized it can be surgically corrected.

Another abnormality that is occasionally seen in the TMJ and can go unrecognized on plain films is synovial osteochondromatosis (Fig. 18–36). This presents as a fullness or swelling in the joint and often goes to biopsy, where it can be confused with a chondrosarcoma. This should be a radiologic diagnosis rather than a histologic one, since it can resemble a sarcoma histologically. CT

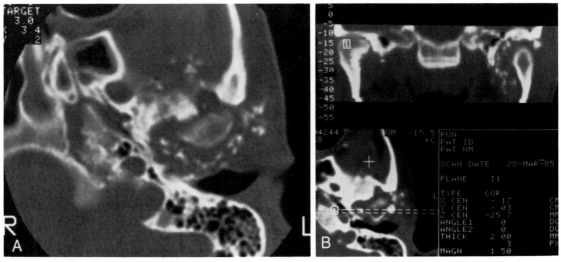

FIGURE 18–36. Synovial osteochondromatosis of the temporomandibular joints. (A) An axial CT through the left temporomandibular joints reveals multiple calcific densities in the joint with some bony erosion of the temporal bone and condylar head. (B) A coronal reformation shows the multiple joint bodies in the left joint and the erosion in the joint, as compared to the normal right joint. This is virtually diagnostic of synovial osteochondromatosis.

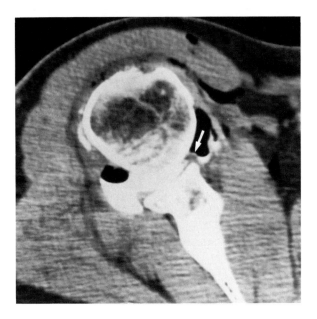

FIGURE 18–37. Normal shoulder CT arthrogram. This CT arthrogram of the shoulder demonstrates a smooth, rounded anterior labrum (arrow). This is a normal appearance. The posterior labrum has a similar appearance in this patient.

of synovial osteochondromatosis in the TMJ is characteristic and should be diagnostic.

CT Arthrography of the Shoulder

CT arthrograms of the shoulder are useful in examining the glenoid labrum in patients with shoulder instability. MRI has replaced the CT arthrogram in many institutions; however, the resolution and clarity of the labra are not nearly as good with MRI as with CT. MRI can also diagnose abnormalities of the rotator cuff such as tendonitis and partial tears, while the CT arthrogram will only tell if there is a full-thickness cuff tear. For many surgeons, that is enough information about the cuff, and the superior imaging of the labrum will make them prefer the CT arthrogram over the MRI exam.

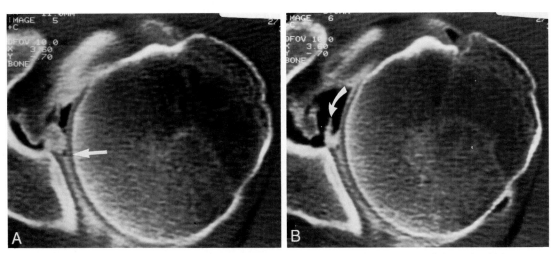

FIGURE 18–38. Torn labrum on CT arthrogram. (*A*) The anterior labrum has a cleft (arrow), which indicates a tear. (*B*) The adjacent CT slice shows the anterior labrum to be completely torn with a frayed piece remaining (arrow).

The technique begins like a routine shoulder arthrogram with a needle placed into the glenohumeral joint near the axillary recess. Instead of the standard 10 ml of contrast placed into the joint, however, only 1.5 to 2 ml are instilled, along with 0.25 ml of 1:10,000 epinephrine and 10 ml of air. The epinephrine will delay absorption of the contrast to allow for possible delays in completing the CT scan. The needle is removed and the patient is instructed to move his shoulder through a full range of motion to adequately coat the joint. Plain films are obtained and reviewed to look for leakage of air or contrast into the subacromial bursa, which would be diagnostic for a rotator cuff tear. The patient is then taken to the CT scanner, and 3-mm-thick contiguous slices through the glenoid are obtained. The normal glenoid has a smooth covering of cartilage, which is slightly thicker and more triangular anteriorly (Fig. 18–37). A torn labrum will have an obvious irregularity (Fig. 18–38) or be absent or small in size.

19

Lumbar Spine

DISC DISEASE

CT has proved to be of immense value in examining the lumbar spine. It gives us the capability of examining in detail not only the discs, but also all the bony and soft tissue structures in and about the spine, including the facets, the neuroforamina, the thecal sac and nerve roots as they exit the thecal sac, the ligamentum flavum, and the vascular structures. This chapter will show how CT can be used to diagnose disc disease and spinal stenosis in the lumbar spine and explain why CT has made myelography obsolete.

Multiple comparison studies of CT and myelography have been published which show that myelography and CT are both roughly 90% accurate in diagnosing disc disease. In fact, most of us who have been interpreting spine CTs for a number of years know that CT is considerably better than myelography. Why doesn't the literature reflect this then? Several reasons account for this discrepancy which I will mention later in this chapter. Suffice it to say that most of those comparison studies were performed in the early days of CT spine work—things have improved considerably since then. Also, more recent studies confirm that CT is around 95% accurate while myelography continues to be around 90% accurate. Even the older studies recommended that CT be the primary study of choice, while myelography be reserved for the nondiagnostic CT exams. The current recommendation is to not perform the myelogram under any circumstances. That's correct. Never! I can think of no clinical situation where a myelogram is warranted. If the CT exam does not answer the question, get the patient to an MRI unit.

How about a myelo/CT exam? Unneccessary. Only a few studies have been performed comparing the accuracy of diagnosis of plain CT and myelographic enhanced CT. These show no statistical differences between the two techniques. If there is no difference why put the patient through the extra expense and morbidity, and, in some centers, hospitalization, when a plain CT will be as effective? There is no good reason for it.

The most common plea for myelography that I hear is that "it's served me well for years, and the CT gives me too much information." It's true that the CT exam is far more sensitive and will give additional information beyond that of the myelogram. I will explain how to deal with that information, and show how to alert the clinician that the findings may or may not be clinically significant. I also hear surgeons who prefer the myelogram because they are fearful of missing tumors of the cauda equina. These do occur, but only rarely do they mimic disc disease. One of the main things to keep in mind with spine CT is that it's just another test and *must* be correlated with the patient's clinical exam.

Multiple papers are now being published comparing CT of the spine with MRI. These are all showing that MRI is just as good as CT. I would certainly agree with that *if* the MRI exam is of high quality. The main point to make is that MRI is *no better* than CT unless it is a post-operative spine. Therefore, there is no good reason to switch from CT to MRI unless the cost of the MRI exam is less (which, of course, it is not). It is interesting to hear many of the MRI proponents claim that myelography is no longer necessary now that MRI is available. In fact, CT made myelography obsolete, but people haven't caught on yet. Several recent review articles on spine imaging concur with these statements (see the four articles listed under Selected Readings at the end of this chapter), but it will take another 10 years or more before myelography is eliminated.

TECHNIQUE

The proper imaging protocol for a diagnostic lumbar spine study is critical to lessen the chances of missing a lesion. The patient should be studied in the supine position with the knees flexed over a pillow or other similar object. An AP and lateral scout film are obtained. The AP scout view will allow the radiologist to determine if transitional vertebrae are present. A significant number of operations are performed at the wrong level because of a mixup with labeling transitional vertebrae. The lateral scout view is used to place the cursors over the intended area of scanning. This should include contiguous slices, no thicker than 5-mm (I prefer 3-mm-thick slices) from the mid-body of L-3 to the top of S-1. Ten percent of disc protrusions occur at the L-3/L-4 level, and they can clinically mimic protrusions from lower levels, therefore L-3/L-4 must be examined.

The early spine protocols recommended several angled–gantry slices parallel to each vertebral body endplate (Fig. 19–1). This is not advised for two

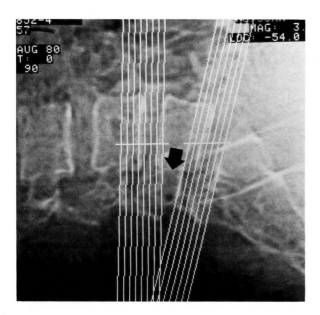

FIGURE 19–1. Inappropriate scanning protocol. This lateral scout view has the gantry angled parallel to the L-5/S-1 endplate with several slices above and below. This is repeated at the L-4/L-5 level. A small but definite space or gap is present between the levels (arrow) where a free fragment or spinal stenosis could be missed. In addition, it is mandatory to study the L-3/L-4 level, since up to 10 percent of disc protrusions occur at that level.

reasons. First, this leaves spaces or gaps in the central canal that are not imaged, which can result in missed free fragments. Second, it is not necessary to angle the gantry parallel to the endplate. I have seen thousands of levels imaged with both angled cuts and straight axial cuts and have yet to see a difference between the two. You simply cannot make a disc impress the thecal sac, or even appear to, with any degree of lordosis or angling of the gantry. Therefore, why spend the extra time and radiation? My recommendation for a complete lumbar spine CT exam is 3-mm-thick slices from the midbody of L-3 to the top of S-1 in a straight axial fashion (Fig. 19–2).

The completed study should be photographed with the images magnified in a manner so they are easily seen at arm's length. Each image should be photographed in a bone and a soft tissue window. I often see radiologists trying to diagnose facet disease or other bony abnormalities from a soft tissue window image, and it can't be done. The AP and lateral scout views should be included on the hard copy film to allow the radiologist and the clinician to anatomically orient each image.

PATHOLOGY

When a disc bulges or protrudes beyond the endplate it takes on several names, some of which have more sinister connotations than others. The terms "herniated nucleus pulposus" (HNP) and "bulging annulus fibrosis" are often mentioned, along with "contained," "extruded," and "sequestered" discs. How do we differentiate these various types of disc protrusions and what are the implications of each? First, radiologists are not very good at differentiating them, and second, except for distinguishing a sequestration (a free fragment) it probably doesn't matter. The surgeons want to know if disc material of any kind is pressing against neural tissue, and even then they know it might not be causing the patient's symptoms.

The early CT literature says that if a disc protrusion or bulge is broadbased in configuration it usually represents a bulging annulus fibrosis, whereas if it is

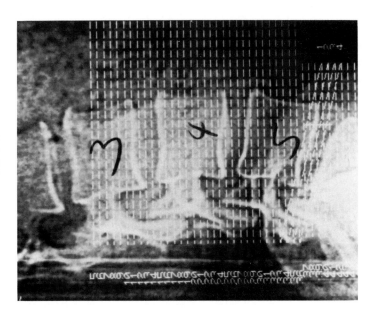

FIGURE 19–2. Proper scanning protocol. This lateral scout view has straight axial 3-mm thick slices from L-3 to S-1 without gaps. This is an adequate examination for disc disease or spinal stenosis.

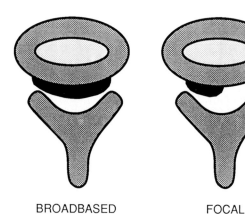

FIGURE 19–3. Schematic of focal versus broadbased disc protrusions. A broadbased disc protrusion has a uniform bulge that extends across the entire central canal. A focal protrusion extends only into a portion of the central canal.

BROADBASED   FOCAL

focal in its configuration it usually represents an HNP (Fig. 19–3). Using the early articles which compared CT to myelography, this morphologic classification was only correct about 85% of the time. It is not unusual to see a focal bulging annulus, or a large, broadbased HNP. Also, most of the investigators did not require the myelogram to differentiate between the two entities—the myelogram only had to note an extradural bulge. Hence, the CT exams were downgraded for accuracy unnecessarily. If this source of error is removed, CT is actually much more accurate at diagnosing disc protrusions than myelography.

If a disc protrusion does not impress the thecal sac or a nerve root it will not be seen on a myelogram, yet it can be seen with CT. It would undoubtedly be asymptomatic and not deserving of treatment. These were called "false positives" in the early comparison studies of CT and myelography, but they are no more false positives than a cervical rib on a chest film is a false positive. They are real findings, but they are not causing any symptoms. These are called grade 1, or mild, disc protrusions (Fig. 19–4) and our surgeons know that they are real but innocuous. If the disc does impress the thecal sac or a nerve root it is called a grade 2, or moderate, disc protrusion (Fig. 19–5). It may or may not be symptomatic, but our surgeons know it has to be matched with the clinical

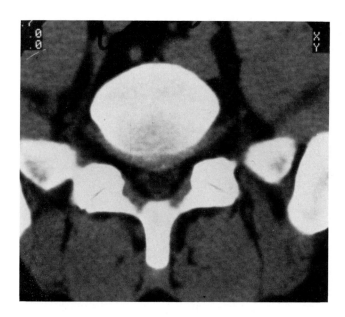

FIGURE 19–4. A grade 1 disc protrusion. This predominantly broadbased disc protrusion is not impressing the thecal sac or nerve roots. It is therefore a grade 1 disc protrusion, which would not be expected to be symptomatic.

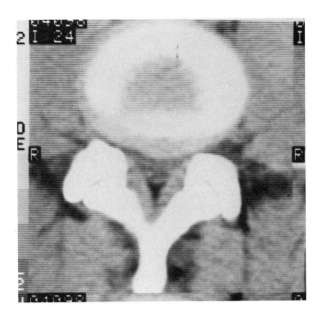

FIGURE 19–5. A grade 2 disc protrusion. This broad-based disc protrusion is impressing the thecal sac moderately. It is therefore a grade 2 disc protrusion which may or may not be symptomatic.

findings. A very large disc protrusion is termed a grade 3 disc (Fig. 19–6) and they are almost always symptomatic.

A large or grade 3 disc should make one very suspicious for a sequestration or free fragment. The most common cause for failure of a percutaneous discectomy procedure and a not infrequent cause for failed surgical discectomy procedures is a missed free fragment. A free fragment should be suggested any time disc material is identified in the cut above or below the disc level (Fig. 19–7). If a soft tissue density is identified above or below the disc space it should be determined if it is of a similar density as the thecal sac or if it is of a higher density. If it is clearly a higher density it is disc material and should be considered a free fragment.

There are three methods to examine the density of the suspect tissue: (1) a region of interest (ROI) box or cursor can be placed over the suspect area and

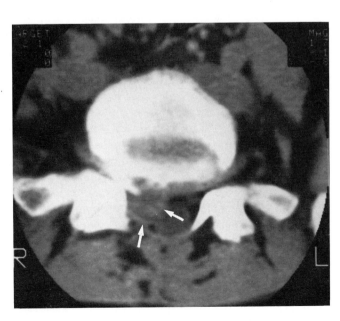

FIGURE 19–6. A grade 3 disc protrusion. This is an extremely large, focal, right-sided disc protrusion (arrows), which is impressing the right-sided nerve root and thecal sac. This disc also has a broadbased component that is not touching the thecal sac or nerve roots.

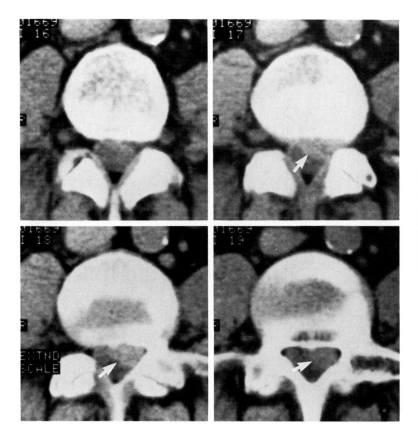

FIGURE 19–7. Free fragment.
These four contiguous slices show a large, focal, left-sided disc protrusion on at least three adjacent cuts (arrows). The lowest cut (#19) is below the disc space level and extends into the lateral recesses. This is consistent with a free fragment.

the actual CT attenuation number can be compared to that of the thecal sac (Fig. 19–8); (2) the identity mode or "blink mode" can be set at disc density and compared to the questionable tissue (Fig. 19–9); the "blink mode" is a button on the scanner console that, when pressed, highlights in white all the tissue densities of a chosen CT number, allowing easy distinction of subtle density differences; (3) the window width can be reduced to a very low setting and the density differences of various tissues will stand out. If a soft tissue density cannot be clearly distinguished visually as to its density compared to the thecal sac, one of these three methods should be tried.

If the soft tissue density above or below the disc space is isodense to the thecal sac, it is not a free fragment and is either a Tarlov cyst or a conjoined nerve root. A Tarlov cyst is merely an enlarged nerve root sheath. It is a normal variant and not a cause of any symptoms. It can get quite large and because of persistent pulsations from the cerebrospinal fluid can cause bony erosion (Fig. 19–10). It has also been termed a "perineural" cyst.

A conjoined root is a congenital anomaly of two nerve roots exiting the thecal sac together instead of separately (Fig. 19–11). The two roots run in the lateral recess together and appear as a soft tissue mass on CT (Fig. 19–12). A free fragment can have the same appearance but will have an increased density as compared to the thecal sac, whereas a conjoined root will be isodense to the thecal sac (Fig. 19–13). The roots will invariably exit through their appropriate foramina, hence it is very unusual to have an "empty" foramen. Also, the conjoined roots are always associated with a slightly wider lateral recess than the opposite side. Conjoined roots occur in 1 to 3% of all patients and are incidental findings with no reported symptomatology.

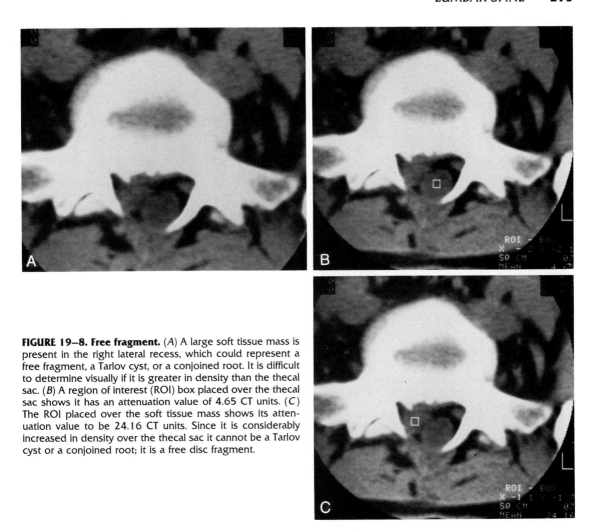

FIGURE 19–8. Free fragment. (*A*) A large soft tissue mass is present in the right lateral recess, which could represent a free fragment, a Tarlov cyst, or a conjoined root. It is difficult to determine visually if it is greater in density than the thecal sac. (*B*) A region of interest (ROI) box placed over the thecal sac shows it has an attenuation value of 4.65 CT units. (*C*) The ROI placed over the soft tissue mass shows its attenuation value to be 24.16 CT units. Since it is considerably increased in density over the thecal sac it cannot be a Tarlov cyst or a conjoined root; it is a free disc fragment.

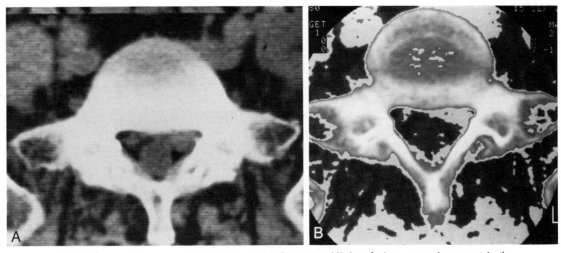

FIGURE 19–9. "Blink mode" identifying a free fragment. (*A*) A soft tissue mass is present in the left lateral recess, which could represent a free fragment, a Tarlov cyst, or a conjoined nerve root. It is difficult to tell visually if the mass is greater in density than the thecal sac. (*B*) With the "blink mode" set at a level that allows the ligamentum flavum to light up, there is highlighting of the mass in the left lateral recess. This is diagnostic of a free fragment, because a conjoined root and a Tarlov cyst would be lower in density than a free fragment. The ligamentum flavum is the same density as disc material and can be used to set the blink mode when the disc is not visible.

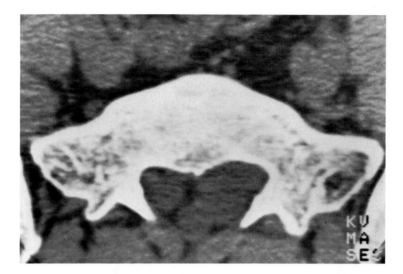

FIGURE 19–10. Tarlov cyst. Large dilatations of the nerve root sheaths are present, causing some erosion into the vertebral body. The cysts are filled with cerebrospinal fluid and are the same density as the thecal sac.

FIGURE 19–11. Drawing of a conjoined root. Two nerve roots have arisen from the thecal sac on the right side in an asymmetric manner as compared to the left. When a CT cut is made at the level of the cursor (*C*), two roots are visualized on the axial cut on the right side, one of which could be confused with a free fragment. They will be lower in density than disc material, however.

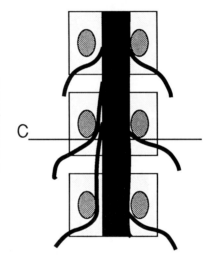

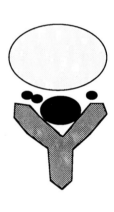

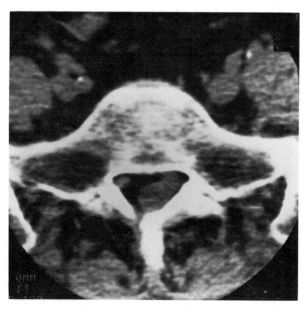

FIGURE 19–12. Conjoined root. A soft tissue density, which appears to be contiguous with the thecal sac, is present in the left lateral recess. This is characteristic of a conjoined root. Note that it appears isodense with the thecal sac.

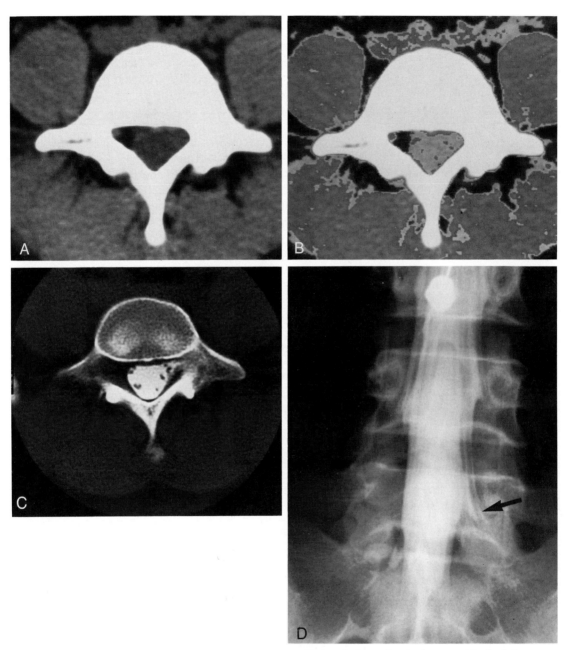

FIGURE 19–13. Conjoined root with blink mode. (*A*) A soft tissue density is present in the left lateral recess, it appears isodense to the thecal sac. (*B*) The blink mode highlights the soft tissue mass at the same time the thecal sac is highlighted; therefore, this is isodense to the thecal sac and cannot be a free fragment. (*C*) A CT myelogram shows the conjoined root sleeve filled with metrizamide in the left lateral recess. (*D*) An anteroposterior view of the conventional myelogram shows two roots arising from the thecal sac on the left side at the L-5 pedicle level (arrow).

Many patients have had neural damage at surgery due to failure to recognize two roots in an area where there is normally only one. Also, many patients have had explorations for "free fragments" when there was a conjoined root mimicking a free fragment. Since percutaneous discectomy is contraindicated in the presence of a free fragment and an open procedure requires a diligent search if a free fragment is suspected, it is critical for the radiologist to differentiate between a free fragment and a conjoined root or a Tarlov cyst. This is easily done by noting the density differences between the mass and the thecal sac. Therefore, it is inappropriate to list a differential diagnosis of free fragment, conjoined root, and Tarlov cyst when a soft tissue mass is found in a lateral recess.

A lateral disc is a disc protrusion that occurs lateral to the neuroforamen (Fig. 19–14). It is one of the most commonly missed disc protrusions simply because it is overlooked. The usual search pattern examines the thecal sac/disc interface and not the area lateral to the foramen. A lateral disc has huge implications for the surgeon. First, a lateral disc will irritate a nerve root that has already exited the neuroforamen and will therefore mimic a disc protrusion at a more cephalad level (Fig. 19–14C). For instance, if a disc protrudes posteriorly at the L-4/L-5 level it will usually press against the L-5 root; therefore, if a patient presents with signs and symptoms of an L-5 root irritation the L-4/L-5 level is usually the surgical level. However, the L-5 root can also be irritated from a lateral disc protrusion at L-5/S-1. Therefore, if overlooked, it can result in surgery at the wrong level, especially in a patient with disc abnormalities at multiple levels, in whom the clinical presentation is relied on to determine which level should be operated. Also, a lateral disc does not require a laminectomy, since it can be approached from outside the bony central canal. A myelogram will not

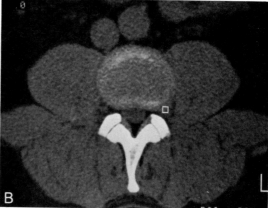

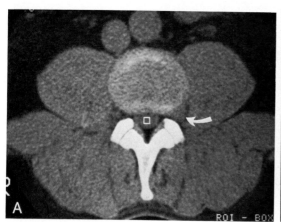

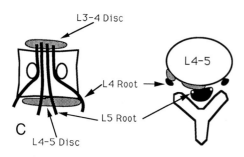

FIGURE 19–14. Lateral disc. (A) A soft tissue mass that appears contiguous with the disc is present on the left side just lateral to the neuroforamen (arrow). An ROI box placed on the thecal sac gives a density of 9 CT units. (B) An ROI box placed on the soft tissue mass shows its density to be 20.6 CT units. The increased density makes this mass diagnostic of a lateral disc. (C) This drawing demonstrates how a posterior disc protrusion at L-4/L-5 typically affects the L-5 root, yet a lateral disc at the same level affects the L-4 root. Because the L-4 root is typically affected by a posterior L-3/L-4 disc protrusion, a lateral disc at L-4/L-5 could result in the L-3/L-4 disc's being inappropriately surgically removed.

demonstrate a lateral disc, and an "exploration" is not likely to discover a lateral disc because it is not in an area the surgeon would normally explore. Lateral discs occur in less than 5% of cases but should be searched for in every case at each disc level.

SPINAL STENOSIS

Spinal stenosis has been classically divided into two types: congenital and acquired. Congenital stenosis includes achondroplasia, Morquio's disease, and idiopathic. Acquired stenosis includes degenerative joint disease (DJD), posttraumatic, postsurgical, Paget's disease, and calcification of the posterior longitudinal ligament. In reality, almost nobody ever presents clinically with spinal stenosis unless some component of acquired stenosis is present. Even the most severe form of congenital stenosis, achondroplasia, does not have clinical signs and symptoms until DJD ensues in early adulthood secondary to an accentuated lordosis (Fig. 19–15).

A preferred classification for spinal stenosis would be on an anatomic basis. This divides stenosis into central canal stenosis, neuroforaminal stenosis, and lateral recess stenosis. In each of these areas the most common cause is DJD.

Central Canal Stenosis

For many years radiologists have been asked to measure the central canal to diagnose spinal stenosis. Many different histograms have been published to show which measurements are within normal limits for each anatomic level (Fig. 19–16). These do not take into account the fact that most people with small bony canals also have small neural structures and are, therefore, asymptomatic. We often encounter patients with bony measurements that are small but who have small neural components as well (Fig. 19–17). For stenosis to be clinically manifest there must be a discordance in the size of the bony canal and the thecal sac. Simply measuring the central canal will not address the "fit" of the thecal sac in that canal, hence measurements are virtually worthless. Currently, very few surgeons require measurements for diagnosing central canal stenosis.

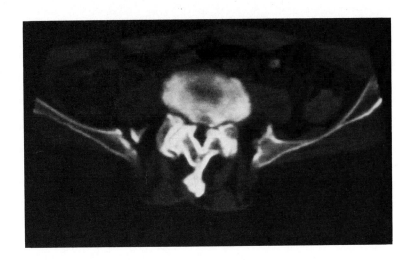

FIGURE 19–15. Achondroplasia with severe stenosis. Severe central canal stenosis occurs in patients with achondroplasia owing to their congenital stenosis combined with severe degenerative facet disease.

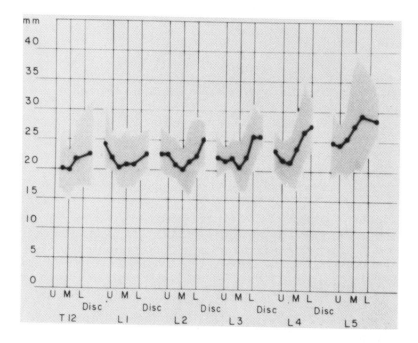

FIGURE 19–16. Spinal stenosis histogram. The normal interpediculate distance at each spinal level is marked with a heavy line, and a standard deviation above and below is shaded in gray. For example, the average L-5 interpediculate measurement near the midbody would be 25 mm.

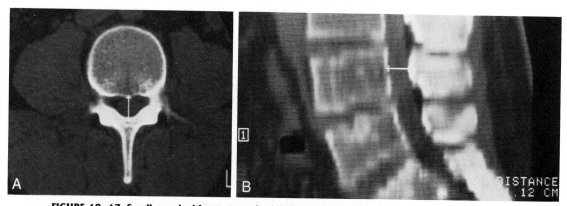

FIGURE 19–17. Small canal without stenosis. (*A*) The anteroposterior diameter of the canal in this patient measures 11.5 mm, which is extremely small. Note that the thecal sac is not compressed and that the epidural fat is not obliterated. (*B*) The anteroposterior measurement taken on a sagittal reformatted image is 11.2 mm. This patient had no clinical findings of spinal stenosis in spite of a very small central canal. The patient has a small thecal sac that is not compressed by the small bony canal, hence no symptoms are present. This patient has no spinal stenosis clinically, and measurements are not enough to make the diagnosis.

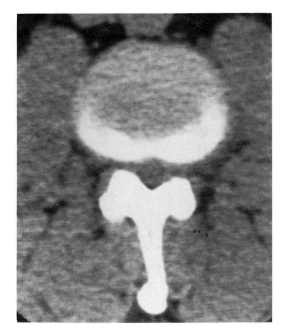

FIGURE 19–18. Obliteration of epidural fat. This patient has central canal stenosis that is compressing the thecal sac. The thecal sac is not visualized because the epidural fat has been obliterated. When the epidural fat is absent one should be suspicious for spinal stenosis.

The most useful criteria for diagnosing central canal stenosis are obliteration of the epidural fat (Fig. 19–18) and flattening of the thecal sac (Fig. 19–19). Both of these findings can be present without symptoms of spinal stenosis; therefore, stenosis can only be *proposed* by the radiologist, with clinical correlation required.

The most common cause of central canal stenosis is facet degenerative disease, which results in hypertrophy of the facets and encroachment of the central canal and the lateral recesses (Fig. 19–20). As mentioned previously, even the most severe example of congenital spinal stenosis, achondroplasia,

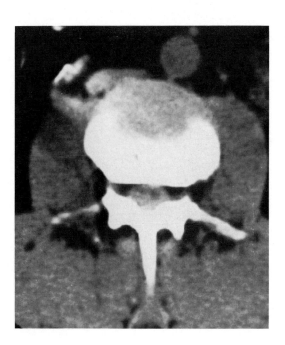

FIGURE 19–19. Flattening of the thecal sac. The best CT sign for central canal stenosis is flattening of the thecal sac, as in this example. The patient may not have clinical signs or symptoms of stenosis, but the diagnosis must be suggested.

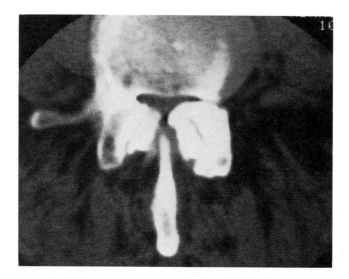

FIGURE 19–20. Facet hypertrophy. The most common cause of spinal stenosis is facet degenerative disease with hypertrophy, as in this example. This is best seen with bone windows, since soft tissue windows can be very misleading and make normal facets appear hypertrophied.

rarely presents with clinical complaints until marked facet degenerative disease occurs.

Another very common cause of central canal stenosis is hypertrophy of the ligamentum flavum (Fig. 19–21). This is a misnomer, as the ligamentum flavum does not actually hypertrophy but buckles inward due to facet slippage and disc space narrowing. Since this is a soft tissue encroachment, measurements of the size of the bony canal would not reflect this process—another reason measurements are not reliable in detecting spinal stenosis.

Paget's disease with enlargement of the vertebral body can occasionally

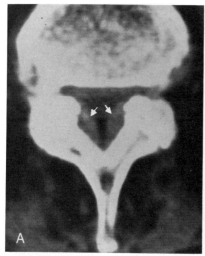

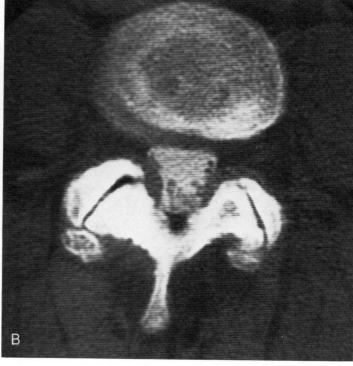

FIGURE 19–21. Ligamentum flavum hypertrophy. (*A*) The ligamentum flavum (arrows) is bowing inward and encroaching on the central canal, causing spinal stenosis. The facets are hypertrophied, although this is a soft tissue window and does not show them well. (*B*) This metrizamide CT scan shows a large impression on the right side of the thecal sac from ligamentum flavum hypertrophy. Note the facet DJD.

cause central canal stenosis (Fig. 19–22), as can ossification of the posterior longitudinal ligament (OPLL) (Fig. 19–23). Reportedly, up to 25% of the patients with diffuse idiopathic skeletal hyperostosis (DISH), a very common ailment of people over the age of 50, will have OPLL. Additional uncommon causes of central canal stenosis would include trauma and postoperative changes.

Neuroforaminal Stenosis

The causes of neuroforaminal stenosis, as in central canal stenosis, can be diverse but are usually due to DJD. Osteophytes off the vertebral body (Fig. 19–24) or off the superior articular facet (Fig. 19–25) are most often the cause, but disc herniation and post-operative scar can also occur in the foramen.

The nerve root exits the central canal in the superior aspect of the neuroforamen; therefore, encroachment in the inferior aspect, near the disc space, is an infrequent cause of clinical problems. The nerve root is immobile in the neuroforamen, rather than free to move about; hence, even a small amount of stenosis in the superior aspect of the foramen can cause severe clinical symptomatology, whereas severe stenosis of the inferior aspect of the foramen may elicit no symptoms at all. For these reasons, the amount of narrowing of the neuroforamen often does not correlate clinically.

Although many feel that sagittal reformations through the neuroforamen are the best way to identify stenosis, axial images are by far the most reliable in fully demonstrating the degree of neuroforaminal stenosis and its cause. The neuroforamen and the nerve root can be seen in its entirety with the axial images, whereas a sagittal reformation will show only a 3- to 5-mm slice (depending on the thickness of the reformation).

A frequent cause of failed back surgery is failure to preoperatively note neuroforaminal stenosis in a patient undergoing disc surgery, which results in an

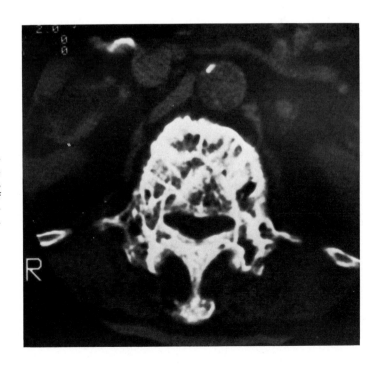

FIGURE 19–22. Paget's disease. Bony overgrowth secondary to Paget's disease has caused central canal stenosis in this patient. This is a typical appearance of Paget's disease in a vertebral body, although it does not always cause stenosis.

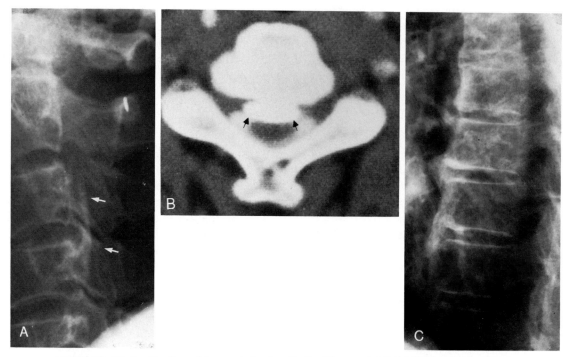

FIGURE 19–23. Ossification of the posterior longitudinal ligament. (*A*) Calcification behind the C-3 and C-4 vertebral bodies (arrows) is seen on the plain film. (*B*) A metrizamide CT scan at the C-3 level shows a spherical calcific mass (black arrows) impressing the cord. This is a characteristic appearance of ossification of the posterior longitudinal ligament. (*C*) A lateral thoracic spine plain film reveals hyperostosis consistent with diffuse idiopathic skeletal hyperostosis (DISH). Up to 25 percent of the patients with DISH are said to have ossification of the posterior longitudinal ligament.

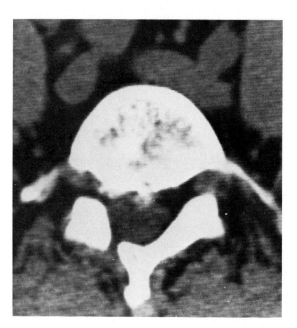

FIGURE 19–24. Neuroforaminal stenosis. An osteophyte off the vertebral body is extending into the right neuroforamen causing neuroforaminal stenosis. The left neuroforamen is normal.

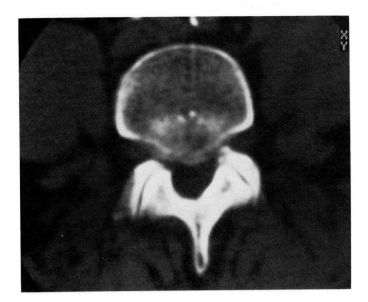

FIGURE 19–25. Neuroforaminal stenosis. An osteophyte off the left superior articular facet is extending into the left neuroforamen, causing neuroforaminal stenosis.

inadequate procedure being performed. It cannot be stressed enough that disc disease and stenosis, in any of its forms, often occur together and addressing only the disc often results in a case of failed back surgery.

Lateral Recess Stenosis

The lateral recess is the bony portion of the central canal that is both caudal and cephalad to the neuroforamen. When the neuroforamen ends as one proceeds caudally, the lateral recess begins. It is also called the nerve root canal because the nerve roots, after they leave the thecal sac and before they exit the central canal through the neuroforamina, run in this bony triangular space. In the bony lateral recess the nerve roots are vulnerable to being impinged by osteophytes (Fig. 19–26), disc fragments, and scar tissue from prior surgery.

Although measurements exist which define the normal lateral recess, they are very difficult to apply and have little practical meaning. As with the neuroforamen, the amount of stenosis often does not correlate with the clinical picture; therefore, it is best to just note that the lateral recess is or is not normal in appearance. Any narrowing should be correlated clinically.

SPONDYLOLYSIS AND SPONDYLOLISTHESIS

Spondylolysis can cause low back pain and sciatica, but only rarely causes spinal stenosis. As discussed in the chapter on musculoskeletal CT, on rare occasions a fibrocartilaginous mass builds up around a pars break which can extend into the central canal and impress on the thecal sac or nerve roots (Fig. 19–27). Although this is unusual, it should be looked for in every case with a pars break so as not to have an unfortunate example of a fusion being performed without removal of the offending soft tissue mass in the central canal.

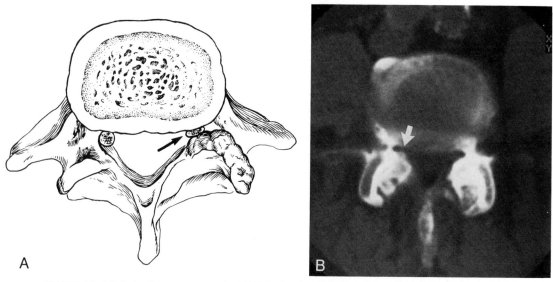

A

B

FIGURE 19–26. Lateral recess stenosis. (*A*) This drawing illustrates how a nerve root (arrow) can become impinged in the lateral recess by bony overgrowth. (*B*) The right lateral recess (arrow) is narrowed from bony overgrowth. The nerve root lies in the lateral recess and may or may not be impinged enough by this process to cause symptoms.

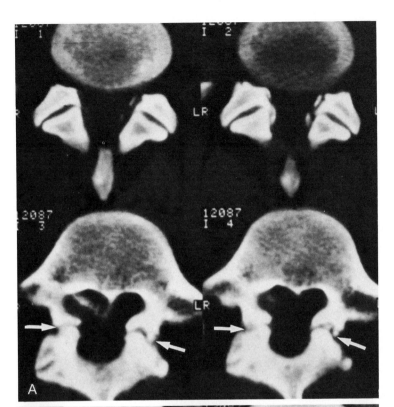

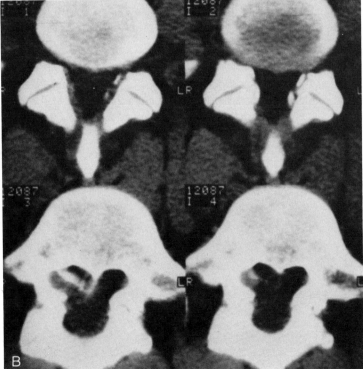

FIGURE 19–27. Spondylolysis with fibrocartilaginous mass. (*A*) Bone windows through the L-4/L-5 disc and the L-5 body reveal a pars break (arrows) bilaterally. (*B*) Soft tissue windows of the same slices show a large, partially calcified soft tissue mass in the right lateral recess, which at surgery was found to arise from the pars break. This has been likened to callus around a fracture that increases when inadequate immobilization occurs.

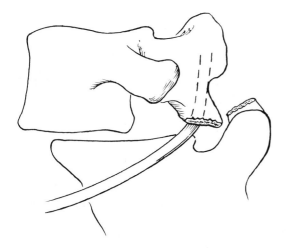

FIGURE 19–28. Spondylolisthesis. This drawing shows how the broken ends of the pars interarticularis can extend into the neuroforamen with spondylolisthesis and impinge a nerve root.

Spondylolisthesis can cause central canal stenosis or neuroforaminal stenosis. When one vertebral body slides forward on another the thecal sac can be squeezed at the level of the slip. This rarely occurs with a grade 1 spondylolisthesis but is not uncommon with the more advanced grades. Occasionally the broken pars will extend into the neuroforamen and impinge the nerve root (Fig. 19–28).

SUMMARY

CT has replaced myelography for diagnosing lumbar spine disc disease. It can demonstrate disc protrusions that are central, lateral, and sequestered. The ability to fully evaluate both the bony and soft tissue structures is one of CT's greatest assets and has helped diminish the incidence of failed back surgery.

Spinal stenosis has many causes, congenital and acquired, yet almost all clinically significant cases have DJD as the overriding etiology. Measurements are not helpful in the lumbar spine and do not reflect the clinical picture in most instances. Spinal stenosis includes the neuroforamina and the lateral recesses as well as the central canal, and is often present concomitantly with disc disease. Failure to note coexisting stenosis and disc disease is one of the leading causes of failed back surgery.

SUGGESTED READING

Dillon W: Myelography: In memoriam. Perspect Radiol, 1:131–147, 1988.
Hesselink JR: Spine imaging: History, achievements, remaining frontiers. Am J Roentgenol, 150:1223–1230, 1988.
Jackson RP, Becker GJ, Jacobs AR, et al.: The neuroradiologic diagnosis of lumbar herniated nucleus pulposus (I): A comparison of computed tomography, myelography, CT-myelography, and CT-discography. Spine, 14:1356–1361, 1989.
Modic MT, Masaryk TJ, Ross JS, et al.: Imaging of degenerative disk disease. Radiology, 168:177–186, 1988.

Index

Note: Page numbers in *italics* refer to illustrations, page numbers followed by (t) refer to tables.